Psychiatric Genetics

Psychiatric Genetics

A Primer for Clinical and Basic Scientists

Edited by

Thomas G. Schulze, MD
Professor and Director
Institute of Psychiatric Phenomics and Genomics (IPPG)
Medical Center of the University of Munich
München, Germany

Francis J. McMahon, MD
Chief
Human Genetics Branch
National Institute of Mental Health Intramural Research
    Program
Bethesda, MD

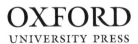

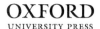

Oxford University Press is a department of the University of Oxford. It furthers
the University's objective of excellence in research, scholarship, and education
by publishing worldwide. Oxford is a registered trade mark of Oxford University
Press in the UK and certain other countries.

Published in the United States of America by Oxford University Press
198 Madison Avenue, New York, NY 10016, United States of America.

Library of Congress Cataloging-in-Publication Data
Names: Schulze, Thomas G., editor. | McMahon, Francis J., editor.
Title: Psychiatric genetics : a primer for clinical and basic scientists /
edited by Thomas G. Schulze, Francis J. McMahon.
Other titles: Psychiatric genetics (Schulze)
Description: New York, NY : Oxford University Press, [2018] |
Includes bibliographical references.
Identifiers: LCCN 2017042084 | ISBN 9780190221973 (paperback : alk. paper)
Subjects: | MESH: Mental Disorders—genetics | Mental Disorders—epidemiology |
Epigenomics | Genome-Wide Association Study | Genetic Research
Classification: LCC RC455.4.G4 | NLM WM 140 | DDC 616.89042—dc23
LC record available at https://lccn.loc.gov/2017042084

9 8 7 6 5 4 3 2

Printed by Webcom, Inc., Canada

Contents

Preface

The quest to understand the hereditary basis of major psychiatric disorders is almost as old as psychiatry itself. Family, twin, and adoption studies carried out over the past 50 years have demonstrated a strong genetic basis for schizophrenia, bipolar disorder, and autism. A weaker but still significant genetic basis has also been shown for major depression and anxiety disorders. The use of ever more sophisticated molecular tools in recent years has led to an explosion of new findings pointing toward numerous genes that influence risk for most of these psychiatric disorders. These findings have deepened our understanding of the genetic complexity of mental illness, provided some of the first solid clues about pathogenesis, and have even begun to influence clinical care.

What are we to make of these developments? Psychiatrists and other mental health care professionals are now confronted with vital questions concerning the contribution of genetics to psychiatric illness and the clinical applications of new genetic findings. Basic scientists involved in psychiatric genetics research are also seeking guidance as to the most clinically relevant research questions. There is an urgent need to educate clinicians and scientists about psychiatric genetics. This has always been one of the primary missions of the International Society of Psychiatric Genetics (IPSG) and is the main goal of this book, *Psychiatric Genetics: A Primer for Clinical and Basic Scientists*.

This primer is meant to provide medical students, psychiatric residents, psychiatrists, and neuroscience researchers with an introduction to the fundamental concepts of psychiatric genetics, complementing more comprehensive textbooks already available that can seem overwhelming for those new to the field. With this primer, we aim to provide a straightforward introduction to the essentials of psychiatric genetics. We hope *Psychiatric Genetics* will also be a valuable tool for educating the educators of the next generation of mental health professionals.

The book covers all major aspects of psychiatric genetics, ranging from basic epidemiology to recruitment for human studies, phenotyping strategies, formal genetic and molecular genetic studies, statistical genetics, bioinformatics and genomics, pharmacogenetics, the most relevant animal models, and biobanking. Each chapter is structured with a summary of the main "take-home" points, followed by a brief overview of current knowledge, with suggestions for further reading.

We hope that our readers will find this primer of value for resident education, research design, preparation of grant applications, continuing education, and clinical care. Psychiatric genetics is changing fast—this book should be an essential tool for everyone who wants to get caught up with the exciting advances in this field.

The editors are grateful for the support and encouragement of the ISPG and Parthenon Management Group, LLC, and have agreed to assign any royalties to benefit the educational mission of the ISPG.

Contributors

Schahram Akbarian, MD, PhD
Friedman Brain Institute
Departments of Psychiatry and
    Neuroscience
Mount Sinai School of Medicine
New York, NY

Nirmala Akula, PhD
Human Genetics Branch
National Institute of Mental Health
    Intramural Research Program
National Institutes of Health
Bethesda, MD

Laura Almasy, PhD
Department of Genetics
Perelman School of Medicine
University of Pennsylvania
Department of Biomedical and
    Health Informatics
Children's Hospital
    of Philadelphia
Philadelphia, PA

Till F. M. Andlauer, PhD
PostDoc
Department of Translational
    Research in Psychiatry
Max Planck Institute of Psychiatry
    (MPI)
Munich, Germany

John Blangero, PhD
South Texas Diabetes
    and Obesity Institute
University of Texas Rio Grande
    Valley School of Medicine
Brownsville, TX

**Sevilla D.
Detera-Wadleigh, PhD**
Human Genetics Branch
National Institute of Mental
    Health Intramural Research
    Program
National Institutes
    of Health
Bethesda, MD

Luanna Dixson, MSc
Department of Psychiatry and
    Psychotherapy
Systems Neurosciences in Psychiatry
    (SNiP)
Central Institute of Mental Health
    (CIMH)
Mannheim, Germany

Gökcen Eraslan, MSc
Institute of Computational
    Biology
Helmholtz Zentrum
    München
Neuherberg, Germany

David C. Glahn, PhD
Department of Psychiatry
Yale University School
    of Medicine
New Haven,
    CT
Olin Neuropsychiatric
    Research Center
Institute of Living,
    Hartford Hospital
Hartford, CT

Tobias B. Halene, MD, PhD
Friedman Brain Institute
Departments of Psychiatry and
    Neuroscience
Mount Sinai School of Medicine
New York, NY
Mental Illness Research
    Education and Clinical
    Center (MIRECC)
James J. Peters VA Medical Center
Bronx, NY

Gregor Hasler, MD
Friedman Brain Institute
Departments of Psychiatry
    and Neuroscience
Mount Sinai School
    of Medicine
New York, NY
Division of Molecular Psychiatry
Translational Research Center
University Hospital of Psychiatry
    and Psychotherapy
University of Bern
Bern, Switzerland

Liping Hou, PhD
Human Genetics Branch
National Institute of Mental
    Health Intramural
    Research Program
National Institutes of Health
Bethesda, MD

Layla Kassem, PsyD, PhD
Malachite Institute for Behavioral
    Health Corp.
Washington, DC

Tadafumi Kato, MD, PhD
Laboratory for Molecular Dynamics
    of Mental Disorders
RIKEN Brain Science Institute
Wako, Japan

George Kirov, PhD
MRC Centre for Neuropsychiatric
    Genetics and Genomics
Institute of Psychological Medicine
    and Clinical Neurosciences
Cardiff University School of Medicine
Cardiff, Wales

Ivan Kondofersky, PhD
Institute of Computational Biology
Helmholtz Zentrum München
Neuherberg, Germany
Department of Mathematics
Technische Universität München
Garching, Germany

Gonzalo Laje, MD
Director
Washington Behavioral Medicine
    Associates, LLC
Chevy Chase, MD

Jun Z. Li, PhD
Department of Human
    Genetics
University of Michigan
Ann Arbor, MI

Francis J. McMahon, MD
Chief
Human Genetics Branch
National Institute of Mental
    Health Intramural Research
    Program
Bethesda, MD

Alison K. Merikangas, MPH, PhD
Postdoctoral Fellow
Neuropsychiatry Program
Department of Psychiatry
Perelman School
    of Medicine
University of Pennsylvania
Philadelphia, MI

Kathleen R. Merikangas, PhD
Senior Investigator and Chief
Genetic Epidemiology
   Research Branch
Intramural Research Program
National Institute of Mental Health
National Institutes of Health
Bethesda, MD

**Andreas Meyer-Lindenberg,
MD, PhD**
Director
Central Institute of Mental Health
   (CIMH)
Department of Psychiatry and
   Psychotherapy
Systems Neurosciences in Psychiatry
University of Heidelberg
Medical Faculty Mannheim
Mannheim, Germany

Amanda Mitchell, PhD
Friedman Brain Institute
Departments of Psychiatry
   and Neuroscience
Mount Sinai School of Medicine
New York, NY

Jennifer C. Moore, PhD
Department of Genetics
The Human Genetics Institute of
   New Jersey
RUCDR Infinite Biologics®
Rutgers, the State University of
   New Jersey
Piscataway, NJ

Bertram Müller-Myhsok, MD
Research Group Leader
Statistical Genetics
Max Planck Institute
   of Psychiatry (MPI)
Munich, Germany

Nikola S. Mueller, PhD
Institute of Computational Biology
Helmholtz Zentrum München
Neuherberg, Germany

Bertram Müller-Myhsok, MD
Max Planck Institute of Psychiatry
München, Germany
Institute of Translational Medicine
University of Liverpool
Liverpool, UK

James B. Potash, MD, MPH
Department of Psychiatry and
   Behavioral Sciences
Johns Hopkins School of Medicine
Baltimore, MD

Shweta Ramdas, BSc
Program in Bioinformatics
University of Michigan
Ann Arbor, MI

Elliott Rees, PhD
MRC Centre for Neuropsychiatric
   Genetics and Genomics
Institute of Psychological
   Medicine and Clinical
   Neurosciences
Cardiff University School of
   Medicine
Cardiff, Wales

John P. Rice, PhD
Department of Psychiatry
Washington University
St. Louis, MO

Stephan Ripke, MD, PhD
Group Leader
Laboratory for Statistical Genetics
The Charité University of Berlin
Berlin, Germany

xi

Michael Sheldon, PhD
Department of Genetics
The Human Genetics Institute of
    New Jersey
RUCDR Infinite Biologics®
Rutgers, the State University
    of New Jersey
Piscataway, NJ

Thomas G. Schulze, MD
Professor and Director
Institute of Psychiatric
    Phenomics and
    Genomics (IPPG)
Medical Center of
    the University
    of Munich
München, Germany

Michael Sheldon, PhD
Department of Genetics
The Human Genetics
    Institute of New Jersey
RUCDR Infinite Biologics®
Rutgers, the State University
    of New Jersey
Piscataway, New Jersey

Julia C. Stingl, MD
Centre for Translational Medicine
University of Bonn, Medical
    School Bonn
Federal Institute for
    Drugs and Medical
    Devices (BfArM)
Bonn, Germany

Subha Subramanian, MS
University of Iowa Carver College
    of Medicine
Iowa City, IA

Fabian J. Theis, MSc, PhD
Institute of Computational Biology
Helmholtz Zentrum München
Neuherberg, Germany
Department of Mathematics
Technische Universität München
Garching, Germany

Jay A. Tischfield, PhD
Department of Genetics
The Human Genetics Institute of
    New Jersey
RUCDR Infinite Biologics®
Rutgers, the State University of
    New Jersey
Piscataway, NJ

Heike Tost, MD, PhD
Group Leader
Systems Neurosciences in Psychiatry
    (SNiP)
Department of Psychiatry and
    Psychotherapy
Central Institute of Mental Health
    (CIMH)
Mannheim, Germany

Karolina Worf, MS
Institute of Computational Biology
Helmholtz Zentrum München
Neuherberg, Germany

Chapter 1

Contribution of Epidemiology to Our Understanding of Psychiatric Genetics

Alison K. Merikangas and Kathleen R. Merikangas

Take-Home Points

1. The role of epidemiology will be increasingly important in designing future case-control studies for genome-wide analyses, moving beyond categorical diagnosis by incorporating phenotypical subtypes and their dimensional underpinnings.
2. Future studies that incorporate the role of environmental exposures in genetic risk estimates will be critical for closing the gap between phenotypical and genotypic heritability estimates, and elucidating understanding of the etiology and prevention of mental disorders.
3. The importance of epidemiology to the future of genetics will involve moving beyond clinical samples to biobanks, health systems, and other registries that have sufficiently large samples of diseases and comprehensive information on clinical phenotypes, environmental exposures, health behaviors, laboratory measures, treatment patterns, and genetic data.

Introduction

During the past decade, the descriptive mission of the field of psychiatric epidemiology has reached its maturity. Psychiatric epidemiology has made several major contributions to our understanding of mental disorders in the general community, including: (1) development of standardized tools that operationalize diagnostic criteria in order to obtain reliable estimates of psychiatric disorders; (2) estimation of the magnitude and correlates of disorders; (3) documenting patterns of comorbidity; (4) quantification of disability attributable to mental disorders; and (5) identification of risk and protective factors for mental disorders. Perhaps the most basic finding from these diverse investigations is the high prevalence of psychiatric disorders in community residents, which range from 20–57%. Despite the high prevalence of disorders across the lifetime, only a small proportion (approximately 5%) actually suffers from chronic disorders across the lifetime. Community surveys have also provided information on the sociodemographic correlates of mental disorders, and environmental and genetic risk factors and correlates.[1,2]

With the growing success in identifying genetic risk factors for chronic human disorders, the field of epidemiology will play an important role in defining study designs, appropriate samples, population generalizability, and statistical tools that will facilitate our ability to identify the joint influence of genetic and environmental factors on the susceptibility to mental disorders.

Overview

Epidemiology

Epidemiology is the study of the distribution and determinants of diseases in human populations. Epidemiological studies examine the extent and types of illnesses in groups of people and the factors that influence their distribution. Epidemiologists investigate the interactions that may occur among the host, agent, and environment (the classic epidemiological triangle) to produce a disease state. The chief aim of epidemiology is to identify the etiology of a disease in order to intervene in its progression or to prevent the disorder. To achieve this goal, epidemiological research proceeds from studies that specify the distribution of a disease within a population by person, place, and time (i.e., *descriptive* epidemiology), to more focused studies of the determinants of disease in specific groups (i.e., *analytical* epidemiology).

Differences in prevalence rates by particular characteristics (e.g., sex, age, ethnicity, urban vs. rural) provide clues regarding potential underlying etiological factors. Case-control designs compare the association between a particular risk factor or disease correlate and the presence or absence of a given disease, after controlling for relevant confounding variables. Lack of appropriate selection of controls is often the chief threat to validity of these studies; controls should be chosen from the same population, and have the same characteristics of cases, with the exception of the major independent variable. Case-control designs generally employ either cross-sectional or retrospective studies of associations between risk factors among cases compared to controls. Risk factors identified in case-control studies can then be tested in prospective cohort studies in large samples of unaffected individuals. Prospective studies can yield information on the attributable risk and temporal direction of risk factors on disease incidence.

The core measure in epidemiology is estimation of the magnitude of a disease in a defined population over a specific time period (i.e., lifetime, one year, current). Measures include *incidence*—the number of new cases of disease that occur during a specified time period in a defined population at risk, and *prevalence*—the number of affected persons in the population at a particular time divided by the number of persons in the population at that time period. Prevalence estimates must be anchored in time, ranging from over a lifetime to the current time period. These approaches yield a range of risk estimates, including *relative risk*, the magnitude of the association between an exposure and disease incidence; *absolute risk*, the overall probability of a disease developing in an individual or in a particular population; *attributable risk*, the difference in the risk of the disease in those exposed to a particular risk factor compared to the background risk of a disease in a population (i.e., in the unexposed); and *population attributable risk*, the risk of a disease in a total population (exposed and unexposed), indicating the amount the disease can be reduced in a population if an exposure is eliminated. The *odds ratio* (OR), defined as the ratio of the odds that cases were exposed to a risk factor to the odds that the controls were exposed, is an approximation of the relative risk that is employed in cross-sectional or retrospective case-control studies that do not yield incidence rates because of their reliance on retrospective assessment of exposures.

There are several criteria for assessing the extent to which a risk factor is causally associated with a trait or disease. These include strength of the association, a dose–response effect, and a lack of temporal ambiguity. Broader criteria that can be applied to a set of studies on a putative etiological risk factor include consistency of the findings across studies, biological plausibility of the hypothesis, and the specificity of association.[3] Criteria for causal inference in epidemiological studies have been clearly articulated by Rothman and Greenland.[4]

The field of epidemiology, which is intricately tied to biostatistics, has employed increasingly sophisticated analytical methods to investigate risk factors for disease while simultaneously accounting for confounders, effect mediation, interactions, and varying time periods of observation of both disease and covariates to test associations in order to build causal models. During the past decade, there has been increasing recognition of the danger of false-positive findings based on multiple testing in population studies in medical research.[5] Increased scrutiny of publication bias, false positives, and failure to replicate has been particularly evident in studies of genetic risk factors,[6] but these sources of lack of validity are also common in other types of research. The field of epidemiology has played a leading role in identifying approaches, increasing reliability of measurement and analytical approaches to increase the reproducibility and validity of psychiatric research.

Psychiatric Epidemiology

Contributions of Psychiatric Epidemiology

The term *psychiatric epidemiology* was first used during the second half of the 20th century, following the revival of interest in psychiatric disorders and the emergence of chronic disease epidemiology that came about after World War II.[7] For the next 25 years, the "second generation" of psychiatric epidemiology was dominated by sociologists and social psychiatrists, who applied newly developed household survey techniques to the problem of estimating the prevalence of mental problems, and who studied causal factors such as socioeconomic stratification, social integration, and social stress. Awareness of the weak reliability of psychiatric diagnoses, and increasing work on empirical diagnostic methods, led to the development of structured diagnostic interviews and a focus on diagnostic utility.

As summarized in Table 1.1, the major contributions of epidemiology of mental disorders have been: (1) developing standardized tools that operationalize diagnostic criteria in order to obtain reliable estimates of psychiatric disorders; (2) estimating the magnitude and correlates of disorders; (3) documenting patterns of comorbidity; (4) quantifying disability attributable to mental disorders; and (5) identifying risk and protective factors for mental disorders.

The early application of the tools of epidemiology to psychiatry chiefly involved methodological developments, including the introduction of structured and semi-structured diagnostic interviews, statistical methods for estimating prevalence and correlates of mental disorders, and the focus on population-based samples to obtain estimates of the magnitude and correlates of mental disorders unbiased by treatment-seeking behavior. Over the past 30 years, a series of national population-based studies has generated information on the widespread prevalence of mental disorders, their sociodemographic and clinical correlates, systematic data on impairment and disability associated with mental disorders, and service patterns and correlates. Diagnostic tools that were developed for large-scale epidemiological studies include the Diagnostic Interview Schedule,[8] which tapped *Diagnostic and Statistical Manual of Mental Disorders* (DSM)-III-R and subsequently DSM-IV[10] criteria, and the Composite International Diagnostic Interview (CIDI)[9] that collected information to apply diagnostic criteria for DSM-IV and the *International Classification of Diseases* (ICD)-10. The development of the CIDI strongly facilitated international comparability of epidemiological studies.[11] These fully structured interviews were developed to maximize reliability, or consistency of measurement, through extensive field-testing of the specific queries regarding the core features of each disorder, followed by questions regarding symptoms, duration, and impairment. These interviews provided common methods for ascertaining the targeted diagnostic criteria for mental disorders that could be administered by lay interviewers in community surveys. As described later in this chapter, these studies have demonstrated the

Table 1.1 Chief Contributions and Findings from Psychiatric Epidemiological Studies

- Standardized assessments of mental disorders
- Magnitude of mental disorders in the general population
- Patterns of comorbidity
- Disability associated with mental disorders
- Risk and protective factors for psychopathology

difficulty in applying the diagnostic nomenclature in non-clinical samples, in terms of the extent to which these conditions are manifest on a spectrum without clear-cut distinctions between a case and a non-case as specified in the diagnostic criteria.[12–14]

The lack of validity of psychiatric phenotypes—the extent to which a diagnostic concept represents a true entity, based solely on clinical manifestations without pathognomonic markers or laboratory tests—has been the chief impediment to our identification of their causes.[15] Widespread agreement regarding the lack of validity of the psychiatric classification system has led to substantial efforts to study the dimensional manifestations of the core domains underlying psychiatric disorders.[16–19] The Research Domain Criteria (RDoC) initiative established by the National Institute of Mental Health (NIMH) was designed to develop new ways of classifying mental disorders based on behavioral dimensions and neurobiological measures for research purposes (http://www.nimh.nih.gov/research-priorities/rdoc/index.shtml).

Implementation of dimensional underpinnings of complex disorders has long been recognized in population genetics as represented by models, such as the threshold liability model, that assume multifactorial additive etiology with an underlying quantitative distribution of liability for a condition. Thresholds that distinguish disorder from non-disorder are defined by the population prevalence or prevalence in relatives of affected individuals (Figure 1.1). The application of these models for family studies of psychiatric disorders has informed the spectra of expression of many psychiatric disorders, including alcoholism,[20] mood disorders,[21] and schizophrenia.[22] However, whether these dimensional domains are more valid than traditional categorical domains in psychiatry, according to the classic formulation of diagnostic validity by Robins and Guze,[23] is still to be determined.

Prevalence of Mental Disorders

Numerous studies across the world over the past 40 years have generated information on the prevalence of mental disorders. Results of several surveys of mental disorders in the United States,[12,24–28] as well as numerous studies worldwide, have yielded population-specific estimates of the magnitude of disease. The World Mental Health Survey Initiative sponsored by the World Health Organization[25] was the largest contemporary international collaborative study of mental disorders and included more than 85,000 participants in 18 countries. Aggregate estimated lifetime prevalence of the major classes of disorders from the World Mental Health Survey[25] are: mood disorders (20.8%); anxiety disorders (16.9%); substance use disorders (10.5%); and impulse control disorders (i.e., intermittent explosive disorder, conduct disorder, oppositional disorder) (5.2%). The total lifetime prevalence of any disorder of 36.4% indicates that, on average, about one-third of the general population will have at least one mental disorder during their lifetime. The most recent U.S. population-based data were collected in the National

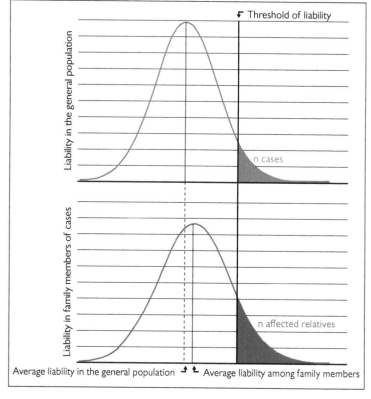

Figure 1.1 Hypothetical distribution of liability in the general population, and in family members of cases with a complex genetic disorder.

Epidemiologic Survey on Alcohol and Related Conditions (NESARC), which conducted three waves of interviews. Aggregate prevalence rates from Waves 1 and 2 of NESARC are comparable for all conditions, with the exception of substance use disorders, which were substantially greater in the United States than in the international data.[27]

Perhaps the most basic finding from these diverse investigations is the high prevalence of psychiatric disorders in community residents, ranging from 20%[12] to 57%.[29] The high prevalence rates across sites underscores the magnitude of psychopathology in non-clinically derived samples. However, despite the high prevalence of disorders across the lifetime, only a small proportion (approximately 5%) actually suffers from chronic disorders across the lifetime.[30]

Community surveys have also provided information on the sociodemographic correlates of mental disorders, including gender, age, education, income, marital status, ethnicity, urbanicity and geographic region, etc., of different classes of mental disorders. They have also identified characteristics of clinical samples (i.e., comorbidity with other mental and physical conditions, severity, suicidal behavior) that differ from people with the same disorders in population samples.[31]

As with adults, there have been numerous population-based studies of children and adolescents across the world that have provided information on the magnitude, correlates, and treatment patterns for mental disorders in youth.[32] The only nationally representative surveys of the full spectrum of disorders in U.S. youth are the National Comorbidity Survey–Adolescent Supplement,[33] and the National Health and Nutrition Examination Survey (NHANES).[34] There have also been several longitudinal population-based studies of children and adolescents in the United States and in international settings,[35–40] as well as more recent studies of youth that have also provided information on the developmental stages, order of onset of disorders, indicators of impairment, and course of childhood disorders. Population studies of adult and child cohorts, such as the Zurich Cohort Study,[41] and the Early Development Stages of Psychopathology (ESDP)[42,43] study, have been particularly informative in documenting the spectra of expression of particular conditions, as well as deconstructing psychiatric phenotypes by their component features or subtypes.[44]

Comorbidity

One of the most salient findings from epidemiological research has been the evidence for the pervasive magnitude of comorbidity among the major mental disorders. The striking overlap across different mental disorders was first highlighted by findings from the Epidemiologic Catchment Area study, which showed that comorbidity between mental disorders occurred for nearly every pairwise set of conditions.[45] Although comorbidity is in part induced by the classification system that fails to distinguish discrete boundaries between disorders, there is also evidence for developmental-specific manifestations of some disorders, such as links between anxiety in childhood and depression in adolescence and adulthood, as well as causal associations between primary conditions such as bipolar disorder and substance abuse as a consequence.[46]

Burden of Illness

One of the major advances in epidemiology during the past decade has been the growing focus on the impact and burden of mental disorders. The importance of role disability has become increasingly recognized as a major source of indirect costs of illness because of its high economic impact on ill workers, their employers, and society.[47] The introduction of the concept of *disability-adjusted life years* (DALYs), which estimate the disease-specific reduction in life expectancy attributable to disability and increased mortality, has highlighted the dramatic public health impact of mental disorders.[48]

Risk Factors and Correlates of Mental Disorders

One of the major goals of epidemiology is to identify clues to etiological factors underlying diseases based on differential distribution of disorders across population strata. Differences in the sex ratios of several psychiatric disorders are among the most consistent findings across studies. Whereas women have greater rates of anxiety, affective, and eating disorders, men report more substance-related and other behavioral disorders. Although the sex ratio for schizophrenia and other psychotic disorders is approximately equal, research has revealed gender differences in the age of onset of schizophrenia.[49,50] Furthermore, prospective research has shown that the sex differences in the affective and emotional disorders tend to emerge during adolescence,[51] whereas the male predominance in behavior and attention problems manifests throughout life.[52,53] Risk factor research has also included designs that can discriminate between environmental and genetic risk factors.

Environmental Risk Factors

There is now compelling evidence for a range of environmental exposures that are associated with an elevated risk of psychiatric disorders. The bulk of the work on environmental risk factors has been based on retrospective and ecological data; however, there is now growing information from prospective studies and national registries that has identified both risk factors and early manifestations of adult mental disorders. Longitudinal studies are critical in order to evaluate the order of onset of putative risk factors and diseases, as well as to characterize the evolution, course, and consequences of psychiatric disorders. However, the lack of identified specific environmental factors that play an etiological rather than provocative role in mental disorders is a major gap.

Both distal and proximal stressful life events are associated with an elevated risk of mood disorders; however, prospective research has demonstrated that these events tend to be provocative rather than causal. Most of the environmental risk factors for mental disorders (e.g., life stress, infections, birth complications) have been non-specific in that they are associated with a range of disorders.[54] Early environmental risk factors, including obstetrical complications, childhood trauma, and prenatal factors such as nutritional deficiencies, increased paternal age, maternal infections, maternal cytokines, and cannabis use, have been consistently associated with an elevated risk of psychotic disorders. When taken together with genetic risk factors that have been recently elucidated, schizophrenia is now widely viewed as a neurodevelopmental disorder comprising a confluence of vulnerability genes and environmental exposures.[55,56] Similar progress has emerged from research on autism spectrum disorder (ASD) that has demonstrated that increased prenatal and perinatal complications and exposures are strongly associated with the subsequent development of ASD and other neurodevelopmental disorders.[57]

One valuable source of identification of environmental risk factors is cross-cultural studies that elucidate cultural differences in rates and patterns of disorders. These studies can provide clues regarding the context, assessment, and risk factors for the major categories of psychopathology. Recent studies of migrants have also demonstrated the importance of environmental exposures to schizophrenia. Numerous studies have reported an increased risk for the development of schizophrenia among immigrants in several different countries.[58] Although selective migration may be one explanation, there is converging evidence that socially disrupted environments may trigger the onset of schizophrenia in susceptible individuals.[56,59]

Genetic Risk Factors

There is a wide range of estimates of the magnitude of familial aggregation of the most common mental disorders from controlled studies. The risk ratios comparing the proportion of affected relatives of cases versus controls are greatest for ASD (50–100), bipolar disorder (7–10), and schizophrenia (8–10); intermediate for substance dependence (4–8) and subtypes of anxiety (4–6), particularly panic (3–8); and lowest for major depression (2–3). The estimates of heritability (i.e., the proportion of variance attributable to genetic factors) derived from twin studies, which compare rates of disorders in monozygotic and dizygotic twins, demonstrate that a substantial proportion of the familial aggregation of mental disorders can be attributed to genetic factors. Heritability estimates are greatest for ASD (.90) and schizophrenia (.80), followed by bipolar disorder (.65) and panic disorder (.60), followed by substance dependence (.40), anxiety disorders (.35), and major depression (.30). Furthermore, adoption and half-sibling studies also support a genetic basis for the observed familial aggregation.[60]

The major impediments to gene identification for psychiatric disorders are the lack of validity of the classification of psychiatric disorders (e.g., phenotypes, or observable aspects of diseases) and the complexity of the pathways from genotypes to psychiatric phenotypes. Recent studies have attempted to identify more valid phenotypical constructs for genetic studies. Phenotypical traits or markers that may represent intermediate forms of expression between the output of underlying genes and the broader disease phenotype have been termed *endophenotypes*.[61,62] Studies of the role of genetic factors involved in these systems may be more informative than studies of the aggregate psychiatric phenotypes because they may more closely represent expression of underlying biological systems. However, a recent meta-analysis of psychiatric endophenotypes,[63] and a review of the genetic architecture of traits in model organisms do not provide evidence that currently identified endophenotypes are superior to current phenotypical disease definitions.[64]

Genetic Epidemiology

The sub-discipline of genetic epidemiology focuses on identification of the role of genetic factors and their joint influence with environmental factors in disease etiology.[1,65] Genetic epidemiology employs traditional epidemiological study designs, including case-control and cohort studies, to evaluate the aggregation in groups as closely related as twins or as loosely related as migrant cohorts. Prior to the molecular genetic era, studies in genetic epidemiology were designed to infer genetic causation by controlling for genetic background while letting the environment vary (e.g., migrant studies, half-siblings, separated twins) or conversely, controlling for the environment while allowing variance in the genetic background (e.g., siblings, twins, adoptees, non-biological siblings).[66] Measures of risk in genetic epidemiology include *familial relative risk* (disease risk in relatives of cases versus controls), and *genetic attributable risk* (the proportion of a particular disease that would be eliminated if a particular gene or genes were not involved in the disease). As described later in this chapter, sophisticated methods have been developed to compare combinations of genetic markers between cases and controls (e.g., polygenic risk scores), and genome-wide complex trait analysis (GCTA), which estimates the proportion of phenotypical variance explained by genetic variants (typically single-nucleotide polymorphisms [SNPs]) for complex traits.[67]

Family Studies

Familial aggregation is generally the first source of evidence that genetic factors may play a role in a disorder. The most common indicator of familial aggregation is the *relative risk ratio*, computed as the rate of a disorder in families of affected persons divided by the corresponding rate in families of controls. The patterns of genetic factors underlying a disorder can be inferred from the extent to which patterns of familial resemblance adhere to the expectations of Mendelian laws of inheritance. The degree of genetic relatedness among relatives is based on the proportion of shared genes between a particular relative and an index family member or proband. On average, first-degree relatives share 50% of their genes, second-degree relatives share 25% of their genes, and third-degree relatives share 12.5% of their genes. If familial resemblance is wholly attributable to genes, there should be a 50% decrease in disease risk with each successive decrease in relatedness. This information can be used to derive estimates of familial recurrence risk within and across generations as a function of population prevalence (λ).[68] Whereas λ tends to exceed 20 for most autosomal-dominant diseases, values of λ derived from family studies of many complex disorders tend to range from 2 to 5. Decrease in risk according to the degree of genetic relatedness can also be examined to detect interactions between several loci. If the risk to second- and third-degree relatives decreases by more than 50%, this implies that more than a single locus must contribute to disease risk, and that no single locus can largely predominate.

The major advantage of studying diseases within families is that etiological factors are more likely to be homogeneous than those studied between families that may result from heterogeneous etiology. In fact, the family study approach is particularly valuable when sources of heterogeneity are unknown. Evidence for specificity of familial aggregation of diagnostic subgroups and core features of disorders can inform both phenotypical and etiological heterogeneity. Phenotypical heterogeneity is suggested by variable expressivity of symptoms and diseases within families, whereas etiological heterogeneity is demonstrated by similar phenotypes manifesting between families. Moreover, the family study method permits assessment of associations between disorders by evaluating specific patterns of co-segregation of two or more disorders within families.[69]

Systematic family studies of both clinical and community samples have shown that spouses of people with mental disorders often manifest either the same or another mental disorder.[70] Assortative mating has been found for numerous psychiatric disorders, including depression,[71] alcoholism,[72,73] and schizophrenia.[74] Concordance for mental disorders could be partly attributable to widespread similarity between couples for other numerous traits and disorders aside from psychiatric disorders such as physical/somatic characteristics (e.g., blood pressure, height, weight, eye color, race), sociocultural and behavioral patterns (e.g., religious affiliation/attendance, education, diet, smoking, exercise, other health habits), and personality and cognition (e.g., extroversion/introversion, IQ).[75-84]

Non-random mating has rarely been considered in genetic studies of psychiatric disorders, despite its major impact on the distributions of diseases and alleles in the general population. In general, assortative mating increases the population variance of a given trait and the proportion of individuals who are homozygous for the trait. Therefore, studies of genetic risk should incorporate the tendency for assortative mating, which may influence the distribution of susceptibility alleles in both clinical and population samples. The importance of assortative mating in recent polygenic analyses (as described later) has received increasing attention.[85,86]

Twin Studies

The twin family design is one of the most powerful study designs in genetic epidemiology because it yields estimates of heritability, but also permits evaluation of multigenerational patterns of expression of genetic and environmental risk factors.[87] Twin studies that compare concordance rates for monozygotic twins (who share the same genotype) with those of dizygotic twins (who share an average of 50% of their genes) provide estimates of the degree to which genetic factors contribute to the etiology of a disease phenotype. Path-analytic approaches that estimate the proportion of variance attributable to additive genes, common, and unique environments have been the standard method of data analysis from large twin studies. Twin studies can also provide information on the genetic and environmental sources of sex differences in a disease through investigation of sex-specific concordance rates. Environmental exposures may also be identified through comparison of differential exposures among discordant monozygotic twins. Twin studies may also inform the genetic mode of transmission of a disease by inspecting the degree of adherence of the difference in risk between monozygotic and dizygotic twins to the Mendelian ratio of 50%. Finally, twin studies may inform the spectrum of expression of diseases and disease subtypes through identifying the components of the phenotypes that are most heritable.[88–91]

Adoption Studies

Adoption studies have been the major source of evidence regarding the joint contribution of genetic and environmental factors to disease etiology. Adoption studies either compare the similarity between an adoptee and his or her biological versus adoptive relatives, or the similarity between biological relatives of affected adoptees with those of unaffected, or control, adoptees. The latter approach is more powerful because it eliminates the potentially confounding effect of environmental factors. Similar to the familial recurrence risk, the genetic contribution in adoption studies is estimated by comparing the risk of disease to biological versus adoptive relatives, or the risk of disease in biological relatives of affected versus control adoptees. These estimates of risk are often adjusted for sex, age, ethnicity, and other factors that may confound the links between adoption status and an index disease.

With the recent trends towards selective adoption and the diminishing frequency of adoptions in the United States, adoption studies are becoming less feasible methods for identifying genetic and environmental sources of disease etiology.[92] However, the increased rate of *reconstituted families* (families composed of both full and half siblings) may offer a new way to evaluate the role of genetic factors in the transmission of complex disorders.[93] Genetic models predict that half siblings should have a 50% reduction in disease risk compared to that of full siblings. Deviations from this risk provide evidence for polygenic transmission, gene–environment interaction, or other complex modes of transmission.

Genetic Epidemiology in the Molecular Era

With advances in molecular biology, there has been a flood of information on the contribution of genetic risk factors to complex diseases. This has transformed the sub-discipline of genetic epidemiology that previously relied solely on inferences based on phenotypical disease manifestations in relatives. Genome-wide association studies (GWAS), designed to compare common genetic variants (i.e., SNPs with >1% population frequency) between large samples of cases and controls, have had increasing success in identifying markers of small effect for diverse complex diseases.[94] The high *a priori* statistical significance threshold of 5×10^{-8} protects against the false-positive error that has plagued studies of individual specific genes.[95] Similar studies have also been used to investigate structural variation, such as segmental duplications and deletions, or copy number variants (CNVs). These have led to the development of new study designs and statistical approaches in genetic epidemiology, as described later.

Designs and Statistical Methods

Mendelian randomization was one of the first approaches to incorporate identification of specific susceptibility alleles with known effects on specific phenotypes in epidemiological analyses.[96,97] Since genotypes are randomly transmitted across generations according to Mendel's laws, these genotypes may be used to identify influences of modifiable environmental exposures by defining "caseness" via the genotype. This approach can yield unbiased estimates of causal influences on diseases without formally conducting a randomized trial. The genetic randomization eliminates the effects of confounding and reverse causation that require consideration in observational epidemiological studies.[98] A major limitation of this design is the requirement of *a priori* identification of a susceptibility gene with influence on the disease or outcome of interest, which has not been forthcoming for psychiatric disorders.

Several statistical approaches that take advantage of markers identified in GWAS have also advanced our understanding of the genetic architecture of psychiatric disorders, notably genomic profile (or polygenic) risk scores, and Genome-wide Complex Trait Analysis (GCTA). Polygenic scores summarize genetic effects in a GWAS by computing a weighted sum of associated "risk" alleles within each subject. Initially, markers (typically SNPs) are selected based on their evidence for association, typically their p-values, using a training sample, and the weighted score is then constructed in an independent replication sample.[99] If an association is found between a trait/disorder and the polygenic score, one assumes that a genetic signal is present among the selected markers. Later, this score can be used to predict individual trait values.[100] The original use of polygenic scores has now been extended to include detecting shared genetic etiology among traits or to infer the genetic architecture of a trait, to establish the presence of a genetic signal in underpowered studies, and can act as a biomarker for a phenotype.[101] The first polygenic score analysis that was applied to schizophrenia provided molecular genetic evidence for a substantial polygenic component to the risk of schizophrenia involving thousands of common alleles of very small effect.[102] Figure 1.2 shows the polygenic model of disease susceptibility, wherein the distribution of risk alleles in both cases and controls follows a normal distribution; however, cases have a shift towards a higher number of high-risk alleles. This approach has also been used to examine the shared genetic effect between purportedly distinct disorders, notably schizophrenia and bipolar disorder.[103]

GCTA, which estimates the proportion of phenotypical variance explained by genetic variants (typically SNPs) for complex traits, is another method that can be used to characterize the genetic architecture of complex disorders.[67] Contrary to standard behavioral genetics studies that define relatedness by pedigree structure, GCTA estimates genetic relatedness directly from the SNP data.[104] In addition to defining the genetic relationship from genome-wide SNPs, GCTA can also be used to predict the genome-wide additive genetic effects for individual subjects and for individual SNPs, to estimate the linkage

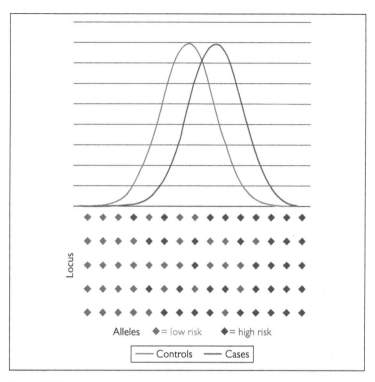

Figure 1.2 Polygenic model of disease susceptibility. The distribution of risk alleles in both cases and controls follows a normal distribution. However, cases have a shift towards a higher number of risk alleles.

disequilibrium structure encompassing a list of target SNPs, and to estimate the genetic correlation between two traits or diseases by using a bivariate SNP-based model that estimates the average genome-wide relationship between two disorders.[105] Application of GCTA has been applied to psychiatric disorders,[106] such as attention-deficit hyperactivity disorder (ADHD),[107] major depressive disorder,[108] bipolar disorder,[109] anxiety-related behaviors,[110] and ASD.[111]

Estimates of SNP-based heritability (h^2_{SNP}) tend to be substantially lower than those for phenotypical heritability.[112] For example, the SNP-based heritability for bipolar disorder and schizophrenia is about one-third that of phenotypical heritability (e.g., $h^2_{phenotype}$ = .70 vs. h^2_{SNP} = .20, and $h^2_{phenotype}$ = .80 vs. h^2_{SNP} = .30, respectively). Moreover, in contrast to the much greater heritability of bipolar disorder compared to major depression, the estimates of SNP-based heritability for bipolar disorder and major depression are nearly equal (i.e., .25 for bipolar and .21 for major depression).[112] Whereas the SNP-based estimate for major depression is nearly equal to the phenotypical heritability, there is a large discrepancy between these estimates for bipolar disorder.

Differences between phenotypical and SNP-based heritability have important implications for risk prediction. There has been increasing concern regarding the low attributable risk of GWAS "hits" because few of the molecular genetics findings have improved our ability to predict risk. For example, the variance explained by GWAS for bipolar disorder is .02 and for schizophrenia is .01.[113] This disparity can in part be attributed to the fact that GWAS do not examine the full range of genetic variation, such as rare or structural variants.[114] Furthermore, they do not reflect sources of complexity of the genetic architecture of the diseases such as pleiotropy (multiple phenotypical effects of single variants),[115] or the dichotomous classification of disease, which may lead to misclassification of cases with sub-threshold manifestations of disease as controls. Recent studies have also begun to use genetic markers to dissect phenotypes; for example, a recent study examined variants that are both specific and non-specific to particular neurodevelopmental disorders such as ASD.[116]

Expanding Samples: Population Registries and Biobanks

One of the most important sources of future data for psychiatric genetic epidemiology will be systematic data from population samples, disease, medical, or population registries, and biobanks that have sufficiently large samples of diseases coupled with comprehensive information on clinical phenotypes, environmental exposures, health behaviors, laboratory measures, treatment patterns, and genetic data. Population-based registries and data collection have made a growing contribution to epidemiological research because of their large sample size, representativeness of their target populations, and the reduced likelihood of bias due to recall, or non-response. The availability of genotype information in population registries such as the Scandinavian administrative registries, which have been used for decades at the phenotype level to examine the genetic architecture of mental disorders, are now being increasingly used to estimate genotypic heritability for mental disorders.[117] Analysis of registry data as a retrospective cohort study can provide insight into important associations that can be tested in prospective and far more expensive study designs.

Epidemiologists have also become engaged in developing *biobanks*, repositories for biological samples (typically including blood and extracted DNA, but also other tissues and cells) that can be used to examine associations between genetic and other biomarkers with mental disorders. The observational and retrospective nature of opt-in biobanks and registries is perhaps the most serious impediment to generalizability of the findings.[118] Likewise, ethical concerns such as informed consent, reporting of incidental findings, and confidentiality will continue to be important considerations in biobanks and registry settings.[119] The most powerful studies of the future will require large numbers of participants with in-depth assessment of both phenotypes and potential risk factors for these diseases, particularly cohort studies that can detect incident cases who are followed prospectively over time.

Future Directions

The importance of epidemiology to the future of genetics has been increasingly evident, as the application of GWAS has led to the identification of literally thousands of genes that comprise risk factors for chronic disorders, particularly for the major mental disorders. It is likely that population-based studies will assume increasing importance in translating the products of genomics to public health.[120] To obtain accurate risk estimates, it will be necessary to move beyond samples identified through individuals who are affected, to the population as a whole to obtain estimates of the risk of specific genetic variants for the population. Epidemiology will be increasingly involved in the establishment and analysis of population and clinical registries that include genetic, biological, and phenotypical data. Epidemiologists can employ the same measures used to test the predictive value of traditional risk factors (i.e., specificity, sensitivity) to quantify the effect of genetic markers at both the levels of the individual and the population.[121] With the growing success in identifying genetic risk factors for chronic human disorders, the field of epidemiology will play an important role in defining study designs, appropriate samples, population generalizability, and statistical tools that will facilitate our ability to identify the joint influence of genetic and environmental factors on the susceptibility to mental disorders.[122]

References

1. Burton, P. R., Tobin, M. D., & Hopper, J. L. (2005). Key concepts in genetic epidemiology. *Lancet*, *366*(9489), 941–951.

2. Davey Smith, G., et al. (2005). Genetic epidemiology and public health: hope, hype, and future prospects. *Lancet*, *366*(9495), 1484–1498.

3. Hill, A. B. (1965). The environment and disease: Association or causation? *Proceedings of the Royal Society of Medicine*, *58*, 295–300.

4. Rothman, K. J., & Greenland, S. (2005). Causation and causal inference in epidemiology. *American Journal of Public Health*, *95*(S1), S144–S150.

5. Ioannidis, J. P. (2005). Why most published research findings are false. *PLoS Medicine*, *2*(8), e124.

6. Ioannidis, J. P. (2007). Limitations are not properly acknowledged in the scientific literature. *Journal of Clinical Epidemiology*, *60*(4), 324–329.

7. Eaton, W. W., & Merikangas, K. R. (2000). Psychiatric epidemiology: progress and prospects in the year 2000. *Epidemiologic Reviews*, *22*(1), 29–34.

8. Robins, L. N., et al. (1981). National Institute of Mental Health diagnostic interview schedule. Its history, characteristics, and validity. *Archives of General Psychiatry*, *38*(4), 381–389.

9. Wittchen, H. U., et al. (1991). Cross-cultural feasibility, reliability and sources of variance of the Composite International Diagnostic Interview (CIDI). The Multicentre WHO/ADAMHA field trials. *British Journal of Psychiatry, 159,* 645–653, 658.

10. American Psychiatric Association. (1994). *Diagnostic and Statistical Manual of Mental Disorders DSM-IV* (4th ed.). Washington, DC: American Psychiatric Association.

11. Kessler, R. C., et al. (2004). The US National Comorbidity Survey Replication (NCS-R): design and field procedures. *International Journal of Methods in Psychiatric Research, 13*(2), 69–92.

12. Regier, D. A., Burke, J. D., & Bruke, K. C. (1990). Comorbidity of affective and anxiety disorders in the NIMH Epidemiologic Catchment Area (ECA) program. In J. D. Maser and R. Cloninger (Eds.), *Comorbidity of Mood and Anxiety Disorders* (pp. 113–122). Washington, DC: American Psychiatric Press.

13. Kessler, R. C., et al. (1994). Lifetime and 12-month prevalence of DSM-III-R psychiatric disorders in the United States. Results from the National Comorbidity Survey. *Archives of General Psychiatry, 51*(1), 8–19.

14. First, M. B., et al. (2004). Clinical utility as a criterion for revising psychiatric diagnoses. *American Journal of Psychiatry, 161*(6), 946–954.

15. Kendell, R. E. (1989). Clinical validity. *Psychological Medicine, 19*(1), 45–55.

16. Angst, J. (1997). The bipolar spectrum. *British Journal of Psychiatry, 190,* 189.

17. Angst, J., & Merikangas, K. (1997). The depressive spectrum: diagnostic classification and course. *Journal of Affective Disorders, 45*(1–2), 31–39; discussion 39–40.

18. Judd, L. L., et al. (1998). A prospective 12-year study of subsyndromal and syndromal depressive symptoms in unipolar major depressive disorders. *Archives of General Psychiatry, 55*(8), 694–700.

19. Kendell, R., & Jablensky, A. (2003). Distinguishing between the validity and utility of psychiatric diagnoses. *American Journal of Psychiatry, 160*(1), 4–12.

20. Murray, R. M., & Gurling, H. M. (1982). Alcoholism: polygenic influence on a multifactorial disorder. *British Journal of Hospital Medicine, 27*(4), 328, 331, 333–334.

21. Tsuang, M. T., et al. (1985). Transmission of affective disorders: an application of segregation analysis to blind family study data. *Journal of Psychiatric Research, 19*(1), 23–29.

22. Faraone, S. V., & Tsuang, M. T. (1988). Familial links between schizophrenia and other disorders: application of the multifactorial polygenic model. *Psychiatry, 51*(1), 37–47.

23. Robins, E., & Guze, S. B. (1970). Establishment of diagnostic validity in psychiatric illness: its application to schizophrenia. *American Journal of Psychiatry, 126*(7), 983–987.

24. Eaton, W. W., et al. (1994). Panic and panic disorder in the United States. *American Journal of Psychiatry, 151*(3), 413–420.

25. Kessler, R. C., et al. (2007). Lifetime prevalence and age-of-onset distributions of mental disorders in the World Health Organization's World Mental Health Survey Initiative. *World Psychiatry, 6*(3), 168–176.

26. Grant, B. F. (1997). Prevalence and correlates of alcohol use and DSM-IV alcohol dependence in the United States: results of the National Longitudinal Alcohol Epidemiologic Survey. *Journal of Studies in Alcoholism, 58*(5), 464–473.

27. Hasin, D. S., & Grant, B. F. (2015). The National Epidemiologic Survey on Alcohol and Related Conditions (NESARC) Waves 1 and 2: review and summary of findings. *Social Psychiatry and Psychiatric Epidemiology*, *50*(11), 1609–1640.

28. Takayanagi, Y., et al. (2015). Antidepressant use and lifetime history of mental disorders in a community sample: results from the Baltimore Epidemiologic Catchment Area Study. *Journal of Clinical Psychiatry*, *76*(1), 40–44.

29. Kessler, R. C., et al. (2003). Comorbid mental disorders account for the role impairment of commonly occurring chronic physical disorders: results from the National Comorbidity Survey. *Journal of Occupational and Environmental Medicine*, *45*(12), 1257–1266.

30. Paksarian, D., et al. (2016). Latent trajectories of common mental health disorder risk across 3 decades of adulthood in a population-based cohort. *JAMA Psychiatry*, *73*(10), 1023–1031.

31. Khazanov, G. K., et al. (2015). Treatment patterns of youth with bipolar disorder: results from the National Comorbidity Survey–Adolescent Supplement (NCS-A). *Journal of Abnormal Child Psychology*, *43*(2), 391–400.

32. Merikangas, K. R., Nakamura, E. F., & Kessler, R. C. (2009). Epidemiology of mental disorders in children and adolescents. *Dialogues in Clinical Neuroscience*, *11*(1), 7–20.

33. Merikangas, K., et al. (2009). National Comorbidity Survey Replication–Adolescent supplement (NCS-A): I. Background and measures. *Journal of the American Academy of Child and Adolescent Psychiatry*, *48*(4), 367–369.

34. Merikangas, K. R., et al. (2010). Prevalence and treatment of mental disorders among US children in the 2001–2004 NHANES. *Pediatrics*, *125*(1), 75–81.

35. Copeland, W. E., Brotman, M. A., & Costello, E. J. (2015). Normative irritability in youth: Developmental findings from the Great Smoky Mountains Study. *Journal of the American Academy of Child and Adolescent Psychiatry*, *54*(8), 635–642.

36. Copeland, W. E., et al. (2015). Increase in untreated cases of psychiatric disorders during the transition to adulthood. *Psychiatric Service*, *66*(4), 397–403.

37. Costello, E. J. (2010). Grand challenges in child and neurodevelopmental psychiatry. *Frontiers in Psychiatry*, *1*, 14.

38. Costello, E. J., Copeland, W., & Angold, A. (2016). The Great Smoky Mountains Study: developmental epidemiology in the southeastern United States. *Social Psychiatry and Psychiatric Epidemiology*, *51*(5), 639–646.

39. Briere, F. N., et al. (2014). Comorbidity between major depression and alcohol use disorder from adolescence to adulthood. *Comprehensive Psychiatry*, *55*(3), 526–533.

40. Wittchen, H. U., et al. (1998). Early Developmental Stages of Psychopathology study (EDSP): objectives and design. *European Addiction Research*, *4*(1–2), 18–27.

41. Angst, J., et al. (2016). The epidemiology of common mental disorders from age 20 to 50: results from the prospective Zurich Cohort Study. *Epidemiology and Psychiatric Sciences*, *25*(1), 24–32.

42. Beesdo-Baum, K., et al. (2009). The structure of common mental disorders: a replication study in a community sample of adolescents and young adults. *International Journal of Methods in Psychiatric Research*, *18*(4), 204–220.

43. Lieb, R., et al. (2000). The Early Developmental Stages of Psychopathology study (EDSP): a methodological update. *European Addiction Research*, *6*(4), 170–182.

44. Merikangas, K. R., et al. (2012). Mania with and without depression in a community sample of US adolescents. *Archives of General Psychiatry, 69*(9), 943–951.

45. Regier, D. A., et al. (1990). Comorbidity of mental disorders with alcohol and other drug abuse. Results from the Epidemiologic Catchment Area (ECA) study. *Journal of the American Medical Association, 264*(19), 2511–2518.

46. Merikangas, K. R., et al. (2008). Specificity of bipolar spectrum conditions in the comorbidity of mood and substance use disorders: results from the Zurich Cohort Study. *Archives of General Psychiatry, 65*(1), 47–52.

47. Whiteford, H. A., et al. (2016). Global burden of mental, neurological, and substance use disorders: An analysis from the Global Burden of Disease Study 2010. In V. Patel, et al. (Eds.), *Mental, Neurological, and Substance Use Disorders: Disease Control Priorities* (3rd ed., Vol. 4; pp. 29–40). Washington, DC: The International Bank for Reconstruction and Development/The World Bank.

48. Lopez, A. D., & Mathers, C. D. (2006). Measuring the global burden of disease and epidemiological transitions: 2002–2030. *Annals of Tropical Medicine and Parasitology, 100*(5–6), 481–499.

49. Thorup, A., et al. (2007). Young males have a higher risk of developing schizophrenia: a Danish Register study. *Psychological Medicine, 37*(4), 479–484.

50. Hafner, H., et al. (1993). Generating and testing a causal explanation of the gender difference in age at first onset of schizophrenia. *Psychological Medicine, 23*(4), 925–940.

51. Costello, E. J., Foley, D. L., & Angold, A. (2006). 10-year research update review: the epidemiology of child and adolescent psychiatric disorders: II. Developmental epidemiology. *Journal of the American Academy of Child and Adolescent Psychiatry, 45*(1), 8–25.

52. Broidy, L. M., et al. (2003). Developmental trajectories of childhood disruptive behaviors and adolescent delinquency: a six-site, cross-national study. *Developmental Psychology, 39*(2), 222–245.

53. Loeber, R. (1991). Antisocial behavior: more enduring than changeable? *Journal of the American Academy of Child and Adolescent Psychiatry, 30*(3), 393–397.

54. Hultman, C. M., et al. (1999). Prenatal and perinatal risk factors for schizophrenia, affective psychosis, and reactive psychosis of early onset: case-control study. *British Medical Journal, 318*(7181), 421–426.

55. Dean, K., & Murray, R. M. (2005). Environmental risk factors for psychosis. *Dialogues in Clinical Neuroscience, 7*(1), 69–80.

56. Morgan, C., & Fisher, H. (2007). Environment and schizophrenia: environmental factors in schizophrenia: childhood trauma—a critical review. *Schizophrenia Bulletin, 33*(1), 3–10.

57. Abdallah, M. W., et al. (2012). Infections during pregnancy and after birth, and the risk of autism spectrum disorders: a register-based study utilizing a Danish historic birth cohort. *Turkish Journal of Psychiatry, 23*(4), 229–235.

58. Cantor-Graae, E., et al. (2003). Migration as a risk factor for schizophrenia: a Danish population-based cohort study. *British Journal of Psychiatry, 182*, 117–122.

59. Morgan, C., et al. (2010). Migration, ethnicity, and psychosis: toward a sociodevelopmental model. *Schizophrenia Bulletin, 36*(4), 655–664.

60. Merikangas, K. R., & Karayiorgou, M. (2014). Genetic epidemiology and molecular genetics of psychiatric disorders. In T. A., et al. (Eds.), *Psychiatry*. New York: Wiley.

61. Gottesman, I. I., & Erlenmeyer-Kimling, L. (2001). Family and twin strategies as a head start in defining prodromes and endophenotypes for hypothetical early-interventions in schizophrenia. *Schizophrenia Research, 51*(1), 93–102.

62. Gottesman, I. I., & Gould, T. D. (2003). The endophenotype concept in psychiatry: etymology and strategic intentions. *American Journal of Psychiatry, 160*(4), 636–645.

63. Flint, J., & Munafo, M. R. (2007). The endophenotype concept in psychiatric genetics. *Psychological Medicine, 37*(2), 163–180.

64. Valdar, W., et al. (2006). Genome-wide genetic association of complex traits in heterogeneous stock mice. *Nature Genetics, 38*(8), 879–887.

65. Smith, G. D., et al. (2005). Genetic epidemiology and public health: hope, hype, and future prospects. *The Lancet, 366*(9495), 1484–1498.

66. Hopper, J. L., Bishop, D. T., & Easton, D. F. (2005). Population-based family studies in genetic epidemiology. *The Lancet, 366*(9494), 1397–1406.

67. Yang, J., et al. (2011). GCTA: a tool for genome-wide complex trait analysis. *American Journal of Human Genetics, 88*(1), 76–82.

68. Risch, N. (1990). Linkage strategies for genetically complex traits. I. Multilocus models. *American Journal of Human Genetics, 46*, 222–228.

69. Merikangas, K. R. (1990). Comorbidity for anxiety and depression: review of family and genetic studies. In C. R. Cloninger (Ed.), *Comorbidity of Mood and Anxiety Disorders* (pp. 331–348). Washington, DC: American Psychiatric Press.

70. Maes, H. H., et al. (1998). Assortative mating for major psychiatric diagnoses in two population-based samples. *Psychological Medicine, 28*(6), 1389–1401.

71. Mathews, C. A., & Reus, V. I. (2001). Assortative mating in the affective disorders: a systematic review and meta-analysis. *Comprehensive Psychiatry, 42*(4), 257–262.

72. Grant, J. D., et al. (2007). Spousal concordance for alcohol dependence: evidence for assortative mating or spousal interaction effects? *Alcoholism, Clinical and Experimental Research, 31*(5), 717–728.

73. Low, N., Cui, L., & Merikangas, K. R. (2007). Spousal concordance for substance use and anxiety disorders. *Journal of Psychiatric Research, 41*(11), 942–951.

74. Parnas, J. (1988). Assortative mating in schizophrenia: results from the Copenhagen High-Risk Study. *Psychiatry, 51*(1), 58–64.

75. Merikangas, K. R. (1982). Assortative mating for psychiatric disorders and psychological traits. *Archives of General Psychiatry, 39*(10), 1173–1180.

76. Merikangas, K. R., & Brunetto, W. (1996). Assortative mating and psychiatric disorders. *Balliere's Clinical Psychiatry International Practice and Research, 2*(1), 175–185.

77. Mascie-Taylor, C. G. (1989). Spouse similarity for IQ and personality and convergence. *Behavior Genetics, 19*(2), 223–227.

78. Mascie-Taylor, C. G., & Gibson, J. B. (1979). A biological survey of a Cambridge suburb: assortative marriage for IQ and personality traits. *Annals of Human Biology, 6*(1), 1–16.

79. Farley, F. H., & Davis, S. A. (1977). Arousal, personality, and assortative mating in marriage. *Journal of Sex and Marital Therapy, 3*(2), 122–127.

80. Farley, F. H., & Mueller, C. B. (1978). Arousal, personality, and assortative mating in marriage: generalizability and cross-cultural factors. *Journal of Sex and Marital Therapy, 4*(1), 50–53.

81. Heun, R., & Maier, W. (1993). Morbid risks for major disorders and frequencies of personality disorders among spouses of psychiatric inpatients and controls. *Comprehensive Psychiatry, 34*(2), 137–143.

82. Dubuis-Stadelmann, E., et al. (2001). Spouse similarity for temperament, personality and psychiatric symptomatology. *Personality and Individual Differences, 30*, 1095–1112.

83. Feng, D., & Baker, L. (1994). Spouse similarity in attitudes, personality, and psychological well-being. *Behavior Genetics, 24*(4), 357–364.

84. Mascie-Taylor, C. G., & Boldsen, J. L. (1984). Assortative mating for IQ: a multivariate approach. *Journal of Biosocial Science, 16*(1), 109–117.

85. Plomin, R., Krapohl, E, & O'Reilly, P. F. (2016). Assortative mating: A missing piece in the jigsaw of psychiatric genetics. *JAMA Psychiatry, 73*(4), 323–324.

86. Peyrot, W. J., et al. (2016). Exploring boundaries for the genetic consequences of assortative mating for psychiatric traits. *JAMA Psychiatry, 73*(11), 1189–1195.

87. Harvey, P. D., et al. (2010). Cognition and disability in bipolar disorder: lessons from schizophrenia research. *Bipolar Disorder, 12*(4), 364–375.

88. Lichtenstein, P., et al. (2006). The Swedish Twin Registry in the third millennium: an update. *Twin Research and Human Genetics, 9*(6), 875–882.

89. McGuffin, P., et al. (2003). The heritability of bipolar affective disorder and the genetic relationship to unipolar depression. *Archives of General Psychiatry, 60*(5), 497–502.

90. van Beijsterveldt, C. E., et al. (2013). The Young Netherlands Twin Register (YNTR): longitudinal twin and family studies in over 70,000 children. *Twin Research and Human Genetics, 16*(1), 252–267.

91. Verhulst, B., Neale, M. C., & Kendler, K. S. (2015). The heritability of alcohol use disorders: a meta-analysis of twin and adoption studies. *Psychological Medicine, 45*(5), 1061–1072.

92. U.S. Department of Health and Human Services, Administration for Children and Families, Administration on Children, Youth and Families, Children's Bureau. (2017). *Trends in Foster Care and Adoption: FY 2007-FY 2016.* Available from: https://www.acf.hhs.gov/sites/default/files/cb/trends_fostercare_adoption_07thru16.pdf.

93. Risch, N., et al. (2014). Familial recurrence of autism spectrum disorder: evaluating genetic and environmental contributions. *American Journal of Psychiatry, 171*(11), 1206–1213.

94. Psychiatric GWAS Consortium Coordinating Committee, et al. (2009). Genome-wide association studies: history, rationale, and prospects for psychiatric disorders. *American Journal of Psychiatry, 166*(5), 540–556.

95. Moonesinghe, R., et al. (2008). Required sample size and nonreplicability thresholds for heterogeneous genetic associations. *Proceedings of the National Academy of Sciences of the U S A, 105*(2), 617–622.

96. Smith, G. D. (2010). Mendelian randomization for strengthening causal inference in observational studies: Application to gene x environment interactions. *Perspectives on Psychological Science, 5*(5), 527–545.

97. Smith, G. D., & Ebrahim, S. (2003). "Mendelian randomization": can genetic epidemiology contribute to understanding environmental determinants of disease? *International Journal of Epidemiology, 32*(1), 1–22.

98. Thomas, D. C., & Conti, D. V. (2004). Commentary: the concept of "Mendelian Randomization." *International Journal of Epidemiology, 33*(1), 21–25.

99. Wray, N. R., et al. (2014). Research review: Polygenic methods and their application to psychiatric traits. *Journal of Child Psychology and Psychiatry, 55*(10), 1068–1087.

100. Dudbridge, F. (2013). Power and predictive accuracy of polygenic risk scores. *PLoS Genetics, 9*(3), e1003348.

101. Euesden, J., Lewis, C. M., & O'Reilly, P. F. (2015). PRSice: Polygenic Risk Score software. *Bioinformatics, 31*(9), 1466–1468.

102. Purcell, S. M., et al. (2009). Common polygenic variation contributes to risk of schizophrenia and bipolar disorder. *Nature, 460*(7256), 748–752.

103. Hamshere, M. L., et al. (2011). Polygenic dissection of the bipolar phenotype. *British Journal of Psychiatry, 198*(4), 284–288.

104. Benjamin, D. J., et al. (2012). The genetic architecture of economic and political preferences. *Proceedings of the National Academy of Sciences of the U S A, 109*(21), 8026–8031.

105. Lee, S. H., et al. (2012). Estimating the proportion of variation in susceptibility to schizophrenia captured by common SNPs. *Nature Genetics, 44*(3), 247–250.

106. Cross-Disorder Group of the Psychiatric Genomics Consortium, et al. (2013). Genetic relationship between five psychiatric disorders estimated from genome-wide SNPs. *Nature Genetics, 45*(9), 984–994.

107. Yang, L., et al. (2013). Polygenic transmission and complex neuro developmental network for attention deficit hyperactivity disorder: genome-wide association study of both common and rare variants. *American Journal of Medical Genetics, Part B: Neuropsychiatric Genetics, 162b*(5), 419–430.

108. Ferentinos, P., et al. (2015). Familiality and SNP heritability of age at onset and episodicity in major depressive disorder. *Psychological Medicine, 45*(10), 2215–2225.

109. Huo, Y. X., et al. (2016). Identification of *SLC25A37* as a major depressive disorder risk gene. *Journal of Psychiatric Research, 83*, 168–175.

110. Trzaskowski, M., et al. (2013). First genome-wide association study on anxiety-related behaviors in childhood. *PLoS One, 8*(4), e58676.

111. Klei, L., et al. (2012). Common genetic variants, acting additively, are a major source of risk for autism. *Molecular Autism, 3*(1), 9.

112. Wray, N. R., & Gottesman, I. I. (2012). Using summary data from the Danish national registers to estimate heritabilities for schizophrenia, bipolar disorder, and major depressive disorder. *Frontiers in Genetics, 3*, 118.

113. Visscher, P. M., et al. (2012). Evidence-based psychiatric genetics, AKA the false dichotomy between common and rare variant hypotheses. *Molecular Psychiatry, 17*(5), 474–485.

114. Wray, N. R., Goddard, M. E., & Visscher, P. M. (2008). Prediction of individual genetic risk of complex disease. *Current Opinion in Genetics and Development, 18*(3), 257–263.

115. Visscher, P. M., et al. (2012). Five years of GWAS discovery. *American Journal of Human Genetics, 90*(1), 7–24.

116. Merikangas, A. K., et al. (2015). The phenotypic manifestations of rare genic CNVs in autism spectrum disorder. *Molecular Psychiatry, 20*(11), 1366–1372.

117. Gudbjartsson, D. F., et al. (2015). Large-scale whole-genome sequencing of the Icelandic population. *Nature Genetics, 47*(5), 435–444.

118. Krumholz, H. M. (2009). Registries and selection bias: the need for accountability. *Circulation: Cardiovascular Quality and Outcomes, 2*(6), 517–518.

119. Gottweis, H., & Lauss, G. (2010). Biobank governance in the post-genomic age. *Personalized Medicine, 7*(2), 187–195.

120. Weissman, M. M., Brown, A. S., & Talati, A. (2011). Translational epidemiology in psychiatry: linking population to clinical and basic sciences. *Archives of General Psychiatry, 68*(6), 600–608.

121. Yang, Q., et al. (2000). On the use of population-based registries in the clinical validation of genetic tests for disease susceptibility. *Genetics in Medicine, 2*, 186–192.

122. Hunter, D. J. (2005). Gene–environment interactions in human diseases. *Nature Reviews Genetics, 6*(4), 287–298.

Chapter 2

Recruitment of Human Subjects

An Overview of Techniques and Methods Used in Psychiatric and Other Clinical Studies

Layla Kassem

Take-Home Points

1. Recruitment invariably requires more time than anticipated: be realistic when planning.
2. Prepare clear recruitment material.
3. Train recruiters well and comprehensively.
4. Establish trust.
5. Have a clear plan for follow up and feedback to participants.

Introduction

Success of psychiatric and other clinical research studies depends on several factors: the understanding of the disease and its natural course, the research team, the clarity of questions to be addressed, the science behind it, the *participants* and how they are recruited, and finally, being realistic. While these factors are important when one is recruiting for any clinical research study, they are doubly important when recruiting for psychiatric studies. Psychiatric disorders continue to carry a fair amount of stigma and appear to be typically misunderstood by the general public. The stigma, coupled with misinformation at times, renders participants unwilling to declare themselves or their families as carriers of the disease.

Years of experience, and a 2009 report from the Agency for Healthcare Research and Quality (AHRQ), demonstrate that recruitment of participants is a challenging activity that "often takes longer than anticipated, incurs higher costs than expected, and that participation rates typically range between 3–20% of the eligible participant pool." Recruitment rates may vary for a variety of reasons, starting with the nature of the disease under investigation, potential recruits' mistrust of research and researchers, a general lack of interest in research, disappointment in researchers, potential volunteers' limited knowledge of research and its implications, and limited information about the disease under investigation, its treatment, and possibly its inheritance patterns. This chapter will address techniques, methods, and points to consider when recruiting participants, and approaches for addressing participants' apprehension or reluctance to volunteer for research studies.

Study Design, Recruitment, and Retention

Recruitment is an essential dialogue occurring between researchers and participants; it forms the foundation of any study, and has three main goals: recruiting a sample that is a representative of the target populations, recruiting sufficient participants to meet the power requirements of a study, and retention of participants.[1]

Factors to consider when recruiting participants include sample size requirements, the type of study design, data collection methods, and geographic locations. Sample size is a critical issue involving power calculations to be addressed during the design stage. Hence the first question to address prior to recruitment is: How many participants are needed? followed by: What are we collecting? What for? And who are the target populations?

How Many Participants Are Needed? What Are We Collecting? And What Is It For?

These first three questions are addressed by the nature and design of the study. Clinical data and biomaterials (blood, sputum, cerebrospinal fluid, brain, skin, hair, urine) to be collected influence, and at times limit, recruitment. Which clinical data and biomaterials collected and how they are collected follow strict ethical and humanistic guidelines. The study team, funding sources, and the Internal Review Board (IRB) share in the responsibility of upholding and reinforcing the guidelines; and share in creating effective and safe recruitment environments.

Whom Are We Collecting?

This fourth question is determined by the study design and the research questions to be addressed. Case-control studies, family-based studies, longitudinal studies, genetic studies, and randomized clinical trials each have a set of requirements that guide recruitment efforts. Each of the study designs poses different recruitment challenges, and at times demands different recruitment methods. In other words, each study design imposes a different set of requirements when it comes to recruitment.

Preparing for Recruitment

Guided by the study design, study questions and hypotheses, and the materials to be collected, potential populations are identified and the process of generating interest in the research and participating in it begins.

How Do We Generate Interest?

Designing brochures, recruitment letters, and fliers that are simple, attractive, and informative to be distributed in strategic areas known to your targeted population is the first step. Successful written material typically includes: information on the purpose and usefulness of the study, description of participation, the voluntary and confidential nature of the research, possibly how personal data will be used, incentives, opt-out options, principal investigators and collaborators, and recruitment personnel's contact information.

In addition to written materials, advertising in key newspapers and radio stations, having an online presence, developing a website, and having a 24-hour free telephone line enhance recruitment and increase study exposure. Interest-generation is further enhanced through presentations at key institutions in different communities. Presentations typically address the communities' concerns regarding the diseases being investigated, and concerns surrounding participating in research, its confidentiality, and its importance. Presentations also allow participants to interact with the researchers and see them as "human" and accessible.

Finally, studies that require large sample sizes and/or a variety of analysis methods benefit greatly, and increase their efficiency, through collaborating with others. Collaboration with others is a two-step process. The initial step occurs pre-study and involves promotion of the study, clear agreements, documentation, and the demonstration that the study will not interfere with, or burden the referring institutions, clinicians, and administrative staff. The initial step is also marked by the development of clear understanding and mutually agreed-upon procedures. The second step entails maintaining the collaborations. Maintenance of collaborative relationships requires reciprocity, appreciation, and sharing of and follow-up on overall study results and findings.

Ethical Concerns

Once a population has been identified, researchers need to attend to the following: establishing recruitment methods that guarantee equitable and fair selection of participants. All participants who meet criteria for a study should have an equal chance of participating in the study. Age, gender, orientation, religion, or geographic location, unless otherwise specified, are typically not used as exclusion criteria.

Participants' privacy is to be respected. For example, when mailing out fliers and thank-you letters, or letters requesting more information, or when leaving telephone messages for a participant, recruiters ought to attend to the details and make sure that envelopes and cards do not identify the nature of the study, and that voice messages left are neutral and do not have language that would compromise participants' privacy.

Participation in studies is a voluntary action; hence, when presenting a study to potential participants, the presentation has to be free of pressure and unbiased. Pressure may come in the form of incentives that are too attractive to turn down, the use of key personalities in a participant's life or treatment, or offering favors in return for participation. Biased presentations may come in the form of misleading and incomplete information. Recruiters need to make sure that the information imparted is accurate, complete, and presented in a manner that provides participants with options and the right to refuse.

Clinical and genetic studies face an added challenge; namely, therapeutic misconception: potential participants may at times believe or expect that research proposed by health care professionals will benefit them in some immediate way. It is imperative that recruiters address this expectation clearly, repeatedly, and prior to recruitment.

Recruitment

Methods

Advertising
As mentioned earlier in this chapter, acceptable recruitment methods include the generation of interest and advertising. IRB-approved brochures, fliers, information sheets, recruitment letters, Internet postings, radio advertisements, and community connections are necessary, and enhance recruitment efforts. When you are designing advertisement materials, the recruitment settings need to be considered, and vulnerable populations—i.e., populations who can be harmed, coerced, or deceived because of their diminished knowledge or competence, or because of disadvantaged status—need to be protected. Sutton et al.[2] suggest that collaboration between health care providers, participants, and community leaders enhances recruitment of vulnerable populations while protecting the rights of the participants. Advertising material needs to be presented in clear and complete language, and be free of all misleading language.

Direct Recruitment, Random or Opportunistic Sampling, and Referrals
Direct recruitment includes face-to-face contact with potential participants, and it can occur in the community, at hospitals, in clinics, and at community meetings/activities. Mathos et al.[3] in a study assessing recruitment methods for a study investigating the genetics of psychotic illness, found that the success of face-to-face recruitment depends on several factors: positive reports by other research participants, family support for research participation, and the support of health care providers. Fuqua et al.[4] (p. 00), when discussing the recruitment of African Americans in a heart study, suggested that successful

face-to-face recruitment is highly dependent on strategies "built on a foundation of community partnerships that assured possibilities for community-wide benefit." Taylor[5] states that, when attempting to recruit non-majority populations (e.g., African Americans or others), "understanding of, and sensitivity to" their culture is an important starting point. Having a knowledge of a population's history with the health system, research, and organizations in general is necessary in order to develop the appropriate communication methods.

When recruiting face-to-face, recruiters need to pay considerable attention to their communication and to attend to perceived or actual pressure when approaching participants. Given that this is face-to-face interaction, and at times includes participants' physicians and caregivers, there is a possibility that participants may experience pressure, or feel shy about declining participation.

Face-to-face recruitment has distinct benefits; mainly that it allows for rapidly establishing rapport with study participants, defusing in real time their concerns or questions about the research or their data. Multiple types of data can be collected during a single meeting. Questions, or errors regarding consent and questionnaires (when used) can be reviewed and corrected immediately. Drawbacks to this method of recruitment are the expenses involved in staff training and traveling; and standardizing the research protocol.

Random sampling and referrals typically come from other professionals, family members, and other participants. Taylor et al. (2009), Mathos et al. (2006), and Fuqua et al. (2005) all found that the highest number of participants came from health care providers, family members, and registries. While health care providers, registries, and family members are good referral sources, in these instances, recruiters have to wait for the participants to contact them, and referring individuals (unless otherwise specified) are not at liberty to provide personal identifiers of any potential participant.

Participant Pools

Participant pools include participants who have been or are active participants in studies and have consented to having their information shared with other researchers. These pools are characteristically available to collaborators and non-collaborators. However, they cannot be accessed by non-collaborators in the absence of an IRB-approved, signed, informed consent by the participant.

Establishing and Maintaining Collaborations; Methods of Collaboration

Collaborations are an essential component of any recruitment effort. Collaborations with other researchers are sometimes an efficient way for increasing sample sizes. Collaborating with institutions and organizations is essential for recruitment and follows ethical and humanistic guidelines. When recruiting at different institutions and treatment facilities, recruiters first seek permission from the organization, followed by providing complete information to the staff, and finally guaranteeing that recruitment efforts will not burden the participants, the institution, or its staff.

Collaborative relationships are designed to be a win–win situation for all involved and are developed through organizing meetings, presentations, and possibly offering workshops for the staff and different professionals involved with potential participants. Maintenance of collaborations is as important as the collaborations themselves. It is important to have reasonably frequent contact, find appropriate opportunities to reciprocate, and to offer information on overall results and findings and their possible benefit to the referring organizations and professionals.

Who May Recruit?

The initial contact with participants is the starting point of successful recruitment; first contact is both delicate and sensitive and is ideally conducted by an individual who is thoroughly knowledgeable about the study and the science behind it: well educated on the disease being investigated, and fully trained on the study protocol. Those involved with the first contact also need to be trained on the voluntary nature of participation; need to have knowledge of, and a deep appreciation for, ethical standards; and should be well able to answer questions honestly and completely, and fully able to attend to the needs of the participants before the needs of the study. Finally, they should be able to present the pros and cons of participation, and provide options.

Family Member Recruitment

At times, family members volunteer to recruit other family members or are asked to recruit other members. In such cases, researchers are obligated to establish methods by which privacy is maintained, and undue pressure is minimized.

Recruitment Models

There are several recruitment models; here we will address to two main ones.

Model A: Advertisement Driven—Participant Initiated

This is a paradigm where awareness of and accessibility to a study are established through advertisements, press releases, and posters placed at community centers, libraries, religious centers, treatment facilities, hospitals, clinics, and health care management organizations (HMOs). Participants find the studies through the advertisements, fliers, mailings, other volunteers, presentations, or the Internet, or through organizations focused on the disease of interest. Participants make the initial contact.

While efficient and at times cost-effective, this paradigm is not free of challenges. Primarily, when participants come to the research teams, there are assumptions made on both sides. Participants may assume that because they made contact, they will be automatically enrolled. Recruiters at times make the assumption that potential participants understand research and the disease, are eager and ready to enroll, and understand their rights. While some of the assumptions may bear some truth, it is best to treat all individuals contacting the teams as novices both on research protocols, and on participation in studies. It is also important to be sensitive to the possibility that participants do not fully understand their or their family member's disease.

A second challenge may be that participants experience research materials as an intrusion into their places of safety; for example, the clinic, hospital, place of worship, treating professional, or favorite radio station. A third challenge is participants' being reluctant to show interest in a posting lest others find out that they suffer from a disease. This last situation is especially true for individuals dealing with mental health issues. Mental illness, unlike other diseases, still appears to carry a fair amount of stigma and social undesirability. It also remains shrouded in mystery and is little understood; as a result, it could be surrounded by fear, confusion, and concern. Hence, it is highly recommended that prior to embarking on recruitment, researchers should give serious consideration and attention to the social, personal, and familial implications of participation. Recruiters need to be sensitive to the participants' needs and concerns.

Model B: Community Driven—Personnel Initiated

In this paradigm, recruiters go into participants' communities. This model of recruitment is more involved, more labor intensive, and more challenging. When following Model B, recruiters can make no assumptions about potential recruits or communities. This model is best perceived as having three phases, starting with the question—*How best to collect data?*

Experience working with isolated populations, vulnerable populations, and individuals out of mainstream culture has demonstrated that, while the method is time-consuming, best results are achieved when data are collected in person, using interviews and community facilitators. In order to complete this form of recruitment, the following three phases are necessary.

Phase I: Trust Building

This phase is the most crucial and most sensitive when working with Model B across cultures. Trust-building requires the following: patience, educating recruiters on populations and cultures of interest, flexibility, and at times, modification of expectations. On the human level, trust building requires authenticity, honesty, and openness in communication. It also requires sensitivity to the individuals and their communities, and recognition that, at times, the community and its needs come before the research. And finally, trust building requires giving back to the community. Phase I may take time and resources and may add to the time allotted to recruitment, however, it is necessary, and studies need to take that into consideration when embarking on transcultural recruitment efforts.

Phase II: Data Collection

The data collection phase starts with screening of potential participants, and is followed by obtaining informed consent from willing and appropriate participants. Screening materials are typically a structured template addressing the enrollment criteria for a study. Informed consent follows IRB regulations, and consent documents are IRB-approved. While all studies have some form of consent process, recruiters have to be educated on the consent process and have to develop an understanding of the cultures within which they are working prior to recruiting consenting participants. Why is this so? The consenting stage is the participants' entry point into any study—if consents are not appropriately explained, participants could be intimidated by the process and discourage others from participating, and the study could potentially be compromised.

Consent forms are sensitive documents that need to use language that is accessible to most educational levels, and sensitive to the disease and culture it is being used within. Consent language has to be clear, simple, and inclusive, and it must address the limits and boundaries of the study. Consent documents explain the study, its procedures, its implications for the participant, the compensation (when applicable); and must fully explain confidentiality and the participant's right of withdrawal from the study. And, when applicable, consent documents also address how the study deals with incidental findings and follow-up.

Phase III: Termination and Follow-up
The final phase of recruitment activities is termination and follow-up. The challenge faced by most clinical studies is that many potential recruits have experienced some form of distress and are seeking relief that is not immediately available through participating in a study. The issue of termination is dealt with at the time of enrollment. Participants are informed about when their enrollment is considered terminated. Follow-up is a more complicated matter—different studies address follow-up differently. However, when working cross-culturally and with vulnerable populations, having an annual newsletter that covers the latest developments, some findings, and information that could be useful to the target population is a recommended form of follow-up.

Through their participation in studies, some participants view research teams as a useful source of information, and as a resource. Part of giving back to communities may involve the establishment of a system through which participants are able to call when they have questions or need advice on resources available for the disease in question.

Finally, potential participants need to be informed clearly about when their participation is considered terminated, and informed on what happens upon termination of a study.

Conclusion

Participant recruitment is a challenging task that involves a number of activities—identifying potential participants, explaining the study, recruiting an adequate sample based on study goals and design, obtaining informed consent, maintaining ethical standards, and retaining participants until study completion.

Recruiters aim to minimize inconvenience to participants, are cognizant of participants' needs and limits, and recognize that external factors may sometimes affect participants' willingness and ability to participate.

While there are many different ways to recruit participants, it is often necessary to use more than one recruiting approach. Screening and eventually getting the consent of participants are the most sensitive and crucial part of any recruitment effort.

Finally, multisite collaborations, especially these involving multiplex families, require recruitment methods that are well defined and uniformly applied. While these requirements appear intuitive to any researcher, in practice, they entail extensive planning, training, and effort.

References

1. Patel, M., Doku, V., & Tennakoon, L. (2003). Challenges in recruitment of research participants. *Advances in Psychiatric Treatment*, 9, 229–238.

2. Sutton, L. B., Erlen, J. A., Glad, J. M., & Siminoff, L. A. (2003). Recruiting vulnerable populations for research: Revisiting Ethical Issues. *Journal of Professional Nursing*, 19(2), 106–112.

3. Mathos, K. K., Gur, R. E., Lokar, F., Calkins, M. E., & Nimgaonkar, V. (2006). A description of the process of recruitment for research studies investigating the genetics of psychotic illness. *Curr Psychiatry Rep*, 8(4), 307–312.

4. Fuqua, S. R., Wyatt, S. B., Andrew, M. E., Sarpong, D. F., Henderson, F. R., Cunningham, M. F., & Taylor, H. A. (2005). Recruiting African-American Research Participation in the Jackson Heart Study: Methods, Response Rates, and Sample Description. *Ethnicity & Disease*, 15.

5. Taylor, J. Y. (2009). Recruitment of three generations of African American women into genetics research. *Transcultural Nursing*, 20(2), 219–226.

Additional Resources

Calkins, M., Dobie, D. J., Cadenhead, K. S., Kristin, S., Olincy, A., Freedman, R., . . . Braff, D. L. (2007). The Consortium on the Genetics of Endophenotypes in Schizophrenia: Model recruitment, assessment, and endophenotyping methods for a multisite collaboration. *Schizophrenia Bulletin*, 33(1), 33–48.

Callard, F., Broadbent, M., Denis, M., Hotopf, M., Soncul, M., Wykes, T., . . . Stewart, R. (2010). Developing a new model for patient recruitment in mental health services: A cohort study using Electronic Health Records. *BMC Psychiatry*, 4(12), 1–10.

Gupta, C. U., & Kharawala, S. (2012). Informed consent in psychiatry clinical research: A conceptual review of issues, challenges, and recommendations. *Perspectives on Clinical Research*, 3(1), 8–15.

Howard, L., de Salis, I., Tomlin, Z., Thornicroft, G., & Donovanb, J. (2009). Why is recruitment to trials difficult? An investigation into recruitment difficulties in an RCT of supported employment in patients with severe mental illness. *Contemporary Clinical Trials*, 30(1), 40–46.

National Institute of Mental Health. (2005). *Points to Consider About Recruitment and Retention While Preparing a Clinical Research Study.* June 2005.

Sugden, N. A., & Moulson, M. C. (2015). Recruitment strategies should not be randomly selected: Empirically improving recruitment success and diversity in developmental psychology research. *Frontiers in Psychology, 6,* 523.

Sullivan, J. (2004). Subject recruitment and retention: Barriers to success. *Applied Clinical Trials,* Advanstar Communications Inc.

UCLA. (2012). Office of Human Research Protection Program (OHRPP): *Guidance and Procedure: Recruitment and Screening Methods and Materials.* September 28, 1–8.

Woodall, A. (2011). Barriers to participation in mental health research: Findings from the Genetics and Psychosis (GAP) Study. *International Journal of Psychiatry, 23*(1), 31–40.

Woodall, A., Morgan, C., Sloan, C., & Howard, L. (2014). Barriers to participation in mental health research: Are there specific gender, ethnicity and age related barriers? *Health Informatics, 10*(103), 1–10.

Chapter 3

Basic Molecular Genetics Concepts and Tools

From SNPs to Chips

Sevilla D. Detera-Wadleigh, Nirmala Akula, and Liping Hou

Take-Home Points

1. Sequencing of the human genome and genomes of organisms across the evolutionary scale has spawned a remarkable revolution in genetics. Next generation sequencing of whole exome, whole genome and transcriptome has revealed novel functional elements and the vast richness of gene expression.
2. Identification of genome-wide nucleotide variation has provided a framework for high resolution mapping. This, coupled with large sample collections, rapid, high throughput genotyping and novel statistical methods, has bolstered the detection of multiple susceptibility loci in complex diseases and traits.
3. Evolution in genome editing has heightened the potential to alter any nucleotide and discern its biological effect.
4. Taken together, these exceptional advances and innovations plus the ability to generate diverse patient- or individual-specific cells through iPSC technology, in addition to in vivo models, power functional studies that could enhance disease modeling, unravel disease mechanisms and reveal new therapeutic targets.

Introduction: Human Genetics

The breathtaking revolution in the field of genetics traces its beginnings to a few decades ago and continues at an impressive pace. It has bolstered the ambitious goal of identifying and characterizing the biological role of every nucleotide in the human genome in order to understand disease causes and susceptibility factors; prevent, diagnose, and treat disease; and illuminate similarities and dissimilarities between individuals. Ultimately, genetic studies could help minimize the burden of diseases on patients in particular, and on society as a whole.

Genetics aims to define and explain the genetic variation in living organisms. In humans, the unique, multifaceted, and complex inherited characteristics evolve from a genomic DNA sequence, a chain of roughly 3 billion base pairs that is composed, astonishingly, of only four different nucleotides. Although each individual carries her/his own distinctive DNA sequence, most of the genome is shared by all human beings. This suggests that a finite number of sequence variations could distinguish disparate study samples, which on the surface would imply that unraveling the genetic architecture of diseases should be less challenging than it is. However, the variability and multiplicity of combinations of sequence variations, the intricate array of products of individual genetic units, and their interplay with environmental factors magnify the complexity of this problem.

In this chapter, we will present concepts in human genetics, including the evolution of strategies and tools that continue to underpin advances in the field that can lead to the gradual resolution of disease processes. We will focus our discussion on diseases, as the principles are largely applicable to other inherited traits; the important role of de novo variation in central nervous system (CNS) disease will also be discussed. To start, we briefly present examples of large genetics initiatives that continue to be critical to the progress of cogent approaches in genetic studies.

Large Genetics Initiatives

Multinational collaborations launched several large initiatives to tackle fundamental issues in genetics expeditiously and comprehensively. Timely accessibility of data by researchers worldwide was made paramount providing a framework for generating novel strategies, developing improved tools, and hastening discoveries. We have selected some of the immensely impactful international collaborations and briefly present them here.

The Human Genome Project

The Human Genome Project (HGP) was organized and initiated in 1990 with the ambitious goal of sequencing the human genome. HGP may be considered the single most influential venture in the past decades, one that has set the stage for, and driven, the remarkable progress in genetics research. The first draft of the human genome sequence was published in 2001[1,2], and the project was completed in 2003.[3] The workhorse for this early stage of sequencing was the automated DNA capillary sequencer that utilizes the Sanger dideoxy-terminator method (see Genetic Mapping and Analysis). The massive effort revealed exquisite features of the genome, including the number and identity of protein-coding genes, polymorphic sites, and other previously unexplored, distinctive structures. Decoding the human genome spurred the rapid progress in sequencing model organisms, including many eukaryotes and prokaryotes. Extensive amounts of genomic data have been made available publicly and displayed graphically in genome browsers; e.g., University of California Santa Cruz (UCSC) Genome Browser & Ensembl (see Genome Browsers).

Database for Single Nucleotide Polymorphisms

The Database for Single Nucleotide Polymorphisms (dbSNP; http://www. ncbi.nlm.nih.gov/SNP/) is a repository of characterized, validated and mapped SNPs. SNPs are single-nucleotide polymorphisms, and, by convention, each SNP is designated by a unique accession number prefixed by the letters "rs." dbSNP provides detailed information on the nucleotide change, surrounding sequence, location, allele frequency, resultant amino acid or protein sequence change, if any, and other salient features. Since its inception, the database has expanded rapidly, storing millions of variants that populate the genome of humans and other organisms. The vigorous activity in SNP detection was a response to the critical need for high density, high-resolution genetic markers to achieve an efficient and precise survey of the genome for yet undiscovered disease loci and genetic risk factors. SNPs have been key to the progress in genome-wide association studies (GWAS) (see Genetic Mapping Analysis).

1000 Genomes Project

Initially, the 1000 Genomes Project (http://www.1000genomes.org/)[4] planned to determine and assemble exome and whole genome sequences of >1000 different individuals from 14 populations. Progress was fueled by next-generation sequencing (NGS; see DNA Sequencing) technology, which generates enormous amounts of sequence data rapidly, at a relatively low cost. The project has created a detailed depiction of the human genome sequence, including millions of SNPs, indels, copy number variants (CNVs), and their precise chromosomal location. Sequence variations common among diverse populations, in addition to rare variants unique to specific populations, have been revealed. In the final phase of the Project, sequences of >2500 individuals from 26 different populations were determined, out of which >88 million variants were identified.[5] With the benefit of enormous sequence readouts, functional information can be either inferred or predicted. Researchers are provided access to a library of sequences in diverse populations that serves as an indispensable reference for genetic studies.

Encyclopedia of DNA Elements

The Encyclopedia of DNA Elements (ENCODE; https://www.encodeproject.org/) is an international consortium organized in 2003 and funded by National Human Genome Research Institute (NHGRI), the National Institutes of Health (NIH), with the goal of resolving the function of human DNA sequence. The coding region that comprises a minimal portion, ~1%, of the genome was the initial focus; efforts were later extended to cover the entire genome. The wealth of whole genome sequences generated through NGS has delivered vast undefined regions that require annotation. ENCODE analyzed >1,600 data sets from studies of 147 diverse cell types. In 2012, the group reported that >80% of the human genome contains a functional ENCODE element (The ENCODE Project Consortium).[6] The comprehensive annotation brings to the fore the biological relevance of sequences that comprise the bulk of the genome. It is a hugely important and particularly welcome breakthrough post-GWAS, since these studies have disclosed a preponderance of disease-associated variants in intronic and intergenic regions with obscure function. Key findings and data integration are also published in Nature ENCODE Explorer (http://www.nature.com/encode/).

Database for Genotypes and Phenotypes

In 2007, the National Center for Biotechnology Information (NCBI) of the National Library of Medicine (NLM), NIH, reported the creation of the Database for Genotypes and Phenotypes: (dbGaP; http://www.ncbi.nlm.nih.gov/gap), a public repository for data from studies that have examined the interaction between genotypes and phenotypes, including GWAS, medical sequencing and molecular diagnostic assays.[7] To populate dbGaP, investigators are encouraged to submit their data sets with the incentive that all deposited data can be accessed, either freely or on a controlled basis, by researchers worldwide. Analysis on larger cohorts that would otherwise be unattainable in individual laboratories would become feasible, and thus could spawn new breakthroughs.

Genome Browsers

Genome browsers serve as the go-to web-based compendium for manifold features of genes and genomes in humans and other organisms. These websites may be considered the "can't-do-without" reference in genetics. Extensive data on specific loci, variants, or regions of interest, and links to a wide range of genetic sites such as the Online Mendelian Inheritance in Man (OMIM; https://www.ncbi.nlm.nih.gov/omim) can be obtained instantaneously, with just a click of the mouse.

(1) UCSC Genome Browser (https://genome.ucsc.edu/): From its creation at the University of California, Santa Cruz (UCSC), in September 2000, the UCSC Genome Browser has become a vast repository and viewing tool for the human genome and genomes of other organisms. The browser displays a comprehensive annotation of sequences, including all known gene isoforms, regulatory regions, SNPs, secondary structure, tissue expression, and other pertinent information.
(2) Ensembl (http://useast.ensembl.org/index.html): This browser is a joint project of EMBL-EBI and the Wellcome Trust Sanger Institute and has similar genetic content, graphical presentation, and capability as the UCSC Genome Browser.

Goal of Genetic Studies

The fundamental and overarching goal of genetic studies is to understand disease causes and mechanisms and to apply that knowledge to lessen the burden on affected individuals, families, society, and the health care system as a whole. Genetic studies require three essential components: (i) a study sample composed of either a panel of affected pedigrees or parent-offspring trios, or a collection of unrelated cases and controls; (ii) polymorphic markers that could track segregation or transmission in families, or screen for association of genetic variations with diseases or traits; and (iii) statistical methods to analyze and interpret genotype data. In recent years, investigators have driven the exponential growth of marker generation, upsurge in sample collection, and advances in statistical methods that, in combination, expedited the analysis of both monogenic and complex diseases.

The major aims of genetic studies include the following:

- Determine the cause(s) of disease
- Determine genetic risk factors for a complex disease or trait
- Identify markers for early detection
- Identify markers for diagnostic precision
- Generate prognostic markers
- Develop preventive modalities
- Identify novel targets for drug discovery
- Determine environmental factors that trigger disease manifestation

Patterns of Inheritance and Study Samples

Examples of patterns of inheritance in study samples are presented here:

Mendelian Inheritance

Mendelian diseases are rare and are caused by a highly penetrant, segregating single-gene mutation. This distinction suggests that a relatively small size of a well-phenotyped family sample is sufficient to identify the defective locus. The genetic mutation for scores of Mendelian diseases has been identified (OMIM). It is estimated, however, that there are >6,800 rare diseases (https://rare-diseases.info.nih.gov/about-gard/pages/31/frequently-asked-questions), suggesting that the causal mutation for thousands of rare and undiagnosed diseases remains to be determined.

Mendelian diseases display one of the following modes of transmission:

- Autosomal dominant. The disease allele is transmitted from one parent, rendering the affected offspring heterozygous for the mutant allele. Marfan syndrome is an example of an autosomal dominant disease that is caused by mutations in fibrillin (*FBN1*) (OMIM).
- Autosomal recessive. Each parent carries the disease allele, and both transmit that allele; hence, the affected offspring is a homozygote—i.e., it carries two copies of the mutant allele. Mutations in *CFTR* form the molecular basis for cystic fibrosis, an autosomal recessive disease (OMIM).
- X-linked. The mutant allele is located on the X-chromosome and is transmitted from the mother, usually, to male offspring. Hemophilia A is an X-linked disease caused by a deficiency in Factor VIII (OMIM).
    - Anticipation: Disease can be either autosomal dominant or X-linked, and severity is greater with early age of onset and intensifies in succeeding generations. The expansion of triplet repeats in either the coding or untranslated regions accounts for the cause of anticipation. Examples include Huntington's disease, an autosomal dominant disease characterized by expansion of CAG repeats in the huntingtin coding region (OMIM); spinocerebellar ataxia type 1 (*SCA1*), which shows CAG expansion of >39 repeats in *ATXN1* (OMIM); and Fragile X syndrome, where CGG in the *FMR1* gene is repeated >200 times (OMIM).

- Deletion and duplication. Certain diseases are caused by deletion or duplication of a chromosomal region. For example, the majority of Smith-Magenis syndrome (SMS) patients carry a deletion on 17p11.2.[8] This region overlaps with the duplication in Potocki-Lupski syndrome.[9]

Complex Inheritance

It is widely accepted that the etiology of a complex disease involves both genetic and environmental components. Typically, complex diseases show uncertain mode of transmission, incomplete penetrance, variable age of onset, and variability in expression. Common diseases such as bipolar disorder, schizophrenia, diabetes type II, hypertension, and asthma; and common traits, e.g., height and hair color, display these characteristics. Studies have shown that complex diseases are polygenic, which indicates that a combination of multiple minor-effect variants confers the overall genetic risk. Complex disorders are phenotypically and genetically heterogeneous, features that add to the difficulty in defining the full spectrum of loci involved in causation. GWAS on large samples, along with global scale high-resolution markers, have provided the capability to begin to tease out layers of this genetic complexity (see Genetic Mapping Analysis).

Genetic Markers and Genotyping Methods

Genetic markers that interrogate polymorphic loci in the genome include the following.

Single Nucleotide Polymorphism (SNP) or Single Nucleotide Variation (SNV)

Single nucleotide polymorphisms (SNPs) or single nucleotide variations (SNVs) represent nucleotide substitutions that occur at a single position to yield two alleles. They constitute the most abundant sequence alteration in the genome. SNPs arise either through: (i) transition, wherein either a purine is substituted by another purine (A>G or G>A) or a pyrimidine is replaced by another pyrimidine (C>T or T>C); or (ii) transversion, which indicates a change from purine to pyrimidine, or vice versa (e.g., A>T or T>A). Transitions are more common than transversions. Figure 3.1 shows sequence chromatograms of various types of SNPs. *Described here are examples of methods for SNP genotyping:

- Single- or low-throughput SNP genotyping: Among available tools for single SNP genotyping, the TaqMan instrument (Thermo Fisher Scientific) combines simplicity and ease of use. The method is polymerase chain reaction (PCR)-based, and the reagents consist of Taq polymerase, template DNA, forward and reverse primers to amplify the region containing the SNP, and a short minor groove binder (MGB) probe that includes the SNP. The probe is labeled on one end with an allele-specific fluorescent reporter dye, and a quencher is attached to the other end. Elongation of the new chain proceeds during PCR, and if the probe is completely complementary to the target DNA—i.e., no sequence mismatch—the 5'exonuclease activity of Taq polymerase cleaves the probe, releasing the dye from the quencher that then leads to fluorescence.
- Microarray chips and high-throughput genotyping: The ability to immobilize millions of short DNA oligomers representing millions of SNPs on

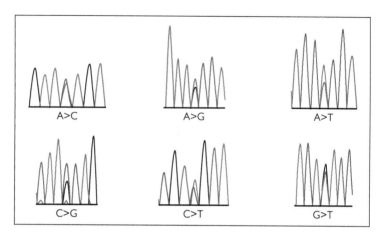

Figure 3.1 Sequence chromatograms of SNPs. Sanger sequencing was performed on a panel of DNA samples and sequences, portions of which are shown here. Each nucleotide is distinguished by a specific colored peak: A = green; C = blue; G = black and T = red. The SNPs are shown where two peaks overlap, indicating heterozygosity. For example, in the third chromatogram on the top row, in the fourth peak from left to right, "A" can be substituted by a "T," or vice versa. In this example, both alleles, "A" and "T" are present, thus the sample is heterozygous at this position.

microarray chips ushered in hybridization-based genotyping at the genome-wide level, and this method has since dominated the genotyping world. At its inception, a SNP microarray chip embedded fewer than a million oligos, permitting a relatively sparse coverage of the genome. The exponential increase in the number of identified and validated SNPs boosted the manufacture of high density, high-resolution SNP arrays that incorporate several million oligos, which, in effect, has achieved a comprehensive and finer coverage of the genome. In addition to SNPs, the chips can assay insertion-deletions (indels) and copy number variants (CNVs) in both coding and noncoding regions.

SNP arrays are commercially available mainly from Affymetrix (www.affymetrix.com/) and Illumina (www.illumina.com/).

The availability of SNP microarray chips has powered genetic screening of thousands of samples to generate millions of genotypes in a matter of a few days. In large part, this advance accounts for the progress of GWAS of many diseases and traits. Arrays designed to query specific targets such as whole genomes, exomes, diverse ethnicities, immune and psychiatric disorders are also commercially available. Likewise, custom arrays can be constructed for specific study designs. A description of these arrays is published in the Illumina website (http://www.illumina.com/).

Microsatellites or Short Tandem Repeat Polymorphisms (STRPs)

Microsatellites or short tandem repeat polymorphisms (STRPs) contain a repeating series of either dinucleotide, trinucleotide, tetranucleotide, or pentanucleotide repeats: e.g., (CT)n, (CTT)n, (CTTT)n, etc. The detection process involves PCR amplification followed by analysis either manually on polyacrylamide gels or by capillary electrophoresis on the ABI sequencer. Genome maps of STRPs generated by Jim Weber's group have been published and periodically updated (http://research.marshfieldclinic.org/genetics). STRPs are highly polymorphic markers that have been prominently used in genetic linkage scans.

Variable Number of Tandem Repeats (VNTR) or Minisatellites

Variable number of tandem repeats (VNTR) or minisatellites: Minisatellites are generally composed of GC-rich 10–60 bp repeats and are highly polymorphic. They have been used popularly in DNA fingerprinting for forensics and paternity assessments. Serotonin-transporter-linked polymorphic region (5-HTTLPR) in the upstream region of the serotonin transporter that has been widely studied and analyzed in neuropsychiatric disorders is an example of a VNTR.[10]

Genetic Mapping Analysis

Genetic Linkage

Linkage mapping evaluates the co-segregation of disease in pedigrees with genetic markers and is the method of choice to identify chromosomal regions that encode major effect and highly penetrant causative genes for monogenic disorders. The likelihood that a disease locus is genetically linked to a marker is reflected in the resulting LOD (logarithm of the odds) score, originally developed by Newton Morton.[11] By convention, a LOD score of ≥3 is taken as evidence of linkage. The genetic distance between marker and disease locus is expressed in centimorgans (cM): 1 cM is approximately equivalent to a physical distance of 1 Mb (million base pairs). Screening for linkage involves genotyping of affected families with mapped markers through either parametric or non-parametric methods. Parametric analysis is used when the mode of transmission, penetrance, and disease population frequency are known. When genetic parameters are uncertain, non-parametric analysis that calculates identity-by-descent (IBD) is used to estimate linkage. A detailed discussion of parametric and non-parametric statistical analyses, particularly as applied to complex diseases, has been presented in Kruglyak et al.[12] In general, linkage regions are large, hence narrowing down the region using various approaches is necessary in order to move toward precise detection of the causative locus.

Transmission Disequilibrium Test (TDT)

The transmission disequilibrium test (TDT)[13] is a test for linkage and association in a panel of trios (two parents + offspring). TDT measures the pattern of transmitted and untransmitted alleles from a heterozygous parent to an offspring. A significant bias in transmission vis-à-vis disease is deemed to represent linkage and association.

Genome-Wide Association Study (GWAS)

Association mapping measures the statistical difference in marker allele frequency in cases versus controls. This analysis can be performed on a limited number of samples with probes for genes of interest or for targeted genomic regions. Here, we will focus our discussion on genome-wide association studies

(GWAS). The development of high-density, high-resolution SNP arrays, coupled with the enormous expansion of large sample collections and vast improvement in statistical methods, has been key to the progress in GWAS. From 2008 up to 2015, >2100 GWASs had been published and collated in the online catalog, NHGRI-EBI Catalog of Published GWAS (http://www.ebi.ac.uk/gwas/). GWAS has identified hundreds of significantly associated risk variants in complex diseases, including neuropsychiatric disorders, such as bipolar disorder (BD),[14] schizophrenia (SCZ),[15] and major depressive disorder (MDD).[16]

- GWAS Pipeline
  - Quality control (QC) in GWAS: The main objective of QC is to ensure that only high-quality variants and samples are used in the final test for association. At the variant level, very rare variants, variants with high rates of missing data, and those that fail the Hardy-Weinberg test are excluded. At the sample level, individuals with discordant sex information, those with high rates of missing genotypes or with anomalous heterozygosity rate, and population outliers are eliminated from the analysis. For case-control GWAS, it is important to assess cryptic relatedness between individuals. Details of QC in GWAS have been previously discussed.[17,18]
  - Imputation. The ability to impute missing genotypes boosts the power of GWAS as it facilitates gaining information and fine mapping of regions not directly assayed by SNPs in chip arrays. The theoretical basis and utility of genotype imputation has been reviewed previously.[19] A number of imputation programs have been developed, including Minimac, IMPUTE, and BEAGLE; and a comparison of these methods has been discussed by Marchini and Howie.[20] Imputation has vastly increased the number of acquired genotypes, circumventing wet lab genotyping and yielding enormous savings in cost, effort, and time.
  - Association tests: PLINK (http://pngu.mgh.harvard.edu/~purcell/plink/)[21] is the major computational resource consisting of a whole-genome association toolset and is widely used in GWAS analysis. Given the multiple tests performed on genotypes generated by millions of SNPs, genome-wide statistical significance is declared when p value $\leq 5 \times 10^{-8}$. A QQ plot is generated from the data as part of the QC. Figure 3.2A shows an example of a good QQ plot versus one that is inflated. Once the QC process is completed, association is computed, and GWA data can be represented graphically as a Manhattan plot that displays the statistical significance achieved by each SNP located along the autosomes (Figure 3.2B).
  - Meta-analysis of association studies: Meta-analysis offers the advantage of "strength in numbers," because risk variants undetectable in individual studies may be revealed in a much more expanded sample. METAL is a commonly used tool to perform meta-analysis of GWAS data, and it provides two different analysis schemes (http://genome.sph.umich.edu/wiki/METAL).[22] In the classical approach (inverse variance-based), effect sizes and standard errors for meta-analysis are used. The sample size–based method uses p-values and direction of effect, weighted by

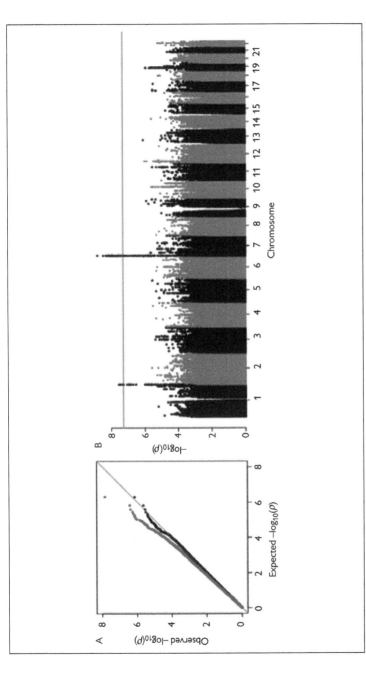

Figure 3.2 Quantile-quantile (QQ) and Manhattan plots. A. The QQ plot shows the expected distribution of association statistics under the null hypothesis of no association compared to observed values. An unbiased QQ plot (black) should approximate the identity line at the lower end. An example of an inflated QQ plot is shown in blue. B. The Manhattan plot shows p values of association across the autosomes with each dot representing a SNP marker. The red line represents the genome-wide significance threshold.

sample sizes. In a study with unequal numbers of cases and controls, the sample size–based method is recommended, and the effective sample size of each study is provided for the final analysis.

DNA Sequencing

Sanger Sequencing Method

Sanger was awarded his second Nobel Prize in Chemistry in 1980 for developing a DNA sequencing technique that utilizes DNA polymerase to copy a DNA template. Extension of the growing chain is terminated when a dideoxynucleotide is incorporated in lieu of the equivalent unmodified dNTP.[23] Radioactively labeled dNTP was used for ease of detection, and the newly synthesized fragments were resolved on polyacrylamide gels and imaged on X-ray films. Years later, this process was automated on a DNA sequencer, e.g., ABI 3730, that resolves newly synthesized fragments by capillary electrophoresis. The reaction proceeds in the presence of four fluorescently tagged dideoxynucleotides, thus precluding the use of a radioactively labeled reagent. A sequence analysis software, e.g., Sequencher, generates the nucleotide sequence and the corresponding chromatogram that depicts each base by a distinctly colored peak (Figure 3.1). The major advantage of this low-throughput sequencing method is its precision and accuracy; hence, it is the standard technique for validating sequencing data generated by NGS (see next section).

Next-Generation Sequencing (NGS)

Next-generation sequencing (NGS) has raised DNA sequencing of whole exomes and whole genomes to stratospheric levels while substantially lowering cost, processing effort, and time of analysis. The enormous benefit derived from NGS is wide- and far-ranging.[24] Goodwin and colleagues published a comprehensive review of NGS platforms that have been used in the last 10 years.[25] Innovative NGS equipment and accompanying protocols have been commercially marketed by various companies, including Illumina, ThermoFisher, Roche, and Pacific Biosciences. So far, Illumina has consistently garnered the biggest market share of equipment and protocols used in exome, whole genome, and other techniques that employ NGS. We refer the reader to the Illumina website for further description and schematic presentation of their NGS pipeline (http://www.illumina.com/technology/next- generation-sequencing.html) as well as reviews on NGS.[26]

It is noteworthy that single-cell genome and transcriptome studies (not discussed here) have begun to flourish, partly because of NGS. Prominent characteristics of individual cells can be assayed and monitored, as opposed to the entire population of heterogeneous cells. *Genome Biology* dedicated a special issue in August 2016 to "Single Cell-Omics."

• Whole-exome sequencing (WES): This sequencing technique aims to capture exons and portions of the 5' and 3' ends of the coding regions (Figure 3.3). Briefly, in whole-exome sequencing, genomic DNA is first cleaved into smaller fragments, onto which sequencing adaptors are attached on both ends. Exon-containing fragments are selectively captured by exonic probes to produce a library. In the Illumina protocol, the fragments are hybridized to flow cells, and each fragment is amplified to generate a clonal cluster. Sequencing proceeds in the presence of DNA polymerase, a mixture of primers, all four nucleotides, each with a blocked 3'OH end and labeled with a specific fluorophore with a distinct emission spectrum, enabling precise identification of the newly incorporated base in the growing chain. After the addition of one base, reaction stops, since the 3'OH end is blocked, and the elongated chain is imaged by fluorescence microscopy. Sequencing proceeds by first cleaving the 3'OH block on the newly attached nucleotide, permitting incorporation of the succeeding base. The sequencing cycle is repeated many times, up to the desired number of reads. Paired-end sequencing—i.e., sequencing in both forward and reverse directions—leads to greater sequencing accuracy. The raw sequencing reads are aligned to a reference genome sequence using bioinformatics software, e.g., (Burrows-Wheeler Aligner (BWA) (http://bio- bwa.sourceforge.net)[27] and analyzed to generate the final exome sequence data. The more reads recorded per region, the more accurate the observed

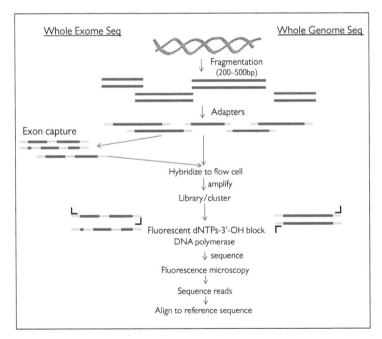

Figure 3.3 A scheme for whole exome and whole genome next-generation sequencing. Blue bars represent a genomic DNA fragment, green bars in the fragment ends are adapter oligos, yellow bars within blue bars represent exons, and black right angles are sequencing primers.

sequence. Variation and mutations that are potentially important must be validated by Sanger sequencing.

- Whole-genome sequencing (WGS): Deep sequencing of the entire genome entails a highly elaborate processing and data analysis because of the level and range of complex and diverse types of sequences. Just as in exome sequencing, fragmented genomic DNA is attached to sequencing adaptors, then the resultant pool of fragments is processed for sequencing (as described under WES) excluding the step of exon capture (Figure 3.3).
- Types of sequence variation:
  - Exonic:
    - Synonymous or silent mutation denotes a base change in a codon that does not result in an amino acid change.
    - Non-synonymous or missense mutation defines a base change in a codon that results in amino acid substitution.
    - Nonsense mutation represents a base change that converts an amino acid specifying-codon into a stop codon.
    - Frameshift mutation is a result of an indel in the coding region producing a new open reading frame specifying a stretch of polypeptide sequence that diverges from the wild type sequence.
  - Copy number variation (CNV) is a structural alteration that indicates either a deletion or duplication of chromosomal segments, encompassing up to several Mb. CNVs originate from errors during recombination and can create either haploinsufficiency or redundancy of functional units that map within the affected region.[28] Genotyping on microarray chips is a rapid and easy method for detecting CNVs in multiple samples, but hybridization to tiling arrays yield higher quality data for clinical use or specialized research applications. Rare de novo CNVs that could impart a role in pathogenesis have been observed in neuropsychiatric diseases such as ASD, schizophrenia, bipolar disorder, and intellectual disability.[28]
  - Indels: Indels occur either in exons or introns and will produce a functional alteration if they occur in exons or regulatory regions. Other chromosomal aberrations such as rearrangements, translocations, and aneuploidy are beyond the scope of this chapter.

Transcriptome and Gene Expression Analysis

Gene activity is under spatial and temporal control, and it reflects gene response to both endogenous and exogenous conditions and stimuli. Disease, age, sex, diet, and xenobiotic exposure are some of the elements that could provoke a prominent impact on gene expression. Listed here are some techniques for examining gene expression.

Northern Blotting

The early method of gene expression analysis, Northern blotting, was conducted by electrophoresis of tissue or cell total RNA on a denaturing gel followed by transfer of RNA onto a membrane, and hybridization of the membrane with a labeled probe for the gene of interest. Northern blotting is slow and has low throughput, but it has the advantage of providing a view of the approximate size and diversity of detectable transcripts.

Microarray Expression Chips
Profiling gene expression using microarray chips embedded with cDNA probes for all known genes provides a snapshot of gene regulation at the global level, under certain conditions and time points. This innovation unleashed gene expression profiling studies in diverse cells and tissues. Microarray chip assay is hybridization-based, and probe redundancy, i.e., each chip contains more than one probe per gene or transcript, ensures target specificity. Sensitivity to low-abundance transcripts remains an issue with microarray chips. The most popularly used expression chip arrays are those manufactured by Affymetrix and Illumina.

RNA Sequencing
RNA sequencing (RNA-seq) is the NGS technique for transcriptome profiling. Because of its wide dynamic range, RNA-seq has the power to reveal the immense complexity and diversity of transcriptome units that had not been previously shown with older technologies. RNA-seq has the demonstrated capability to detect low-abundance transcripts, lncRNA, and alternatively spliced transcripts. Briefly, high-quality total RNA extracted from cells or tissue specimens is subjected to a selective capture of mRNA with oligodT probes. Alternatively, ribosomal RNA, which comprises ~90% of total RNA, is first depleted, leaving the remaining RNA species for further processing. Preserving strandedness during library preparation helps determine the direction of transcription.

RNA is then shorn to a certain size range, reverse transcribed to cDNA using random primers, and second strand synthesis is done. Adaptors and index oligos are attached to the cDNA fragments, then NGS sequencing proceeds, following the same general procedure briefly described under WES (Figure 3.3A). High depth sequencing and inclusion of biological replicates ensure precision and accuracy. At present, there is no optimal pipeline for RNA-seq analysis, and at every step, there are choices of available analysis software. Quality control (QC) check on the raw sequence data is an essential step at the start of the analysis, and one of the bioinformatics tools used is FastQC (http://www.bioinformatics.babraham.ac.uk/projects/fastqc/). Sequence reads are then mapped to a reference genome assembly, and at this stage, several tools can be used, such as TopHat2.[29] Novel transcripts are detected by the latter programs. After sequences are mapped, quantification of transcripts is performed at both gene and transcript levels (Cufflinks; http://cole-trapnell-lab.github.io/cufflinks/),[30] at transcript level (eXpress; http://bio.math.berkeley.edu/eXpress/overview.html), or at the gene level only (HTSeq; http://www-huber.embl.de/HTSeq/doc/overview.html).[31] Differential expression can be scored by Cuffdiff in Cufflinks or by a number of other tools, including DESeq2 (https://bioconductor.org/packages/release/bioc/html/DESeq2.html).[32]

Principal component analysis is done to detect outliers and biases in the experiment. The advantages of using RNA-seq to study the transcriptome are manifold; however, along with them are challenges that remain to be addressed.[33]

Quantitative RT-PCR

Quantitative RT-PCR (qPCR) is used to quantify transcripts and validate gene expression data derived from microarray or RNA-seq. The technique is useful in evaluating low-abundance transcripts. Briefly, total RNA is extracted from a study sample and reversed transcribed to cDNA. PCR amplification of a specific gene is initiated in the presence of gene-specific primers and either a gene-specific or a nonspecific fluorescent probe. Normalization of fluorescence values is done against those of reference housekeeping genes. Fluorescence is proportional to the amount of target, permitting quantification.

Gene Silencing: Knockout and Knockdown

Gene disruption permits examination of the physiological role of that gene at various stages of development and under the influence of diverse stimuli. Gene modification was initiated by the pioneering work of Capecchi, Evans, and Smithies, which earned them a Nobel Prize in 2007. Gene knockout in mouse is well established and cataloged in Mouse Genome Informatics (MGI; http://www.informatics.jax.org/), a resource that provides a wealth of information on known genes, including the availability of mice in which particular genes have been knocked out.

Small interfering RNAs (siRNA)–mediated or short hairpin RNA (shRNA)–mediated gene knockdown rather than knockout of gene activity may be preferred in order to examine the biological effect of diminished expression of a certain gene. This method uses the principle behind RNA interference (RNAi) developed by Fire and Mello (Nobel Prize in Physiology or Medicine, 2006).[34] Their method uses double-stranded RNA to silence a specific gene.[35] siRNAs, oligos designed to bind genes of interest, are transiently transfected into cells to disrupt gene expression. shRNA are siRNA oligos cloned into a vector to create stable transfection in cells. The functional outcome of downregulating multiple specific genes, or globally at genome-wide level by transfecting siRNAs, can be monitored using appropriate phenotype assays.

MicroRNA (miRNA)

MicroRNAs (miRNA) are ~22 bp noncoding RNAs that form base pairs with recognition sites in mRNA molecules resulting in expression silencing. The microRNA database (http://www.mirbase.org/) is a repository of published and annotated miRNAs. A report of the last update was published in 2014.[36] That certain types of microRNA may play a role in risk for schizophrenia and some neurological disorders has been reported, but analysis in larger samples is crucial to achieve well-supported findings.

Expression Quantitative Trait Loci (eQTL)

Expression quantitative trait loci (eQTL) are genomic loci that exert influence on the expression level of a gene(s), and confer the effect either at the level of "cis," i.e., on the same chromosome, or, of "trans," i.e., from a different chromosome. eQTL could help identify regulatory elements and diverse pathways involved in pathogenesis.

Gene Expression Omnibus (GEO)

Gene expression omnibus (GEO; https://www.ncbi.nlm.nih.gov/geo/) is a repository and searchable database that contains expression data derived from microarray chips and RNA-seq.

Genotype–Tissue Expression (GTEx)

(9) Genotype–Tissue Expression (GTEx; https://www.genome.gov/ 27543767/genotypetissue-expression-project-gtex/), launched by NIH in September 2010, has the stated aim of increasing "our understanding of how changes in our genes contribute to common human diseases, in order to improve health for future generations." GTEx has determined and assembled the expression patterns of genes in multiple tissues, organs, and cells, and data can be viewed in the GTEx portal or in theUCSCGenome Browser. For example, the expression of *NR3C1* in >50 different sources is displayed in http://www.gtexportal.org/home/gene/ENSG00000113580.10.

Allen Brain Atlas

The Allen Brain Atlas (http://www.brain-map.org/) is referred to as the "Genetic Geography of the Brain." This project is supported by the Allen Institute for Brain Science and was launched in 2003 through a $100 million donation by Paul G. Allen. The initial focus of the project was to produce detailed facets of gene expression in various parts of the mouse brain; providing huge amount of additional information on studies at the Jackson Laboratory (https://www.jax.org/). Allen Brain pursuits have expanded to generate an intricate expression map of the human brain, and to various other impressive projects, including brain development and connectivity. These resources provide elegant images and workings of the brain and will continue to benefit neuroscience research immensely.

Proteome Databases

Proteins are the workhorses of the cell. A comprehensive description of important properties of a protein, including its expression pattern in conjunction with the unique attributes of the cognate gene, would further illuminate biological pathways and networks in normal and disease states. Protein isoforms encoded by all known genes are presented in the Genome Browsers. Databases focused on the proteome have been developed, including the ProteomicsDB (https://www.proteomicsdb.org/) and the Proteome Map (http://www.humanproteomemap.org/). Kim et al.[37] performed high-resolution mass spectrometry to analyze the protein products of >17,000 human genes expressed in 17 adult tissues, six primary hematopoietic cells, and seven fetal tissues. The ProteomicsDB[38] presents coverage of 80% of the human proteome. In June 2016, the database added a new tool to analyze dose-dependent protein–drug interaction.

Regulatory Landscape and Epigenetics

The linear sequence of genomic DNA coupled with non-genomic or epigenetic factors are principal elements involved in determining the eventual phenotype of an organism. The network of regulatory units and epigenetic structure, including accessibility of DNA regions and the location and propensity of DNA methylation, could be key elements in drug response and pathogenesis. Some of tools used to examine these features are presented next.

ChIPseq

ChIPseq: This technique combines chromatin immunoprecipitation with NGS to identify DNA motifs that interact with specific proteins, particularly transcription factors, at the genome-wide level. Briefly, chromatin is cross-linked, then sonicated, to generate enrichment of between 100–500 bp DNA fragments. Immunoprecipitation with an antibody to a transcription factor is performed. The protein-Ab-DNA complex is reverse cross-linked to recover the ChIPed DNA that is then sequenced through NGS following the same general protocol, as presented in WES (Figure 3.3A) (http://www.illumina.com/techniques/sequencing/dna-sequencing/chip-seq.html).

Assay for Transposase-Accessible Chromatin

Assay for transposase-accessible chromatin (ATAC-Seq)[39] is a method for identifying exposed enhancers, promoters, and other regulatory regions in the genome. It exploits the ability of hyperactive Tn5 transposase to simultaneously cleave genomic DNA and permit insertion of sequencing adapters to any accessible portion of the chromatin. DNA fragments are PCR amplified, and NGS sequencing is performed, permitting a genome-wide assay of exposed chromatin sites and nucleosome position.

DNA Methylation

DNA methylation has been shown to have a profoundly repressive effect on gene activity. A discussion of the methylome as it relates to various aspects of gene regulation and its role in disease has been presented.[40] In adult tissues, the methylated base, 5-methylcytosine, occurs at CpG sites. The genome-wide location and pattern of DNA methylation is evaluated through the use of either methylation chips or methylation sequencing. Methylation chips are commercially available. In methylation sequencing of the whole genome, DNA is first treated with bisulfite, which converts unmethylated cytosine to uracil; methylated cytosines are inert to this treatment. During PCR amplification, DNA polymerase reads uracil as thymine. TruSeq DNA Methylation Assay is a whole-genome methylation sequencing kit available from Illumina (http://www.illumina.com/).

Genome Editing

An exceptionally pivotal development in molecular genetics is the ability to create or repair mutation at specific sites of the genome. Genome editing permits disruption of genes or a stretch of genomic loci to probe their biological role. The ability to create isogenic lines that could be harnessed to analyze contrasting phenotypes between wild type and mutated cells that carry identical genetic backgrounds is exceedingly useful for disease modeling. Cellular therapy is another important potential application of genome editing.

Examples of genome editing methods are briefly presented next.

ZFN and TALEN

Two earlier versions of genome-editing nucleases include Zn finger nuclease (ZFN) and transcription activator-like effector nuclease (TALEN).[41] ZFN consists of a DNA binding domain and a Fok1 restriction enzyme, and TALEN includes a DNA binding domain and a nuclease. ZFN and TALEN methods are reputed to be particularly time consuming.

Clustered Regularly Interspaced Palindromic Repeat

CRISPR: The development of RNA-guided CRISPR (clustered regularly interspaced palindromic repeat)-Cas9 has largely supplanted ZFN and TALEN.[42,43] CRISPR-Cas9, an engineered DNA endonuclease, is derived from the bacterial adaptive immune systems that identify, resist, and degrade viral infection. Cas9 uses a specific guide RNA (gRNA) programmed to bind and cause a double-stranded break (DSB) at the target sequence abutting a protospacer adjacent motif (PAM), 5'-NGG-3'. The cell repairs the damage either through homology-directed repair (HDR) facilitating replacement of the disrupted gene or locus with wild type sequence, or non-homologous end joining (NHEJ) that can effectively delete or knock out a gene or locus. Improving the specificity and reduction of off-target effects of the editing process is being addressed.[44]

Its versatility, potency and relative ease-of-use has elevated CRISPR-Cas9 to the apex of genome editing. The availability of person-specific induced pluripotent stem cells (iPSC) and their derivatives, together with advances in CRISPR, presents a great opportunity to examine effects of genome variation and/or disease mutation carried by particular individuals. The ability to generate neural derivatives, particularly in three-dimensional neural culture, permits modeling studies of neurodevelopmental, neuropsychiatric, and neurological disorders.[45] Single-cell labeling of endogenous protein in neurons using CRISPR-Cas9 has permitted mapping of spatially and temporally controlled subcellular localization of specific proteins.[46] RNA targeting and degradation has been achieved with the discovery of the RNA-guided C2c2 enzyme, a naturally occurring CRISPR system.[47,48] That CRISPR can target both DNA and RNA adds to the impressive power of this gene-editing system.

Biological Processes, Function Predictions, Pathways
Deleteriousness Prediction
Many candidate risk variants have unknown functions, thus a number of predictive programs have been developed to obtain a first-hand view of their potential role in pathogenesis. Dong et al.[49] have recently compared the performance of 18 available predictive programs and two new ensemble prediction methods, including PolyPhen-, SIFT, FATHMM, etc., on three manually curated datasets. They found that "FATHMM and KGGSeq had the highest discriminative power among independent scores and ensemble scores, respectively."

Biological Processes
The biological role of genes that carry disease-associated variants and those that show anomalous expression in disease can be evaluated initially by performing a search analysis in DAVID version 6.8 (https://david.ncifcrf.gov/).[50,51] Enriched biological mechanisms (Gene Ontology (GO) terms), Kyoto Encyclopedia of Genes and Genomes (KEGG) pathways, and multiple salient information can be derived using this bioinformatics tool.

Pathways
Enriched pathways and protein–protein interaction networks for candidate risk genes can be evaluated using available tools, including STRING, a free web-based software (http://string-db.org/) and Ingenuity Pathway Analysis (IPA), for which a license needs to be purchased (http://www.ingenuity.com/). Also, a useful guide for analysis of gene sets following GWAS has been proposed.[52]

Weighted Gene Correlation Network Analysis
Weighted gene correlation network analysis (WGCNA)[53] analyzes co-expression of genes derived from expression profiling studies such as RNA-seq and microarray analysis. The desired outcome of this analysis is to generate modules of co-expressed genes that may be involved in risk or that could be used as targets for drug discovery.

Conclusion

The past decades have experienced a dramatic evolution in genetics. Faced with huge challenges and volumes of unanswered questions in diseases, common and rare, the scientific community came together to formulate novel and ambitious goals. To understand the cause, improve diagnostic precision, and design effective interventions and medications, there needed to be a concerted and collaborative international venture. The large genetics initiatives served to jumpstart the effort, and they spawned new challenges to develop new strategies, develop new tools, to innovate, to encourage collaborations and data sharing, to create fast, high-throughput technologies, and to improve computational and bioinformatics methods. Progress has been palpable, although many of the same questions still remain, foremost of which is directly linking an associated variant to pathogenesis. The genetics researcher now has a panoply of armamentariums, many of which are discussed in this chapter, although more needs to be developed in order to move forward more rapidly to promote health and mitigate the affliction of disease.

Acknowledgments

The authors wish to acknowledge the support of the Intramural Research Program of the National Institute of Mental Health, NIH. We wish to thank T. de Guzman and W. Corona for help with the figures, and C. Song for help with formatting and references.

References

1. International Human Genome Sequencing Consortium. (2001). Initial sequencing and analysis of the human genome. *Nature*, *409*, 860–921.

2. Venter, J. C., Adams, M. D., Myers, E. W., et al. (2001). The sequence of the human genome. *Science*, *291*, 1304–1351.

3. International Human Genome Sequencing Consortium. (2004). Finishing the euchromatic sequence of the human genome. *Nature*, *431*, 931–945.

4. 1000 Genomes Project Consortium. (2012). An integrated map of genetic variation from 1,092 human genomes. *Nature*, *491*, 56–65.

5. 1000 Genomes Project Consortium, Auton, A., Brooks, L. D., et al. (2015). A global reference for human genetic variation. *Nature*, *526*, 68–74.

6. ENCODE Project Consortium. (2012). An integrated encyclopedia of DNA elements in the human genome. *Nature*, *489*, 57–74.

7. Mailman, M. D., Feolo, M., Jin, Y., et al. (2007). The NCBI dbGaP database of genotypes and phenotypes. *Nature Genetics*, *39*, 1181–1186.

8. Smith, A. C., McGavran, L., Robinson, J., et al. (1986). Interstitial deletion of (17) (p11.2p11.2) in nine patients. *American Journal of Medical Genetics*, *24*, 393–414.

9. Potocki, L., Chen, K. S., Park, S. S., et al. (2000). Molecular mechanism for duplication 17p11.2- the homologous recombination reciprocal of the Smith-Magenis microdeletion. *Nature Genetics*, *24*, 84–87.

10. Lesch, K. P., Bengel, D., Heils, A., et al. (1996). Association of anxiety-related traits with a polymorphism in the serotonin transporter gene regulatory region. *Science*, *274*, 1527–1531.

11. Morton, N. E. (1955). Sequential tests for the detection of linkage. *American Journal of Human Genetics*, *7*, 277–318.

12. Kruglyak, L., Daly, M. J., Reeve-Daly, M. P., et al. (1996). Parametric and nonparametric linkage analysis: a unified multipoint approach. *American Journal of Human Genetics*, *58*, 1347–1363.

13. Spielman, R. S., McGinnis, R. E., & Ewens, W. J. (1993). Transmission test for linkage disequilibrium: the insulin gene region and insulin-dependent diabetes mellitus (IDDM). *American Journal of Human Genetics, 52,* 506–516.

14. Psychiatric GWAS Consortium Bipolar Disorder Working Group. (2011). Large-scale genome-wide association analysis of bipolar disorder identifies a new susceptibility locus near ODZ4. *Nature Genetics, 43,* 977–983.

15. Schizophrenia Working Group of the Psychiatric Genomics Consortium. (2014). Biological insights from 108 schizophrenia-associated genetic loci. *Nature, 511,* 421–427.

16. Hyde, C. L., Nagle, M. W., Tian, C., et al. (2016). Identification of 15 genetic loci associated with risk of major depression in individuals of European descent. *Nature Genetics, 48,* 1031–1036.

17. Anderson, C. A., Pettersson F. H., Clarke, G. M., et al. (2010). Data quality control in genetic case-control association studies. *Nature Protocols, 5,* 1564–1573.

18. Winkler, T. W., Day, F. R., Croteau-Chonka, D. C., et al. (2014). Quality control and conduct of genome-wide association meta-analyses. *Nature Protocols, 9,* 1192–1212.

19. Li, Y., Willer, C., Sanna, S., et al. (2009). Genotype imputation. *Annual Review of Genomics and Human Genetics, 10,* 387–406.

20. Marchini, J., & Howie, B. (2010). Genotype imputation for genome-wide association studies. *Nature Reviews Genetics, 11,* 499–511.

21. Purcell, S., Neale, B., Todd-Brown, K., et al. (2007). PLINK: a tool set for whole-genome association and population-based linkage analyses. *American Journal of Human Genetics, 81,* 559–575.

22. Willer, C. J., Li, Y., & Abecasis, G. R. (2010). METAL: fast and efficient meta-analysis of genomewide association scans. *Bioinformatics, 26,* 2190–2191.

23. Sanger, F., Nicklen, S., & Coulson, A. R. (1977). DNA sequencing with chain-terminating inhibitors. *Proceedings of the National Academy of Sciences USA, 74,* 5463–5467.

24. Koboldt, D. C., Steinberg, K. M., Larson, D. E., et al. (2013). The next-generation sequencing revolution and its impact on genomics. *Cell, 155,* 27–38.

25. Goodwin, S., McPherson, J. D., & McCombie, W. R. (2016). Coming of age: ten years of next-generation sequencing technologies. *Nature Reviews Genetics, 17,* 333–351.

26. Mardis, E. R. (2013). Next-generation sequencing platforms. *Annual Review of Analytical Chemistry (Palo Alto, Calif.), 6,* 287–303.

27. Li, H., & Durbin, R. (2010). Fast and accurate long-read alignment with Burrows-Wheeler transform. *Bioinformatics, 26,* 589–595.

28. Malhotra, D., & Sebat, J. (2012). CNVs: harbingers of a rare variant revolution in psychiatric genetics. *Cell, 148,* 1223–1241.

29. Kim, D., Pertea, G., Trapnell, C., et al. (2013). TopHat2: accurate alignment of transcriptomes in the presence of insertions, deletions and gene fusions. *Genome Biology, 14,* R36.

30. Roberts, A., Pimentel, H., Trapnell, C., et al. (2011). Identification of novel transcripts in annotated genomes using RNA-Seq. *Bioinformatics, 27,* 2325–2329.

31. Anders, S., Pyl, P. T., & Huber, W. (2015). HTSeq—a Python framework to work with high-throughput sequencing data. *Bioinformatics, 31,* 166–169.

32. Love, M. I., Huber, W., & Anders, S. (2014). Moderated estimation of fold change and dispersion for RNA-seq data with DESeq2. *Genome Biology, 15*, 550.

33. Wang, Z., Gerstein, M., & Snyder, M. (2009). RNA-Seq: a revolutionary tool for transcriptomics. *Nature Reviews Genetics, 10*, 57–63.

34. Fire, A., Xu, S., Montgomery, M. K., et al. (1998). Potent and specific genetic interference by double-stranded RNA in *Caenorhabditis elegans*. *Nature, 391*, 806–811.

35. McManus, M. T., & Sharp, P. A. (2002). Gene silencing in mammals by small interfering RNAs. *Nature Reviews Genetics, 3*, 737–747.

36. Kozomara, A., & Griffiths-Jones, S. (2014). miRBase: annotating high confidence microRNAs using deep sequencing data. *Nucleic Acids Research, 42*, D68–D73.

37. Kim M-S, Pinto, S. M., Getnet, D., et al. (2014). A draft map of the human proteome. *Nature, 509*, 575–581.

38. Wilhelm, M., Schlegl, J., Hahne, H., et al. (2014). Mass-spectrometry-based draft of the human proteome. *Nature, 509*, 582–587.

39. Buenrostro, J. D., Wu, B., Chang, H. Y., et al. (2015). ATAC-seq: A method for assaying chromatin accessibility genome-wide. *Current Protocols in Molecular Biology, 109*, 21.29.1–9.

40. Jones, P. A. (2012). Functions of DNA methylation: islands, start sites, gene bodies and beyond. *Nature Reviews Genetics, 13*, 484–492.

41. Gaj, T., Gersbach, C. A., & Barbas, C. F. (2013). ZFN, TALEN, and CRISPR/Cas-based methods for genome engineering. *Trends in Biotechnology, 31*, 397–405.

42. Doudna, J. A., & Charpentier, E. (2014). Genome editing. The new frontier of genome engineering with CRISPR-Cas9. *Science, 346*, 1258096.

43. Wang, H., La Russa, M., & Qi, L. S. (2016). CRISPR/Cas9 in genome editing and beyond. *Annual Review of Biochemistry, 85*, 227–264.

44. Wyvekens, N., Topkar, V. V., Khayter, C., et al. (2015). Dimeric CRISPR RNA-guided FokI-dCas9 nucleases directed by truncated gRNAs for highly specific genome editing. *Human Gene Therapy, 26*, 425–431.

45. Muffat, J., Li, Y., & Jaenisch, R. (2016). CNS disease models with human pluripotent stem cells in the CRISPR age. *Current Opinion in Cellular Biology, 43*, 96–103.

46. Mikuni, T., Nishiyama, J., Sun, Y., et al. (2016). High-throughput, high-resolution mapping of protein localization in mammalian brain by in vivo genome editing. *Cell, 165*, 1803–1817.

47. Abudayyeh, O. O., Gootenberg, J. S., Konermann, S., et al. (2016). C2c2 is a single-component programmable RNA-guided RNA-targeting CRISPR effector. *Science, 353*, aaf5573-1-aaf5573-9.

48. East-Seletsky, A., O'Connell, M. R., Knight, S. C., et al. (2016). Two distinct RNase activities of CRISPR-C2c2 enable guide-RNA processing and RNA detection. *Nature, 538*, 270–273.

49. Dong, C., Wei, P., Jian, X., et al. (2015). Comparison and integration of deleteriousness prediction methods for nonsynonymous SNVs in whole exome sequencing studies. *Human Molecular Genetics, 24*, 2125–2137.

50. Huang, D. W., Sherman, B. T., & Lempicki, R. A. (2009a). Bioinformatics enrichment tools: paths toward the comprehensive functional analysis of large gene lists. *Nucleic Acids Research, 37*, 1–13.

52. Huang, D. W., Sherman, B. T., & Lempicki, R. A. (2009b). Systematic and integrative analysis of large gene lists using DAVID bioinformatics resources. *Nature Protocols*, *4*, 44–57.

52. Mooney, M. A., & Wilmot, B. (2015). Gene set analysis: A step-by-step guide. *American Journal of Medical Genetics, Part B: Neuropsychiatric Genetics*, *168*, 517–527.

53. Langfelder, P., & Horvath, S. (2008). WGCNA: an R package for weighted correlation network analysis. *BMC Bioinformatics*, *9*, 559.

Chapter 4

Statistical Genetics

Genome-Wide Studies

Till F. M. Andlauer, Bertram Müller-Myhsok, and Stephan Ripke

---

Take-Home Points

1. Psychiatric disorders are phenotypically heterogeneous and highly polygenic.
2. GWAS on either binary or continuous phenotypes are used for hypothesis-free association analyses of common genetic variants.
3. Analysis of rare variants is more challenging because of decreased statistical power and requires special methods like set-based tests.
4. Careful quality control, conservative statistics, and replication are key elements of GWAS to avoid spurious findings.
5. Large sample sizes are necessary for sufficient power to detect associations with small effect sizes, which are typical for common variants in the genetics of psychiatric disorders. They can be achieved via meta-analysis of different cohorts; e.g., in the context of consortia.

Challenges in Uncovering Genetic Risk Factors for Psychiatric Disorders

For the majority of psychiatric disorders, a family history of disease is a common feature. This is suggestive of a strong genetic component to the underlying disease risk. Epidemiological studies have estimated a high heritability of up to 80% for several common psychiatric disorders, such as autism, schizophrenia, and bipolar disorder.[1] Major depressive disorder, by contrast, has a lower estimated heritability, of up to 40%. Despite this evidence for a strong contribution of genetic factors to disease risk, the actual genes influencing susceptibility for mental disorders have been discovered only at a very slow pace.

One reason for the difficulties in identification of risk genes is the phenotype-based approach used for classification and diagnosis of psychiatric disorders.[2] Diagnostic tests based on quantitative biomarker levels, imaging results, or tissue pathology do not exist yet. Instead, diagnoses are typically made via observation and an assessment of the patient's medical history. At the same time, even the classification of psychiatric disorders and the validity of diagnostic boundaries are still subject to intense debate among psychiatrists and psychologists.[2] As a result, the disorders represent heterogeneous and partly overlapping syndromic concepts.[3] This heterogeneity and uncertainty in diagnosis lead to decreased power in genetic studies. In addition, risk for psychiatric disorders is typically multifactorial or polygenic. This means that a large number of mutations with small individual effect sizes accumulates to confer an overall risk burden. This marked polygenicity hampered discoveries in smaller samples.

Despite these complications, impressive progress has been made in the identification of genetic factors influencing susceptibility for psychiatric disorders in recent years. In the following sections, the most important designs for genetic studies are presented, together with key findings in the field.

General Concepts in Human Genetics

The human genome contains over 3 billion base pairs of DNA. The vast majority of base pairs are invariant between any two individuals. Nevertheless, over 80 million variant sites have been described.[4] Most of these variants are single-nucleotide polymorphisms (SNPs), unique sites in the genome where individuals may differ in their DNA sequence. Typically, these SNPs are biallelic, which means that two different nucleotides can occur at the position. In any given population, one of the alleles is more frequent: the major allele, which in most cases also is the ancestral allele. The other allele is called the minor or derived allele. The minor allele typically arose from a mutation in a human ancestor or within an ancestral species during evolution.

As healthy humans carry two copies of each chromosome, they also have two copies or alleles of each SNP. For any SNP, humans can thus either be homozygous for the minor allele, homozygous for the major allele, or heterozygous; i.e., carry one of each allele. The minor allele frequency (MAF) differs among populations and, in the case of disease-associated SNPs, between cases and controls. SNPs with a MAF ≥5% are considered as commonly occurring; SNPs with lower frequencies, especially with a MAF <1%, as rare. The contribution of common SNPs to disease susceptibility is usually analyzed in genome-wide association studies (GWAS). For the determination of variants assessed via GWAS, inexpensive microarray technology can be used, leading to increasingly large sample sizes. Most currently known genetic risk factors have been discovered with this method. Known rare variants can be determined with specialized genotyping arrays as well. For the discovery of previously unknown rare variations, however, whole-exome and whole-genome sequencing are used. Often, such studies on rare mutations are conducted in families, yet increasingly in the general population as well. In addition to common and rare SNPs, duplications or deletions of either single nucleotides or larger stretches of DNA are relevant for disease. One class of small insertions and deletions are called InDels, while copy number variants (CNVs) encompass larger stretches of repeated DNA sequences. The latter structural variants are often rare and constitute a third focus of genetic studies in psychiatric disorders.

The heritability of a disorder or quantitative trait is determined most accurately in twins. However, the heritability of a trait explained by genotyped variants can readily be estimated in any cohort. A popular method is the estimation of the variance explained using genomic restricted maximum likelihood estimation (REML), as implemented in the tool Genome-wide Complex Trait Analysis (GCTA).[5,6] For larger cohorts, this variance can also be estimated from GWAS test statistics.[7]

Family-Based Studies *vs.* GWAS in Unrelated Individuals

Before the onset of large-scale GWAS and sequencing, linkage analysis was commonly used in genetic epidemiology. Linkage analysis evaluates the co-segregation of well-characterized genetic markers (e.g., microsatellites) with putative disease-associated mutations among affected family members. However, statistical power is higher in GWAS than in linkage analyses.[8] Typical family-based designs involve the analysis of trios; i.e., comparisons of affected children to their unaffected parents. Currently, most GWAS are not performed in families, but in unrelated or only slightly related individuals (less closely related than first-degree cousins). This is the case because in typical, well-behaved and simple study situations, the power per genotyped individual tends to be higher in unrelated samples than in family-based studies.

However, some aspects of genetic information, such as the co-segregation of variants and phenotype, analysis of which is helpful for identifying causative variants, cannot easily be obtained for unrelated samples. If possible at all, severely simplifying assumptions need to be made to allow for the inference of such information. In most current study situations, this is not the focus of analysis. However, it may become more important in studies of more complex dependency patterns. Here, nuisance parameters, confounders, and true signal may not easily be disentangled in unrelated individuals, despite the enormous progress in analytical techniques.

Genome-Wide Association Studies

GWAS on genotyped variants are typically conducted in unrelated individuals. Large GWAS in psychiatric genetics have most often used qualitative, binary phenotypes. In such a study, SNPs are genotyped in cases with a certain disease or trait and healthy controls using commercially available high-throughput genotyping platforms. GWAS constitutes a hypothesis-free analysis method because there is no further requirement for prior biological knowledge of the trait under investigation. It is unbiased because all genotyped variations are analyzed comprehensively for a role in disease, regardless of the genomic location of individual SNPs. Of note, sex chromosomes constitute an exception and require specialized analysis methods.[9,10]

Currently, genotyping platforms measure between 300,000 and 5,000,000 unique variants in each sample. Because nearby SNPs are correlated to one another (a phenomenon called linkage disequilibrium; LD), it is computationally possible to use the genotyped variants for estimation of genotype probabilities of millions of SNPs across the genome using a reference data set. Such reference data are provided by the 1000 Genomes Project[4] and by the Haplotype Reference Consortium.[11] This method of estimating missing genotypes is called imputation and enables meta-analyses across multiple data sets that have used different genotyping platforms.[12] Imputation is a crucial step for collaboration and for combining GWAS data from multiple sources, thereby increasing sample size and thus the power to detect novel genetic associations. Regression analyses on such a large number of variants can be conducted efficiently using highly optimized linear algebra libraries, as implemented in several freely available tools.[13–15]

It is important to point out in this context that GWAS are sensitive to ancestral population differences. If cases originated predominantly from one population and controls from a different one, MAF differences between populations might cause an increase in the rate of false-positive associations. It is therefore considered good practice to pool groups of cases and matched controls both by their ethnic origin and by the genotyping platform used. These cohorts can be refined and validated using principal component analysis (PCA) or multidimensional scaling (MDS) of the genetic relationship matrix (GRM). Moreover, PCA or MDS components are typically used as covariates in the GWAS models to control for residual population stratification. Alternatively, linear mixed models can be employed that include the whole GRM as random effects.[16–19] These methods are especially recommended if related individuals are present in the data set. After running a GWAS in each group separately, cohorts can be pooled using methods for meta-analysis.

In a GWAS, variants showing statistically significant frequency differences between cases and controls point to regions in the genome that harbor mutations with potentially causal links to disease. However, the main drawback of GWAS is a lack of specificity regarding the location of such causal mutations: because of LD among nearby variants, the association signal typically covers a broad chromosomal region, not just a single SNP. In fact, the associated region may span over several hundred thousand base pairs, potentially affecting many genes. Fine mapping of the association signal and prioritization of candidate genes thus typically involves the use of expression data (analysis of expressions quantitative trait loci; eQTL), functional annotation using public databases, and gene-set or pathway analyses.

Unlike an analysis of candidate variants in genes already suspected to be associated with disease susceptibility, GWAS faces a massive multiple testing problem. Millions of variants are analyzed, increasing the chances of finding random, false-positive associations. As a result, GWAS requires much stricter significance thresholds to maintain the type 1 error (false-positive rate) than studies testing specific, predefined hypotheses. However, due to LD between SNPs, the number of independent tests in a GWAS is typically lower than the number of available (imputed) variants. In samples of European descent, application of Bonferroni correction for 1 million tests has emerged as a standard, corresponding to a significance threshold of $\alpha < 5\times10^{-08}$.[20]

Due to this multiple testing burden, GWAS in psychiatric research began—like GWAS in non-psychiatric common diseases—without the discovery of genome-wide significant loci. In case of schizophrenia, it appears that there was a crucial inflection point at sample sizes of around 15,000 cases. Past this point, a seemingly linear relationship between sample size and the number of novel discoveries could be observed. This correlation with sample size appeared to be stronger than with any other variable, including detailed phenotyping, the genotyping platform, or the imputation reference. With a current sample size of 35,000 cases and 45,000 controls, over 100 genome-wide significant hits have been discovered for schizophrenia.[21] Within the framework of the Psychiatric Genomics Consortium (PGC), over 40 centers contributed to this study, encompassing more than 50 distinct datasets. Among the genes identified in this study was the one coding for the DRD2 receptor, the target of all currently marketed antipsychotic drugs, posing an example of retrospective drug target validation.

Special Challenges in the Analysis of Rare Variants

Many common SNPs identified through GWAS to be associated with disease are not located directly within the coding region of a gene. They rather map to intergenic space; i.e., to parts of the genome not containing coding information for any known genes. These variants might play a functional role; for example, by influencing gene expression via enhancers. Instead of applying an entirely hypothesis-free GWAS approach, researchers might be interested in how variants located within exons of protein-coding genes directly contribute to disease risk. Yet many of the variants occurring in exons are rare; i.e., they have a MAF <1%, and require special analysis methods.

Power in an association study scales with the MAF of a variant.[22] The fewer people carry a certain allele, the less information is available for making statistical assumptions. Rare variants within protein-coding regions of the genome, the exome, are thus typically analyzed via set-based tests. Here, information from several variants within a gene is examined jointly. Detailed information on analyses assessing either the combined burden of rare variants or the distribution of aggregated test statistics of variants across a gene is given in the literature.[23]

Nevertheless, analyses of rare variants in psychiatric diseases have often failed to meet significance thresholds, even when using set-based tests. Analyses of *de novo* mutations in families, in contrast, have recently been more successful: when using whole-exome sequencing on trios, rare mutations can be identified that are present in the affected child but not in its healthy parents. This approach led to the identification of the histone methyltransferase *SETD1A* as a novel schizophrenia susceptibility gene.[24,25]

Another class of variants often examined at low frequencies are CNVs. They constitute structural variations in the genome with varying numbers of repeats. Many CNVs can be estimated from genotyping chips. Patients suffering from psychiatric disorders show higher rates of *de novo* CNVs. Moreover, an increasing number of genes is associated with gain or loss of CNVs in psychiatric disorders like schizophrenia.[26,27] In fact, analysis of structural variation within the *complement component 4* constitutes one of the few examples where genetic variation could directly be linked to a functional role in the etiology of psychiatric disorders.[27]

Analysis of Quantitative and Complex Phenotypes

The examples used so far referred to case/control studies; i.e., binary phenotypes. However, the GWAS approach is not limited to qualitative traits and can equally well be conducted on quantitative phenotypes. Mental conditions or treatment response are often assessed on a continuous rating scale. If such data are normally distributed, they can be directly analyzed using linear regression. If this prerequisite is not met, the phenotype can often be transformed; e.g., using *log* or *square root* functions. Alternatively, the phenotype can be transformed into a binary trait using an arbitrary threshold or median split to perform a qualitative case/control GWAS using logistical regression. In case of several, non-continuous phenotype levels, multinomial or ordinal regression might be applied.

As no choice for an arbitrary threshold is required in the analysis of continuous traits, the power of a quantitative GWAS might be higher than in an artificial binary one. The selection whether to treat the phenotype quantitatively or qualitatively is up to the investigator. It goes without saying that many more types of phenotypes can be studied by GWAS, including phenotypes which are actually composed of several other phenotypes or longitudinal and survival-type phenotypes. The GWAS paradigm is sufficiently general to allow for the inclusion of all such settings.

One possibility for analyzing high-dimensional phenotypes is the use of polygenic risk scores (PRS). PRS are a statistical approach designed to predict phenotypical outcome of one dataset with the information derived from an independent dataset. They are especially suited for analysis of the cumulative, polygenic contribution of many small effects collectively associated with disease. Typically, summary test statistics from a large case/control GWAS are employed as a training set. This information is used for calculation of a weighted sum of the number of risk alleles in the independent test set. The resulting quantitative measure of genetic burden, the PRS, can then be used for association analyses of various phenotypes in the test set. Notably, the predictions of the polygenic test usually improve (in terms of the phenotypical variance explained) when more than just the most significant SNPs are considered for the PRS. This observation provides evidence that a further increase in sample size of the training set would lead to additional genome-wide significant signals. However, there is a risk of overfitting when determining the p-value threshold for inclusion of training variants into the PRS in the test set. In case of overfitting, the PRS at a given p-value threshold is ideally suited for analyses in the test set but does not replicate in other data. In order to avoid false-positive associations, it is therefore optimal to choose the p-value threshold in a third, independent data set before application of the PRS on the test set, or to perform cross-validation or nested cross-validation. Of note, PRS can also be used for cross-disorder analyses or for analyses of genetic correlations between disorder susceptibility SNPs and variants influencing quantitative traits; e.g., MRI parameters.[28]

Statistical Power

With the current large number of genome-wide significant findings available for schizophrenia,[21] the distribution of the frequency and effect size of associations can be examined. Except for the top association signal within the major histocompatibility complex, all common variants showed odds ratios <1.2. This suggests that these variants effectively escaped natural selection because of their small individual effects, and that earlier studies were underpowered for detection of these variants.

In case a reasonable estimate for the expected effect sizes exists, it is helpful to conduct power analyses prior to running a GWAS using a sensible choice of parameters. If the estimated power for examining associations is too low, alternative strategies should be applied. These might involve pooling genotype data with other researchers for conducting a collaborative GWAS. In the field of statistical genetics, many methodological discussions have taken place regarding the use of frequentist statistics (i.e., p-values). Bayesian approaches and other more elaborate statistical methods have been brought forward and are applied by some.[13] Nevertheless, the use of a p-value significance threshold of $\alpha < 5 \times 10^{-08}$ is the *de facto* standard in the field.[20] Therefore, power calculations are typically carried out using this criterion of significance.

Power analysis can easily be conducted using online tools; e.g., the genetic power calculator by Shaun Purcell and colleagues (Table 4.1), which offers a very convenient interface to power and sample size analysis for a variety of commonly used tests and study designs.[29] Alternatively, the CaTS power calculator (Table 4.1) is recommended.[30] For researchers familiar with R, the same method is available in the package *twoStageGwasPower*.[30] Several methods for power calculation are also implemented in the R package *gap*.[31] More general power analysis routines stemming from standard statistical analysis can be applied as well, of

Table 4.1 Tools and Publications Useful for Tasks Related to Conducting GWAS on Common Variants

Task	Method or Tool	Reference/URL
Whole GWAS from QC over imputation to association analysis and presentation of results	PGC pipeline Ricopili	https://sites.google.com/a/broadinstitute.org/ricopili/
Quality control (QC)	Several published method papers can act as guidelines	(34–36)
QC and GWAS	PLINK2	https://www.cog-genomics.org/plink2/ (14)
Analysis of the X chromosome	XWAS	http://keinanlab.cb.bscb.cornell.edu/content/xwas/ (9)
Power analysis	Genetic Power Calculator or CaTS	http://zzz.bwh.harvard.edu/gpc/ http://csg.sph.umich.edu/abecasis/CaTS/ (29, 30)
SNP-based heritability	GCTA or LD Score Regression	http://cnsgenomics.com/software/gcta/ https://github.com/bulik/ldsc/ (6, 7)
Genotype imputation	SHAPEIT/ IMPUTE2	https://mathgen.stats.ox.ac.uk/impute/impute_v2.html (37, 38) https://imputation.sanger.ac.uk/ https://imputationserver.sph.umich.edu/
Post-imputation QC	QCTOOL	http://www.well.ox.ac.uk/~gav/qctool/
GWAS using Bayesian statistics	SNPTEST	https://mathgen.stats.ox.ac.uk/genetics_software/snptest/snptest.html (13)

Table 4.1 Continued

Task	Method or Tool	Reference/URL
GWAS using linear mixed models	FaST-LMM or BOLT-LMM	https://github.com/MicrosoftGenomics/FaST-LMM/ https://data.broadinstitute.org/alkesgroup/BOLT-LMM/ (16, 17)
GWAS using logistic mixed models	GMMAT	https://www.hsph.harvard.edu/xlin/software.html#gmmat (18)
Meta-analysis	METAL or METASOFT	http://csg.sph.umich.edu/abecasis/Metal/ http://genetics.cs.ucla.edu/meta_jemdoc/ (39, 40)
Regional association plots	LocusZoom	http://locuszoom.org/ (41)
Automated functional mapping and annotation of GWAS	FUMA	http://fuma.ctglab.nl/
Analysis of linkage disequilibrium	LDlink	https://analysistools.nci.nih.gov/LDlink/ (42)
Polygenic scores	PRSice	http://prsice.info/ (43)

Tools and publications useful for tasks related to conducting GWAS on common variants.

course. Figure 4.1 shows typical plots produced using R. Such plots can be very useful for providing an orientation regarding the sample sizes required.

GWAS generally require quite large sample sizes. Thanks to consortium efforts, samples in the hundreds of thousands can now be achieved quite regularly. While even the largest consortia still face difficulties in meeting such sample sizes in psychiatric genetics, the use of self-reported data or data from electronic health records is currently boosting available sample sizes.[32,33] Discussions are still ongoing whether phenotypes should or may be obtained via clinical or population-based samples and to what extent self-reported data or electronic health records can compete with more classical phenotyping methods. Power for mid-range effects is very high in such large studies, and very small effects can be discovered regularly, making the disentangling of confounders and true signal all the more important. The question of sample size, however, may need to be rephrased in the coming years with more in-depth characterization across various *omics* modalities and dimensions.

Finally, one more distinction in study design should be pointed out in this context. The validity of GWAS findings can be underscored either by conducting a full meta-analysis of all available samples across cohorts or in a

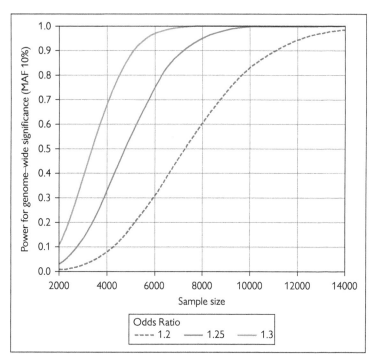

Figure 4.1 The statistical power for reaching genome-wide significance ($p = 5 \times 10^{-8}$) in an association test increases with sample size, the estimated odds ratio of the association, and with the minor allele frequency (MAF) of the variant. The figure visualizes this relationship for a MAF of 10% and three selected odds ratios. The plot has been generated using the function power.prop.test() of the R package pwr.

more conventional discovery and replication setting. Interestingly, a full analysis of all samples has inherently more power than a discovery and replication setting.[30] In previous days, the main advantage of the latter design lay in cost reduction for genotyping. As the cost for genome-wide genotyping has been constantly dropping over the last years, this advantage is constantly diminishing.

Practical Considerations and Conclusions

With the recommendations given throughout the previous sections in mind, Table 4.1 summarizes starting points and tools useful for conducting genome-wide studies on common variants.

References

1. Owen, M. J., Cardno, A. G., & O'Donovan, M. C. (2000). Psychiatric genetics: back to the future. *Molecular Psychiatry, 5,* 22–31.

2. Walter, H. (2013). The third wave of biological psychiatry. *Frontiers in Psychology, 4,* 582.

3. Owen, M. J., Sawa, A., & Mortensen, P. B. (2016). Schizophrenia. *Lancet, 388,* 86–97.

4. 1000 Genomes Project Consortium, Auton, A., Brooks, L. D., Durbin, R. M., Garrison, E. P., Kang, H. M., et al. (2015). A global reference for human genetic variation. *Nature, 526,* 68–74.

5. Yang, J., Lee, S. H., Goddard, M. E., & Visscher, P. M. (2011). GCTA: a tool for genome-wide complex trait analysis. *American Journal of Human Genetics, 88,* 76–82.

6. Lee, S. H., Wray, N. R., Goddard, M. E., & Visscher, P. M. (2011). Estimating missing heritability for disease from genome-wide association studies. *American Journal of Human Genetics, 88,* 294–305.

7. Bulik-Sullivan, B. K., Loh, P.-R., Finucane, H. K., Ripke, S., Yang, J., Schizophrenia Working Group of the Psychiatric Genomics Consortium, et al. (2015). LD Score regression distinguishes confounding from polygenicity in genome-wide association studies. *Nature Genetics, 47,* 291–295.

8. Risch, N., & Merikangas, K. (1996). The future of genetic studies of complex human diseases. *Science (New York, NY), 273,* 1516–1517.

9. Gao, F., Chang, D., Biddanda, A., Ma, L., Guo, Y., Zhou, Z., & Keinan, A. (2015). XWAS: A Software Toolset for Genetic Data Analysis and Association Studies of the X Chromosome. *The Journal of Heredity, 106,* 666–671.

10. König, I. R., Loley, C., Erdmann, J., & Ziegler, A. (2014). How to include chromosome X in your genome-wide association study. *Genetic Epidemiology, 38,* 97–103.

11. McCarthy, S., Das, S., Kretzschmar, W., Delaneau, O., Wood, A. R., Teumer, A., et al. (2016). A reference panel of 64,976 haplotypes for genotype imputation. *Nature Genetics, 48,* 1279–1283.

12. Marchini, J., & Howie, B. (2010). Genotype imputation for genome-wide association studies. *Nature Reviews Genetics, 11,* 499–511.

13. Marchini, J., Howie, B., Myers, S., McVean, G., & Donnelly, P. (2007). A new multipoint method for genome-wide association studies by imputation of genotypes. *Nature Genetics, 39,* 906–913.

14. Chang, C. C., Chow, C. C., Tellier, L. C., Vattikuti, S., Purcell, S. M., & Lee, J. J. (2015). Second-generation PLINK: rising to the challenge of larger and richer datasets. *GigaScience, 4,* 7.

15. Aulchenko, Y. S., Struchalin, M. V., & van Duijn, C. M. (2010). ProbABEL package for genome-wide association analysis of imputed data. *BMC Bioinformatics, 11,* 134.

16. Lippert, C., Listgarten, J., Liu, Y., Kadie, C. M., Davidson, R. I., & Heckerman, D. (2011). FaST linear mixed models for genome-wide association studies. *Nature Methods, 8,* 833–835.

17. Loh, P.-R., Tucker, G., Bulik-Sullivan, B. K., Vilhjalmsson, B. J., Finucane, H. K., Salem, R. M., et al. (2015). Efficient Bayesian mixed-model analysis increases association power in large cohorts. *Nature Genetics, 47,* 284–290.

18. Chen, H., Wang, C., Conomos, M. P., Stilp, A. M., Li, Z., Sofer, T., et al. (2016). Control for Population Structure and Relatedness for Binary Traits in Genetic Association Studies via Logistic Mixed Models. *American Journal of Human Genetics*, *98*, 653–666.

19. Aulchenko, Y. S., de Koning, D.-J., & Haley, C. (2007). Genomewide rapid association using mixed model and regression: a fast and simple method for genomewide pedigree-based quantitative trait loci association analysis. *Genetics*, *177*, 577–585.

20. Sham, P. C., & Purcell, S. M. (2014). Statistical power and significance testing in large-scale genetic studies. *Nature Publishing Group*, *15*, 335–346.

21. Schizophrenia Working Group of the Psychiatric Genomics Consortium. (2014). Biological insights from 108 schizophrenia-associated genetic loci. *Nature*, *511*, 421–427.

22. Zuk, O., Schaffner, S. F., Samocha, K., Do, R., Hechter, E., Kathiresan, S., et al. (2014). Searching for missing heritability: designing rare variant association studies. *Proceedings of the National Academy of Sciences of the United States of America*, *111*, E455–64.

23. Lee, S., Abecasis, G. R., Boehnke, M., & Lin, X. (2014). Rare-variant association analysis: study designs and statistical tests. *American Journal of Human Genetics*, *95*, 5–23.

24. Singh, T., Kurki, M. I., Curtis, D., Purcell, S. M., Crooks, L., McRae, J., et al. (2016). Rare loss-of-function variants in SETD1A are associated with schizophrenia and developmental disorders. *Nature Neuroscience*, *19*, 571–577.

25. Takata, A., Xu, B., Ionita-Laza, I., Roos, J. L., Gogos, J. A., & Karayiorgou, M. (2014). Loss-of-function variants in schizophrenia risk and SETD1A as a candidate susceptibility gene. *Neuron*, *82*, 773–780.

26. CNV and Schizophrenia Working Groups of the Psychiatric Genomics Consortium, Psychosis Endophenotypes International Consortium. (2017). Contribution of copy number variants to schizophrenia from a genome-wide study of 41,321 subjects. *Nature Genetics*, *49*, 27–35.

27. Sekar, A., Bialas, A. R., de Rivera, H., Davis, A., Hammond, T. R., Kamitaki, N., et al. (2016). Schizophrenia risk from complex variation of complement component 4. *Nature*, *530*, 177–183.

28. Franke, B., Stein, J. L., Ripke, S., Anttila, V., Hibar, D. P., van Hulzen, K. J. E., et al. (2016). Genetic influences on schizophrenia and subcortical brain volumes: large-scale proof of concept. *Nature Neuroscience*, *19*, 420–431.

29. Purcell, S., Cherny, S. S., & Sham, P. C. (2003). Genetic Power Calculator: design of linkage and association genetic mapping studies of complex traits. *Bioinformatics (Oxford, England)*, *19*, 149–150.

30. Skol, A. D., Scott, L. J., Abecasis, G. R., & Boehnke, M. (2006). Joint analysis is more efficient than replication-based analysis for two-stage genome-wide association studies. *Nature Genetics*, *38*, 209–213.

31. Zhao, J. H. (2007). gap: Genetic Analysis Package. *Journal of Statistical Software*, *23*. doi:10.18637/jss.v023.i08

32. Hoffmann, T. J., Ehret, G. B., Nandakumar, P., Ranatunga, D., Schaefer, C., Kwok, P.-Y., et al. (2017). Genome-wide association analyses using electronic health records identify new loci influencing blood pressure variation. *Nature Genetics*, *49*, 54–64.

33. Hyde, C. L., Nagle, M. W., Tian, C., Chen, X., Paciga, S. A., Wendland, J. R., et al. (2016). Identification of 15 genetic loci associated with risk of major depression in individuals of European descent. *Nature Genetics, 48*, 1031–1036.

34. Wang, G. T., Peng, B., & Leal, S. M. (2014). Variant association tools for quality control and analysis of large-scale sequence and genotyping array data. *American Journal of Human Genetics, 94*, 770–783.

35. Turner, S., Armstrong, L. L., Bradford, Y., Carlson, C. S., Crawford, D. C., Crenshaw, A. T., et al. (2011). Quality control procedures for genome-wide association studies. *Current Protocols in Human Genetics / Editorial Board, Jonathan L. Haines ... [Et Al.], Chapter 1*, Unit1.19.

36. Weale, M. E. (2010). Quality control for genome-wide association studies. *Methods in Molecular Biology (Clifton, NJ), 628*, 341–372.

37. Howie, B., Fuchsberger, C., Stephens, M., Marchini, J., & Abecasis, G. R. (2012). Fast and accurate genotype imputation in genome-wide association studies through pre-phasing. *Nature Genetics, 44*, 955–959.

38. Delaneau, O., Zagury, J.-F., & Marchini, J. (2013). Improved whole-chromosome phasing for disease and population genetic studies. *Nature Methods, 10*, 5–6.

39. Willer, C. J., Li, Y., & Abecasis, G. R. (2010). METAL: fast and efficient meta-analysis of genomewide association scans. *Bioinformatics (Oxford, England), 26*, 2190–2191.

40. Han, B., & Eskin, E. (2011). Random-effects model aimed at discovering associations in meta-analysis of genome-wide association studies. *American Journal of Human Genetics, 88*, 586–598.

41. Pruim, R. J., Welch, R. P., Sanna, S., Teslovich, T. M., Chines, P. S., Gliedt, T. P., et al. (2010). LocusZoom: regional visualization of genome-wide association scan results. *Bioinformatics (Oxford, England), 26*, 2336–2337.

42. Machiela, M. J., & Chanock, S. J. (2015). LDlink: a web-based application for exploring population-specific haplotype structure and linking correlated alleles of possible functional variants. *Bioinformatics (Oxford, England), 31*, 3555–3557.

43. Euesden, J., Lewis, C. M., & O'Reilly, P. F. (2015). PRSice: Polygenic Risk Score software. *Bioinformatics (Oxford, England), 31*, 1466–1468.

Chapter 5

Human Linkage and Association Analysis

John P. Rice

Take-Home Points

1. Most complex disorders are caused by many genes of small effect, and initial samples were of insufficient size to provide adequate power for detection.
2. Current GWAS (genome-wide association analysis studies) in large samples using standard methods have been successful in identifying hundreds of replicated signals for mental disorders.
3. The challenge for the next decade will be to understand the biology of these GWAS hits. Many identified to date have not been in coding regions, making this harder.
4. In this chapter, we presented the basic genetic concepts and statistical methods needed to understand these exciting advances.

Introduction

In this chapter, we consider statistical approaches for the analysis of human linkage and association data. Linkage analysis has its roots with the seminal paper by Newton Morton[1] where he introduced the logarithm of odds (LOD) score method. The basic idea is that a disease gene will segregate in a family with a close (linked) marker, and typing this marker will lead to the detection of the disease gene. Initially, a whole-genome study consisted of typing a few dozen blood groups and enzymes. This was followed by panels of informative markers Restriction Fragment Length Polymorphism (RFLPs) that covered the whole genome, and then by single-nucleotide polymorphisms (SNPs).

Linkage analysis has been an important approach to the identification of the genetic basis of disease traits such as cystic fibrosis, Duchenne muscular dystrophy, Huntington's disease, and a wide variety of metabolic disorders. The successes using this approach have been largely confined to Mendelian monogenic disorders or complex disorders with Mendelian subforms (e.g., breast cancer and Alzheimer's disease). Although it was natural to apply these methods to complex diseases involving a few to many loci (e.g., schizophrenia, bipolar disorder, major depression, asthma, or diabetes), early applications were not successful and tended to find disparate signals that were not replicated. During the last decade, psychiatric genetics abandoned linkage analysis and moved to case-control studies of association.

Two companies (Affymetrix and Illumina) developed chips to genotype hundreds of thousands of SNPs at an affordable scale. The first GWAS (genome-wide association study) for age-related macular degeneration, in 2005 by Klein and colleagues,[2] was successful; there are now tens of thousands of significant SNPs associated with many diseases[3] (the GWAS Catalog, Welter et al.). The Welcome Trust[4] performed GWAS on several disorders (including bipolar disorder) using a common set of 3,000 controls and 2,000 cases each. This was followed by GAIN (Genetic Association Information Network), which analyzed six disorders (four of which were mental health–related). An important part of GAIN was the requirement that phenotypic and genotypic data be deposited in the public database of Genotypes and Phenotypes (dbGaP) and available to the scientific community after a short embargo period. In the United States, this is now a requirement for all federally funded genetic studies.

It became clear the most complex disorders were caused by many genes of small effect, and that the initial samples were of insufficient size to provide adequate power. The PGC (Psychiatric Genetics Consortium; https://www.med.unc.edu/pgc) began in early 2007 and now includes over 800 investigators from 38 countries. The intent is to conduct meta- and mega-analyses of genome-wide genomic data for psychiatric disorders. There are samples from more than 900,000 individuals currently in analysis. The most recent PGC publication from the Schizophrenia Working Group[5] identified 108 loci using approximately 37,000 cases and over 100,000 controls. The most significant signal was in the human leukocyte antigen (HLA) region on chromosome 6, and this has led to a functional understanding of this signal.[6]

The preceding history covers a few major milestones and, in hindsight, indicates why early candidate gene and linkage were unsuccessful. The reader may ask, "Why bother learning linkage analysis?" There are several answers to this, apart from obtaining an understanding of a fundamental aspect of genetics. We are coming to the end of the GWAS era, and current efforts are now focused on whole-genome sequencing and the discovery of rare variants. We now know that there are many genes of small effect size contributing to our diseases of interest. There will be little power to detect genes of low frequency using a GWAS approach (unless they have large effect size, in which case they would have probably been discovered by linkage). Linkage may be viewed as large-scale detection (about 2,000 independent statistical tests genome-wide); whereas association is fine-grained, with about 1 million independent tests. A combination of linkage to first reduce the size of the genome considered for association would seem warranted. Problems associated with genetic or phenotypic heterogeneity may be helped by studying families, especially using large, densely affected pedigrees or methods that allow for a mixture of linked and unlinked families in a collection of smaller families. Finally, DNA exists on many well characterized families collected for linkage studies. It is too early to know if these hybrid approaches will be successful, but they will certainly be tried.

Linkage Analysis

The best overall and comprehensive reference for methods in linkage analysis remains the book by Ott.[7] We will cover only a small part of this extensive literature.

Linkage: Basic Concepts

"Linkage" describes a physical relationship among loci that are in close proximity of each other along the same a chromosomal strand (chromatid). Mendel's second law of independent assortment predicts that two loci would segregate independently to form gametes, and that is true for loci on different chromosomes or quite far apart on the same chromosome. However, the closer two loci are, the more likely it is that the alleles on each chromatid will segregate together. Consider a doubly heterozygous parent (A1B1/A2B2) at two loci, A and B with alleles A1 and A2 and B1 and B2, respectively. Gametes A1B2, A2B1 are called recombinants, and A1B1, A2B2 are non-recombinants. Then the recombination fraction θ is defined by

$$\theta = \text{Prob (recombinant)}.$$

In linkage analysis, we attempt to find loci for which $\theta < \frac{1}{2}$. The recombination fraction θ is roughly equivalent to the distance between two loci measured in centi-Morgans (cM) for small distances. If $\theta = .01$, A and B are 1 cM apart. The correspondence between genetic distance (in cM) and physical distance (in base-pairs) varies considerably across the genome and by sex,[8] although a rough equivalence is 1 cM ~ 1 megabase (Mb).

In order to estimate the recombination fraction θ and to combine information over families, maximum likelihood theory is used to calculate the probability of observing the data at hand while estimating the recombination fraction. The LOD curve and LOD score are defined by:

$$Z(\theta) = \text{Lod curve} = \log_{10} \frac{L(\theta)}{L(\theta = 1/2)},$$

$$\hat{Z}(\theta) = \text{maximum of } Z(\theta) = \text{lod score}.$$

When Morton defined the LOD score, he selected a cut-off of 3, so the odds of linkage are 1,000 times more likely than non-linkage. However, statistical theory for the likelihood ratio test is based on base e, rather than base 10, so the LOD score yields a chi-square when multiplied by $2/\log_{10} e$. Thus,

$$4.6 \; Z(\theta) \sim \chi_1^2.$$

The cut-off of 3 then corresponds to a chi-square value of 13.8, or p = 0.0001. Morton argued that the prior probability of linkage is low (1/46 for being on the correct arm of a chromosome), so that a conservative p-value is needed to avoid false positive reports of linkage. This cut-off was used for 40 years, until Kruglyak and Lander[9] noted that a LOD score of 3.6 corresponded to a genome-wide significance of 0.05 for an infinitely dense marker map. That is, 1 in 20 linkage screens would yield a LOD score of 3.6 or greater if linkage were not present.

Linkage Analysis with Disease Phenotypes

When linkage analysis is performed between markers, the likelihood is relatively easy to compute. For a disease trait, only the phenotype is observed, and the goal is to locate and identify the underlying trait locus. In order to carry out the linkage analysis, it is usually necessary to make assumptions regarding the mode of inheritance.

Let us assume the disease or trait of interest is caused by a single locus described by the Single Major Locus model (SML) model. That is, for a two-allele locus dichotomous phenotype, we denote the two alleles by "D" and "d," with p the frequency of D, and q = 1–p be the frequency of d. Under the assumption of Hardy-Weinberg equilibrium, the probabilities for the three genotypes DD, Dd, dd, are p^2, $2pq$, q^2, respectively. The penetrances f_{DD}, f_{Dd}, f_{dd} are defined as the probability that individuals of genotype DD, Dd, dd, respectively, are affected. Accordingly, the SML can be described in terms of the four parameters p, f_{DD}, f_{Dd}, f_{dd}. We further assume that all familial resemblance is due to that single locus. Thus, the phenotype of an individual depends only on his/her genotype. That is, if $(X_1 \ldots ,X_m)$ denotes the phenotypes in a family of size m, and $(g_1, \ldots, g_m)$ denotes their genotypes, then $P(X_i| g_1, \ldots, g_m) = P(X_i|g_i)$ and $P(X_i, X_j \mid g_i, g_j) = P(X_i|g_i) P(X_j \mid g_j)$, for individuals i and j, where P() denotes the probability of the event in parentheses. Let θ denote the recombination fraction between the trait locus and a marker M. Then the likelihood of a family depends on the five parameters p, f_{DD}, f_{Dd}, f_{dd}, and θ. Under the assumptions of the SML, the likelihood of large pedigrees can be efficiently calculated using the Elston and Stewart algorithm.[10] This method was implemented in the original LINKAGE package,[11] then Cottington and colleagues[12] developed FASTLINK with more efficient calculations.

Note that in a nuclear family, one parent must be a double heterozygote to provide information for linkage. For example, for a disease locus with alleles

"D" and "d," and a marker locus with alleles "A" and "a," a parent whose genotype is "Ddaa" always transmits "a" to his offspring. Moreover, for a single child, even if a parent is a double heterozygote, there is no information for linkage since the phase of the doubly heterozygous parent is not known. As a special example, for a rare dominant, an affected individual is Dd at the disease locus, so if an affected parent who is heterozygous for a completely linked marker has two affected children who share the same marker allele, the first child determines the phase, and the second contributes 0.3 to the LOD score.

Genetic Maps and Multipoint Analysis

Different types of genetic markers have been used to create a linkage map of the human genome. Early linkage studies were carried out using 300–400 microsatellites uniformly distributed across the genome at a density of 5–10 cM. These markers were favored because of their high polymorphic information content; a large number of alleles assures a high frequency of heterozygosity, which is necessary for informative analysis, as noted before. Given the use of diallelic SNPs, linkage maps are now constructed using these polymorphisms. SNPs are relatively easy and inexpensive to type on dense arrays, and what SNPs lack in polymorphism, they make up for in density. Usually 6,000–10,000 SNPs will provide a map of equal information content to traditional microsatellite maps. However, care must be taken to select a set of markers not in linkage disequilibrium (LD)—an option in the analysis program PLINK, discussed later. When parents are not genotyped, the LOD score as computed by the program LINKAGE, which assumes the markers are in equilibrium, is inflated, and the type I error rate is increased.

Recall that two markers are 1 cM (centi-Morgan) apart if the probability of recombination is 0.01. The human genome is approximately 3,330 cM in length. Under the assumption that crossovers in different intervals are independent (no interference), then Haldane (1919) noted the map distance x is given by $x = -1/2 \ln(1-2\,\theta)$ for $0 \leq \theta < \frac{1}{2}$. The inverse is given by $\theta = \frac{1}{2}[1-\exp(-2|x|)]$. When performing multipoint analyses, the θ's are transformed to distances, so that only N–1 are needed when analyzing N markers, and others are computed using distances and then applying the inverse of the Haldane function. There are several map functions (cf. Ott[7]) that allow for interference. They all have the property that $x \approx \theta$ when θ is small.

Multipoint analysis can be carried out by moving the location of the trait locus across the linear genetic map and calculating LOD scores based on all the marker/haplotype information in the family on the chromosome. Again, the location with the highest LOD score is the most likely location of the trait locus. It should be noted that the extended haplotype information afforded by the multipoint approach allows for the calculation of more accurate odds, and thus provides more information to exclude or confirm linkage. There is a computational challenge associated with multipoint analysis in that while the computer programs such as LINKAGE can analyze pedigrees with hundreds of individuals, it is not practical to do so using hundreds of markers at once. A typical approach for large pedigrees is to use a sliding window of markers. An alternative algorithm, as implemented in MERLIN,[13] can handle hundreds of markers, but only in families of fewer than 20 individuals. The most recent version of MERLIN allows for markers to be in linkage disequilibrium. For larger pedigrees, it is common to thin the markers to eliminate LD among them.

Association Analysis

There is no single reference that covers the background needed to understand association analysis. The books by Sham[14] and Neale and colleagues[15] both give useful background. They also cover linkage analysis. We will first consider a few issues related to an appreciation of current approaches to association analysis.

Preliminary Background

The Scale of the Human Genome

There are 3.3 billion base pairs in the human genome. Recall that a kb is 1,000 base pairs, and a mb is 1,000 kb. Since there are 3,300 cM in the genome, there are 3.3 billion in 3,300 base pairs, so that 1 mb = ~1cM (on average). There are approximately 20,000 protein-coding genes in humans, so that there are, on average, 6 genes per mb and 6 genes per cM. A typical linkage peak is 20–30 cM wide, so it may contain 120–180 genes to interrogate. Linkage is a large-scale phenomenon, whereas linkage disequilibrium as defined later is small-scale.

Hypothesis Testing and Multiple Testing

In statistical testing, we formulate a null hypothesis (such as $\theta = 1/2$ or no association) H_0 and select a significance level α, the Type I error. Under H_0, we have a test statistic X, often a bell-shaped curve centered at 0, and reject the null hypothesis if $|X| > T$, where the probability of extreme values ($|X| > T$) is less than α.

A related concept is that of power. For an alternative hypothesis H_1, the power $1-\beta$ is the probability of rejecting the null hypothesis assuming H_1 is true. B is called the Type II error. Computation of power requires assumptions about the true state of nature, such as effect size, etc. In general, power decreases as the significance level becomes smaller.

For a significance level α, if we perform N independent tests, we expect to reject $N\alpha$ tests if the null hypothesis is true for each test. For example, if $N = 100$ and $\alpha = 0.05$, and x is the number of rejections, then

$$P(x > 1) = 1 - P(x = 0) = 1 - (1 - \alpha)^{100} = .99408.$$

Note that $1 - (1 - \alpha)^N \approx N\alpha$ for α small, so that if we choose $\alpha' = \alpha/N$, then $1 - (1 - \alpha')^{100} = .0488$ in our example. Dividing the intended significance level by N is referred to as the Bonferroni correction.

In GWAS analysis, we assume the equivalent of 1 million independent tests, so to achieve a significance level of 0.05, the standard cutoff is:

$p = .05/1M = 5 \times 10^{-8}$, and a useful, related number is $-\log(5 \times 10^{-8}) = 7.3$.

Definition of LD

Consider the two people here with identical genotypes $A_1 A_2 B_1 B_2$ in the figure

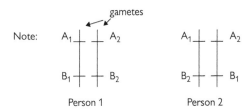

They have different haplotypes, $A_1 B_1/A_2 B_2$ and $A_1 B_2/A_2 B_1$, even though they have the same genotypes. In general, a double heterozygote is ambiguous in terms of haplotypes. Linkage disequilibrium (LD) is defined in terms of haplotypes, rather than genotypes.

D, D′, and r²

For two loci A and B, with alleles A1, . . . Am and B1, . . . , Bn with frequencies p1, . . . , pm and q1, . . . , qn, respectively, there are $m(m + 1)/2 \times n(n + 1)/2$ genotypes and mn haplotypes. For a SNP, there are nine genotypes and four haplotypes. We let h_{ij} denote the haplotype frequencies. The loci A and B are independent if $h_{ij} = p_i q_j$, positively associated if $h_{ij} > p_i q_j$, and negatively associated if $h_{ij} < p_i q_j$. As derived in Sham[14], Chapter 4, the decrease in equilibrium after k generations is given by

$$h_{ijk} - p_i q_j = (1 - \theta)^k \left(h_{ijo} - p_i q_j \right).$$

That is, given an initial amount of LD in a population, the decrease is proportional to $(1-\theta)$ for each generation. Thus, markers that are closely linked remain in LD for many generations. Given genotypic data for two loci, and under the assumption of random mating, the haplotype frequencies may be estimated using the iterative EM algorithm (cf. Sham, Chapter 4), and may be performed using the program HAPLOVIEW.[16]

Following the notation of Neal et al.,[15] we let $P(A_1) = pA_1$, $P(B_1) = pB_1$, and let $P(A_1B_1) = p_{A1B1} = h_{11}$. There is no association if $h_{11} = p_{A1}p_{B1}$. We define D by

$D = h_{11} - p_{A1}p_{B1}$ and say A and B are in w = equilibrium if D = 0.

D tends to take on small values and depends on the marginal gene frequencies. We define D′ by:

$$D' = D/-\max\{-p_{A1}p_{B1}, -p_{A2}p_{B2}\} \text{ if } D < 0$$

$$= D/\min \{p_{A2}p_{B1}, p_{A1}p_{B2}\} \text{ if } D > 0, \text{ and}$$

$$r^2 = D^2 /(p_{A1}p_{A2}\ p_{B1}p_{B2}) = \text{square of usual correlation coefficient.}$$

D′ and r^2 are between −1 and + 1. D′ is ± 1 if and only if one of the cells in the 2x2 table of haplotypes is zero. D′ may be close to ± 1, and r^2 may be close to zero when marginal frequencies are different.

Consider two SNPs, A and B, and suppose there is no variability at locus B, so there are two haplotypes: 11 and 21. Now suppose there is a mutation at B with that chromosome having "2" at A. There are now three haplotypes: 11, 21, 22 (no 12), and D′ is 1. We can get haplotype 12 if there were another mutation (not likely), or a crossover event due to linkage. There are areas of the genome where all pairwise D's are ± 1, and there has been no recombination to create all possible haplotypes. There are recombination "hot spots" that break up these blocks. There is not a direct relationship between LD and physical distance. We don't have a SNP map (in contrast to linkage), and there is no mapping function to reduce the parameter space.

After completion of the Homan Genome Project to provide the complete sequence of the human genome, the International HapMap Consortium[17] produced dense SNPs to provide haplotype blocks to assist association studies in three populations: CEPH (whites), Asians (Japanese and Chinese), and Yorubans in Africa. In a second phase, they complete additional populations. More recently, the 1000 Genomes Project[18] provided many more through sequencings.

Predictability of one SNP by another is best described by r^2. A block is a set of SNPs with all pairwise LD measures of high value. However, if one uses r^2 as the measure, and we insert a SNP with low frequency in between SNPs with frequencies s close to 0.5, then the block breaks up. Scientists from Perlegen[19] defined bins where a tag SNP has r^2 of 0.8 with all other SNPs. Bins need not be contiguous. Blocks using D′ may have a "biological" interpretation (long stretches with |D′| = 1), whereas selection of Tag SNPs is a statistical issue when we want to predict untyped SNPS from those that are typed. r^2 is the natural measure for this.

Case-Control Association Analysis

In case-control analysis, we compare either allele or genotypic frequencies in the two groups. An advantage is that we can use standard statistical approaches based on odds ratios. We will develop analysis based on logistic regression in detail. Here, case/control status is the dependent variable. Advantages include the ability to include covariates and the ability to estimate odds ratios. We assume a dichotomous phenotype; analyses for a quantitative phenotype are based on the standard regression model.

Usual regression requires a dependent variable that can take on any value, $[-\infty,\infty]$. A probability is in the interval $[0,1]$, and would not be a good dependent variable in quantitative regression. If we consider the odds $= p/(1-p)$, it is in the interval $[0,\infty]$. Finally, we consider the logit:

$$\text{Logit} = \log(\text{odds}) \text{ is in the interval } [-\infty,\infty].$$

For a categorical variable with K categories, we can create K-1 "dummy" variables to use that categorical variable as a predictor in a regression equation. A continuous variable may be used directly a covariate.

For a dichotomous outcome Y, let $p = P(Y = 1)$, and let $\Omega = \text{logit}(p) = \log(p/(1-p))$, with

$$\Omega = \alpha + \beta_1 X_1 + \ldots + \beta_N X_N, \text{ for covariates } X_1 \ldots X_N.$$

Then $p/(1-p) = e^{\Omega}$, so that $p = e^{\Omega}/(1 + e^{\Omega})$. e^{β} is the odds ratio, and if $\beta = 0$ then the odds are 1. (Recall $e^0 = 1$ where $2 = 2.7 \ldots$ is the base of the natural logarithms.)

For a SNP, we create a dummy variable X_1 as coded in Figures 5.2 and 5.3:

$$\log(\text{odds}) = \alpha + \beta_1 X_1$$
$$\text{odds} = e^{\alpha} e^{\beta_1 X_1}$$

Genotype	X_1		Genotype	Odds
1/1	0		11	e^{α}
1/2	1		12	$e^{\alpha} e^{\beta_1}$
2/2	2		22	$e^{\alpha} e^{2\beta_1}$

Test $\beta_1 = 0$, all odds $= e^{\alpha}$

Note: No dominance effect

This is the trend test where the SNP effect is coded with one degree of freedom. We note that the full model requires two dummy variables, X_1 and X_2 (since there are three genotypes):

$$\log(\text{odds}) = \alpha + \beta_1 X_1 + \beta_2 X_2$$
$$\text{odds} = e^{\alpha} e^{\beta_1 X_1} e^{\beta_2 X_2}$$

Genotype	X_1	X_2	Genotype	Odds
11	0	0	11	e^{α}
12	1	1	12	$e^{\alpha} e^{\beta_1} e^{\beta_2}$
22	2	0	22	$e^{\alpha} e^{2\beta_1}$

Test $\beta_1 = \beta_2 = 0$, all odds $= e^{\alpha}$
If $\beta_2 = 0$, then have additive model

Common practice is to use the one degree of freedom trend test rather than the full model that requires two degrees of freedom. In a typical GWAS, this test is applied for each SNP.

Table 5.1 100 Observations from Two Populations A and B and the Combined Population

Population A		Population B		Combined	
1	6	25	25	26	34
9	81	25	25	34	106
Odds ratio = 1		Odds ratio = 1		Odds ratio = 2.38	

Important Issues in Testing for Association

We will briefly discuss several areas essential to the analysis of GWAS data.

Population Stratification

Although we would like a significant relationship to indicate the SNP is LD with a disease gene, a potential confounding factor is population stratification. This is a general artifact in the analysis of 2 x 2 contingency tables. For example, if the two populations (each with odds ratios of 1) are combined, the resulting odds ratio is 2.38! (Table 5.1).

The two basic approaches are to use multidimensional scaling or principal component analysis using all the SNP data to produce quantitative covariates to include in the logistic regression analysis. The program EIGENSTRAT[20] is a commonly used tool for this.

Imputation

There is a need to combine many GWAS datasets for the same disorder to achieve increased power, or to compare results from different studies. The different GWAS chips can have very different marker sets and limit these applications. Imputation is now a standard technique to use a reference panel to infer SNPs in the reference panel using the observed SNPs. The results are the probabilities of the predicted SNPs, but these can be used in the standard analysis packages. The program IMPUTE2,[21] using the 1000genome reference panel, is commonly used today. Most recently, McCarthy and colleagues[22] provide a reference panel based on approximately 65,000 haplotypes from whole-genome sequencing to allow accurate imputation for low frequency SNPs. They also describe remote server resources. We will not go into further detail here, but imputed data are now often made available with the primary data available from public databases.

Data Cleaning

In many ways, the cleaning of GWAS is harder than the analysis itself. First, individuals who do not genotype well are removed, and then SNPs with low success rates are removed. With modern platforms, we expect at least 98% of reactions to work. SNPs not in Hardy-Weinberg are usually eliminated. IBD (Identity by Descent) can be estimated and cryptic relatedness between the individuals (or often duplicates) must be detected and removed. Improper cleaning can lead to the top signals v = being due to technical artifacts. The program PLINK[23] allows easy execution of these cleaning steps.

Genomic Inflation Factor

When we test 1 million SNPs, most are not truly associated. When using a chi-square test with 1 df, the median value should be 0.445. The genomic inflation factor λ is the observed median/.445. We expect λ to be 1.0. We can correct the observed chi-squares by dividing by λ. When analyzing data with PLINK[23] (http://pngu.mgh.harvard.edu/purcell/plink/), we obtain the raw p-value, along with the genomic inflation corrected and Bonferroni corrected p-values (as well as several others). A large λ may indicate inadequate cleaning or a bias in the test statistic used. It is always best to control for population admixture, eliminate CNVs, etc., prior to analysis to reduce λ rather than performing this simple correction. A better overall check of validity examines the QQ plot to consider the full range of results, rather than just the median value.

QQ Plots

The quantile-quantile probability (QQ) plot shows observed p-values versus expected p-values assuming no tests are significant. The QQ plot assumes independent tests, so this can be a factor in interpretation. When we perform N independent statistical tests for which all null hypotheses are true, we expect a uniform distribution. That is, 5% should be significant at the 5% level, 1% should be significant at the 1% level, 40% should be significant at the 40% level. If we plot $-\log(p)$ of the expected values under the uniform distribution against the observed values, the plot would be along the diagonal, although we hope a few are above the diagonal. We refer the reader to Figure S1 of Rice and colleagues[24] for a QQ plot for nicotine dependence where $\lambda = 1.02$. This paper considers many of the issues discussed above.

Manhattan Plot

A typical plot related to a GWAS analysis is the Manhattan Plot, where we hope it looks like the landscape of Manhattan with a few skyscrapers. For each SNP, we plot chromosomal location versus $-\log(p)$ for all tests, and values above 7.3 are genome-wide significant. This is a great aid to visualizing the results of a GWAS. Figure 1 of Rice and colleagues[24] shows a significant finding on chromosome 8.

Software

The issues described here may be carried out using the freely available computer program PLINK.[23] The cleaning of GWAS data may be performed, and filters set to form a subset of the data based on these filters. The logistic model may be applied, and results with various corrections applied. The file produced by PLINK may be imported into HAPLOVIEW and the Manhattan Plot produced. There are many options available, and the reader is encouraged to go through the tutorial available.

Discussion

Our aim was to give a non-technical introduction of human linkage and association analysis. Many aspects have not been covered. There is an extensive and elegant literature on the use of affected sibling pairs for linkage. This design has not been useful in psychiatric genetics due to the large number of genes responsible, so that the overall sharing among affected sib pairs is expected to deviate only slightly from the sharing of 50% under the null hypothesis, resulting in very low power.

We have not discussed family-based association analysis. The transmission disequilibrium test TDT uses an affected child and both parents where the alleles in the child are the "case" genotype, and the non-transmitted alleles in the parent are the "control" genotype. The test looks at parents heterozygous and the TDT amounts to testing for a fair coin in the off-diagonal elements of the 2 x 2 table of transmitted and non-transmitted alleles. This design is often seen in studies of childhood disorders such as autism and ADHD. It has the advantage of not being susceptible to population structure, and permits the examination of de novo mutation since the parents are also genotyped. Ironically, genotyping error can inflate the Type I error in the TDT. An error in the child will be detected, whereas an error in the parent may indicate transmission of the other allele. TDT designs tend to find a general overtransmission of the common allele. In a case-control study, the error would affect both groups equally, with a decrease in power, but not Type I error.

We did not cover the analysis of sequence data. The starting point in the analysis of Chip data is usually a binary PLINK file, which is of modest size, and the cleaning and analytical methods are described in this chapter. For sequence data, next generation sequencing (NGS) produces a set of short reads (perhaps 30 base pairs), and the sequence must be aligned to the human genome, with quality scores needed to represent calling and alignment certainty. The file for analysis is a VCF (Variant Call File) containing quality scores and depth of coverage in addition to genotypes.

In standard association analysis, many investigators drop SNPs with frequency under 5%, whereas the focus in sequencing is on rare variants. This often requires collapsing methods to combine rare variants in a genomic region. The power can be greatly decreased by neutral mutation, and the frequencies of variants needs to be considered. Current approaches include the use of SKAT-O[25] and several other tests, as implemented in EPACTS (http://genome.sph.umich.edu/wiki/EPACTS). There are efforts underway for large-scale sequencing of psychiatric phenotypes, and we will be able to assess the impact of rare variants.

The important message is that large samples are needed to find robust signals. The current PGC efforts aim to collect 100,000 cases for each of the major mental disorders. This will provide an important resource that can be applied to studies with smaller sample sizes to address phenotypic and genetic heterogeneity. A recent study[26] by scientists at the company 23andMe reported 15 genes genome-wide significant for major depression using over 75,000 cases. Accordingly, there are other very large samples that will contribute to our knowledge in addition to the PGC samples.

The challenge for the next decade will be to understand the biology of these GWAS hits. The ones identified to date tend not to be in coding regions. This is in keeping with the ENCODE[27] project, where promoters, enhancers, and insulators are catalogued. Understanding relevant pathways may help us understand what all these signals do. Most analyses so far analyze one SNP at a time, and a more comprehensive approach is needed. There are major resources now available that characterize gene expression in multiple tissues and provide another avenue for biological interpretation. Currently, the ExAC[28] database provides frequencies from over 60,000 genomes from exome sequencing, and provides an additional useful resource.

Overall, this is an exciting time to be a psychiatric geneticist.

References

1. Morton, N. E. (1955). Sequential tests for the detection of linkage. *American Journal of Human Genetics*, Sep; 7(3), 277–318.

2. Klein, R. J., Zeiss, C., Chew, E. Y., Tsai, J. Y., Sackler, R. S., Haynes, C., Henning, A. K., et al. (2005). Complement factor H polymorphism in age-related macular degeneration. *Science*, 308(5720), 385–389.

3. Welter, D., MacArthur, J., Morales, J., Burdett, T., Hall, P., Junkins, H., Klemm, A., et al. (2014). The NHGRI GWAS Catalog, a curated resource of SNP-trait associations. *Nucleic Acids Research*, Jan; 42(Database issue); D1001–D1006.

4. Wellcome Trust Case Control Consortium. (2007). Genome-wide association study of 14,000 cases of seven common diseases and 3,000 shared controls. *Nature*, Jun 7; 447(7145), 661–678.

5. Schizophrenia Working Group of the Psychiatric Genomics Consortium. (2014). Biological insights from 108 schizophrenia-associated genetic loci. *Nature*, Jul 24; 511(7510), 421–427.

6. Sekar, A., Bialas, A. R., de Rivera, H., Davis, A., Hammond, T. R., Kamitaki, N., Tooley, K., et al. (2016). Schizophrenia risk from complex variation of complement component 4. *Nature*, Feb 11; 530(7589), 177–183.

7. Ott, J. (1999). *Analysis of Human Genetic Linkage*, 3rd ed. Baltimore, MD: Johns Hopkins University Press.

8. Kong, A., Gudbjartsson, D. F., Sainz, J., Jonsdottir, G. M., Gudjonsson, S. A., Richardson, B., Siqurdardottir, S., et al. (2002). A high-resolution recombination map of the human genome. *Nature Genetics*, 31(3), 241–247.

9. Kruglyak, L., & Lander, E. S. (1995). Complete multipoint sib-pair analysis of qualitative and quantitative traits. *American Journal of Human Genetics*, Aug; 57(2), 439–454.

10. Elston, R. C., & Stewart, J. (1971). A general model for the genetic analysis of pedigree data. *Human Heredity*, 21(6), 523–542.

11. Lathrop, G. M., Lalouel, J. M., Julier, C., & Ott, J. (1984). Strategies for multilocus linkage analysis in humans. *Proceedings of the National Academy of Sciences USA*, Jun; 81(11), 3443–3446.

12. Cottingham, R. W. Jr, Idury, R. M., & Schäffer, A. A. (1993). Faster sequential genetic linkage computations. *American Journal of Human Genetics, 53*, 252–263.

13. Abecasis, G. R., Cherny, S. S., Cookson, W. O., & Cardon, L. R. (2002). Merlin-rapid analysis of dense genetic maps using sparse gene flow trees. *Nature Genetics, 30*(1), 97–101.

14. Sham, P. (1998). *Statistics in Human Genetics*, 1st ed. New York: John Wiley & Sons.

15. Neale, B. M., Ferreira, M. A. R., Medland, S. E., & Posthuma, D. (2008). *Statistical Genetics: Gene Mapping Through Linkage and Association*, 1st ed. New York: Taylor & Francis Group.

16. Barrett, J. C., Fry, B., Maller, J., & Daly, M. J. (2005). Haploview: Analysis and visualization of LD and haplotype maps. *Bioinformatics*, Jan 15; *21*(2), 263–265.

17. International HapMap Consortium. (2005). A haplomap type of the human genome. *Nature, 437*(7063), 1299–1320.

18. 1000 Genomes Project Consortium, Auton, A., Brooks, L. D., Durbin, R. M., Garrison, E. P., Kang, H. M., Korbel, J. O., et al. (2015). A global reference for human genetic variation. *Nature*, Oct 1; *526*(7571), 68–74.

19. Hinds, D. A., Stuve, L. L., Nilsen, G. B., Halperin, E., Eskin, E., Ballinger, D. G., Frazer, K. A., et al. (2005). Whole-genome patterns of common DNA variation in three human populations. *Science*, Feb 18; *307*(5712), 1072–1079.

20. Price, A. L., Patterson, N. J., Plenge, R. M., Weinblatt, M. E., Shadick, N. A., & Reich, D. (2006). Principal components analysis corrects for stratification in genome-wide association studies. *Nature Genetics, 38*(8), 904–909.

21. Howie, B., Marchini, J., & Stephens, M. (2011). Genotype imputation with thousands of genomes. *G3: Genes, Genomes, Genetics (Bethesda)*, Nov; *1*(6), 457–470.

22. McCarthy, S., Das, S., Kretzschmar, W., Delaneau, O., Wood, A. R., Teumer, A., Kang, H. M., et al. (2016). A reference panel of 64,976 haplotypes for genotype imputation. *Nature Genetics, 48*(10), 1279–1283.

23. Purcell, S., Neale, B., Todd-Brown, K., Thomas, L., Ferreira, M. A., Bender, D., Maller, J., et al. (2007). PLINK: A toolset for whole-genome association and population-based linkage analysis. *American Journal of Human Genetics*, Sep; *81*(3), 559–575.

24. Rice, J. P., Hartz, S. M., Agrawal, A., Almasy, L., Bennett, S., Brelau, N., Bucholz, K. K., et al. (2012). CHRNB3 is more strongly associated with Fagerström Test for Cigarette Dependence-based nicotine dependence than cigarettes per day: Phenotype definition changes genome-wide association studies results. *Addiction, 107*(11), 2019–2028.

25. Lee, S., Wu, M. C., & Lin, X. (2012). Optimal tests for rare variant effects in sequencing association studies. *Biostatistics*, Sep; *13*(4), 762–775.

26. Hyde, C. L., Nagle, M. W., Tian, C., Chen, X., Paciga, S. A., Wendland, J. R., Tung, J. Y., et al. (2016). Identification of 15 genetic loci associated with risk of major depression in individuals of European descent. *Nature Genetics, 48*(9), 1031–1036.

27. Kellis, M., Wold, B., Snyder, M. P., Bernstein, B. E., Kundaje, A., Marinov, G. K., Ward, L. D., et al. (2014). Defining functional DNA elements in the human genome. *Proceedings of the National Academy of Sciences USA*, Apr 29; *111*(17), 6131–6138.

28. Lek, M., Karczewski, K. J., Minikel, E. V., Samocha, K. E., Banks, E., Fennell, T., O'Donnell-Luria, A. H., et al. (2016). Analysis of protein-coding genetic variation in 60,706 humans. *Nature*, Aug 17; *536*(7616), 285–291.

Chapter 6

The Role of Copy Number Variation in Psychiatric Disorders

Elliott Rees and George Kirov

Take-Home Points

1. Rare pathogenic CNVs increase risk for schizophrenia, autism, and developmental delay.
2. They are under strong selection pressure but are replaced by new mutations.
3. Their penetrance is high, and psychiatrists should consider how to discuss them with carriers and their families.

Introduction

Copy number variations (CNVs) are structural alterations to chromosomes that constitute a highly prevalent and diverse form of genetic variation.[1] CNVs range in length from ~1,000 bases to several mega-bases, are widely distributed across the genome, and occur across the full frequency spectrum.[2] The most extensively studied class of CNV in psychiatric disorders are large deletions and duplications (Figure 6.1). Given this variability, and the fact that CNVs are abundant among the genomes of healthy individuals,[3] it can be challenging to distinguish between benign and pathogenic CNVs.

Several mechanisms exist for the formation of CNVs. Most CNVs known to cause psychiatric disorders are formed through non-allelic homologous recombination (NAHR).[4] Here, repetitive DNA elements, such as segmental duplications or low copy repeats (LCRs), cause chromosomes to misalign during recombination, leading to unequal chromosomal crossover.[5] This results in recombinant chromosomes containing either a deleted or a duplicated DNA segment (Figure 6.2). Since repetitive DNA elements predispose certain genomic regions to NAHR, CNVs created via this mechanism have relatively high mutation rates and non-random genomic locations.[6] Therefore, CNVs formed through NAHR are termed *recurrent*, as the same (or highly similar)

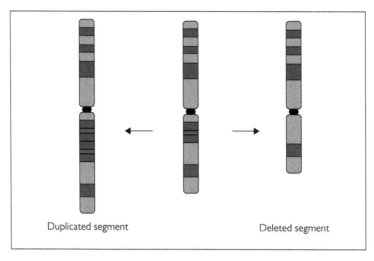

Figure 6.1 Representation of a duplicated and deleted chromosomal segment.

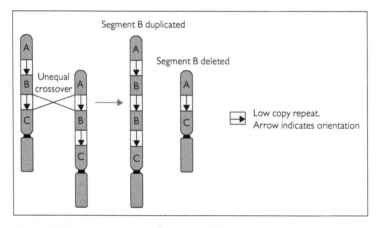

Figure 6.2 Schematic of inter-chromosomal non-allelic homologous recombination.

CNVs among different individuals have arisen by independent mutations. Additional mutational mechanisms leading to CNVs include non-homologous end joining and fork stalling and template switching, which can result from errors in DNA break repair and DNA replication, respectively.[4] CNVs formed through these mechanisms are more likely to be unique in genomic location, and are termed *non-recurrent*.[7]

CNVs in Psychiatric Disorders

In 2008, several large studies reported increased rates of CNVs in SZ, both genome-wide and at specific loci.[8–10] It soon became clear that very large samples of cases and controls were required to identify such associations, due to the rarity of these CNVs. The availability of high-throughput genotyping enabled fast accumulation of data and, as of 2017, according to large-scale analyses involving tens of thousands of patients and controls,[4,11,12,13] there are at least 13 CNVs that are robustly associated with SZ, as they have received sufficient statistical support and replication (Table 6.1).

Several lines of evidence suggest that additional SZ CNVs exist, but their frequencies and/or risk for schizophrenia are too low to allow them to be identified with currently available samples. For example, an excess genome-wide burden of CNVs in SZ is observed after CNVs at known risk loci are removed.[14,13] Additionally, a set of 51 CNVs implicated in intellectual deficit (ID) are found at significantly higher rates in SZ patients than in controls.[12] In fact, all SZ CNVs in Table 6.1 are also risk factors for ID.[15,16]

Given the overlap of risk CNVs between SZ and ID, the question arises as to whether these CNVs are also risk factors for other psychiatric disorders. Due to the requirement of very large sample sizes, this question has been adequately addressed so far only for bipolar affective disorder (BAD) and autism spectrum disorders (ASD). The findings in BAD are based on smaller studies, but they provide a clear conclusion: neurodevelopmental CNVs play a smaller role in BAD.[17] In fact, the rates among BAD patients of some of the CNVs listed in Table 6.1 are closer to those found in controls, and only the 16p11.2 duplication, 1q21.1 duplication, and 3q29 deletions are nominally significantly associated with BAD (Figure 6.3). The possible connection/implication in terms of cognitive impairment will be discussed later.

The frequencies of these CNVs in ID have been provided by studies on tens of thousands of subjects referred to genetics clinics, mostly for developmental delay.[18,15,16] The strongest evidence on the role of CNVs in ASD is summarized by Sanders et al.,[19] based on the rate of de novo occurring CNVs in several thousand ASD subjects whose parents were also available for testing. All significant CNVs in ASD (Table 6.2) are also ID loci, and remarkably, all but three of these are also confirmed SZ susceptibility loci (Table 6.1). The exceptions are *SHANK3* deletions, 16p11.2 deletions, and 22q11.2 duplications. The discrepancy in 22q11.2 duplication is intriguing, as this CNV has been shown to be significantly *depleted* in SZ compared with controls,[20,13] suggesting a potential *protective* association for SZ. The implications of this observation merit further exploration, as it represents the most striking genetic difference between ASD and SZ.

The differences (and similarities) in CNV frequency between the main neurodevelopmental and psychiatric disorders are best visualized when presented together (Figure 6.3). The overall impression is one of a gradient of their

Table 6.1 Rates of the most significant CNVs in SZ patients and controls. The data are according to Rees, Walters, et al. (2014b), except for 16p11.2 distal deletion, reported in the PGC CNV analysis (CNV and Schizophrenia Working Groups of the Psychiatric Genomics, 2017), and 16p12.1 deletion reported in Rees, Kendall, et al. (2016). CNV Coordinates are according to hg19

Locus	Position	Cases	Controls	OR (95% CI)	p-value
1q21.1 del	chr1:146,57-147,39	0.17% (33/19,056)	0.021% (17/81,821)	8.35 (4.65–14.99)	4.1×10^{-13}
1q21.1 dup	chr1:146,57-147,39	0.13% (21/16,247)	0.037% (24/64,046)	3.45 (1.92–6.20)	9.9×10^{-5}
NRXN1 del	chr2:50,15-51,26	0.18% (33/18,762)	0.020% (10/51,161)	9.01 (4.44–18.29)	1.3×10^{-11}
3q29 del	chr3:195,73-197,34	0.082% (14/17,005)	0.0014% (1/69,965)	57.65 (7.58–438.44)	1.5×10^{-9}
WBS dup	chr7:72,74-74,14	0.066% (14/ 21,269)	0.0058% (2/34,455)	11.35 (2.58–49.93)	6.9×10^{-5}
15q11.2 del	chr15:22,80-23,09	0.59% (116/19,547)	0.28% (227/81,802)	2.15 (1.71–2.68)	2.5×10^{-10}
Angelman / Prader-Willi dup	chr15:24,82-28,43	0.083% (12/14,464)	0.0063% (3/47,686)	13.20 (3.72–46.77)	5.6×10^{-6}
15q13.3 del	chr15:31,13-32,48	0.14% (26/18,571)	0.019% (15/80,422)	7.52 (3.98–14.19)	4.0×10^{-10}
16p13.11 dup	chr16:15,51-16,30	0.31% (37/12,029)	0.13% (93/69,289)	2.30 (1.57–3.36)	5.7×10^{-5}
16p11.2 distal del	chr16:28,82-29,05	0.052% (11/21,094)	0.005% (1/20,227)	20.6 (2.6–162.2)	5.5×10^{-5}
16p11.2 dup	chr16:29,64-30,20	0.35% (58/16,772)	0.030% (19/63,068)	11.52 (6.86–19.34)	2.9×10^{-24}
16p12.1 del	chr16:21,95-22,43	0.162% (33/20,403)	0.045% (12/26,628)	3.3 (1.61–7.05)	3.4×10^{-4}
22q11.2 del	chr22:19,02-20,26	0.29% (56/19,084)	0.00% (0/77,055)	NA (28.27–∞)	4.4×10^{-40}

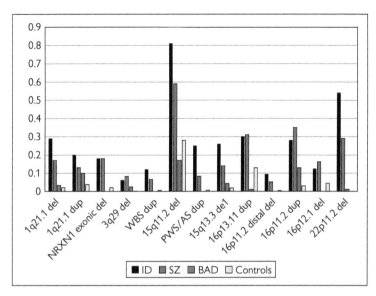

Figure 6.3 Frequencies of SZ-implicated CNVs in ID, SZ, BAD, and controls. Data on BAD are from Green et al. 2016, data on ID are from Dittwald et al., 2013, and Coe et al., 2014, as summarized in Rees, Kendall, et al., 2016.

Table 6.2 Loci identified from studies on de novo occurring CNVs in ASD probands from two collections comprising several thousand families: the Simon Simplex Collection and the Autism Genome Project. The table is adapted from Sanders et al., 2015		
Band	**De novo CNVs (del/dup)**	**q Value (FDR)**
1q21.1 (dup)	(1/8)	2×10^{-9}
2p16.3 *NRXN1* (del)	(7/1)	4×10^{-8}
3q29 (del)	(4/0)	0.02
7q11.23 WBS (dup)	(1/4)	0.0008
15q11.2-13.1 PWS/AS (dup)	(0/10)	$<1 \times 10^{-10}$
16p11.2 (del + dup)	(12/7)	$<1 \times 10^{-10}$
22q11.21 (del + dup)	(4/4)	4×10^{-8}
22q13.33 *SHANK3* (del)	(4/0)	0.02

role, with the highest frequencies reported in ID, followed by SZ, BAD, and controls.

There is evidence that these CNVs also increase susceptibility for additional neuro-psychiatric disorders. For example, an increased genome-wide rate of CNVs, and specifically, 16p13.11 duplications, has been reported in individuals diagnosed with attention-deficit hyperactivity-disorder (ADHD).[21] Several neurodevelopmental CNVs, such as 16p13.11 deletions, 1q21.1 duplications, and Prader-Willi/Angelman syndrome duplications, have also been suggested to increase risk of obsessive-compulsive disorder and Tourette syndrome.[22,23] However, CNV studies of ADHD, obsessive-compulsive disorder, and Tourette syndrome are much smaller than those published for SZ, ASD, and ID. Therefore, larger samples are required to determine the full extent to which CNVs increase risk for these disorders.

Penetrance and Selection Against CNVs

An important question for families and health professionals is what is the penetrance of these CNVs. *Penetrance* is the risk that carriers (for example, children or other relatives of CNV carriers) will develop a disorder, if they have inherited the same CNV. Nearly all CNVs from the list in Table 6.1 have incomplete penetrance (they have been observed in healthy controls). Exact estimates for penetrance are difficult to obtain, as this would involve following up, from birth, large numbers of CNV carriers. We have shown that, with a lot of approximation, one can calculate penetrance figures for these CNVs, using well-established CNV frequencies among disease groups and healthy controls, and using approximate rates of these disease groups in the general population of 1% for SZ and 4% for ID.[24] Table 6.3 shows the estimated penetrance for SZ, for ID, and for the combined SZ/ID penetrance, using data and methods presented in Kirov et al.[24] Although these estimates require many approximations, even large errors in the assumptions lead to only modest changes in the overall conclusions. For example, if we use lower population rates of 0.5% for SZ and 2% for ID, we would only reduce the penetrance estimates by up to half, which are still quite substantial effects.

The penetrance estimates in Table 6.3 suggest that many carriers of these pathogenic CNVs (apart from DiGeorge/Velo-Cardio-Facial Syndrome [VCFS] deletions) should be healthy. However, what is not known is whether these "healthy" persons, who can appear among healthy controls for genetic studies, are completely free of symptoms or disabilities. This is probably not true. Stefansson et al.[25] showed that 144 carriers of 11 pathogenic CNVs, who had no recorded diagnosis of psychiatric or neurodevelopmental disorder, had significant cognitive deficits. Similar results were obtained in the U.K. Biobank,[26] where most carriers of such CNVs (over 1000 of them) had no such diagnoses and probably considered themselves healthy. They also had marginally lower school grades and attained occupations that required less training and academic skills. These differences were subtle, and in fact, just over 30.9% of carriers of neurodevelopmental CNVs held managerial or

Table 6.3 Penetrance and selection coefficients for SZ-associated CNVs. Adapted and updated from Kirov et al. (2014); Rees et al. (2011), and Isles et al. (2016) for maternal duplications at the PWS/AS locus on 15q11-q13. To simplify the presentation, we do not present 95% CI, which are very large in each case

Locus	Selection Coefficient (s)	Penetrance (%)		
		SZ	ID	Total
1q21.1 del	0.24	5.2	35	40
1q21.1 dup	0.19	2.9	18	21
NRXN1 del	0.29	6.4	26	32
3q29 del	0.79	18	53	71
WBS dup	0.59	6.0	44	50
15q11.2 del	0.08	2.0	11	13
PWS/AS maternal dup	0.55	12.3	50	62
15q13.3 del	0.28	4.7	35	40
16p13.11 dup	0.1	2.2	8.4	11
16p12.1 del	0.1	3.4	11	14
16p11.2 distal del	0.29	2.6	23	26
16p11.2 dup	0.27	8.0	26	34
DiGeorge/VCFS del	0.8	12	88	100

professional occupations and about 25% had been at college or university.[26] Clearly, being a carrier of one of these CNVs is compatible with full participation in every aspect of life.

Selection Against CNVs

Table 6.3 also presents the selection pressure that operates against each of these CNVs (expressed as selection coefficients, s). This can be estimated on the basis of the reported rates of de novo occurring CNVs as a proportion of all CNVs observed in the population.[27] This will be made clearer with an example: Let us assume that at a particular locus, all CNVs in the population are found to be de novo occurring mutations. It follows that no carriers of this CNV have transmitted it to any offspring; in other words, the selection pressure against carriers of this CNV should be 100%, or s = 1. Similarly, if 50% of them are transmitted, it follows that half of them get filtered out by selection, and s = 0.5. The selection coefficients for SZ-associated CNVs has been estimated using data from many studies on different disorders that reported the inheritance status of CNVs.[24] The selection pressures against these CNVs are very strong from an evolutionary perspective, and these CNVs would

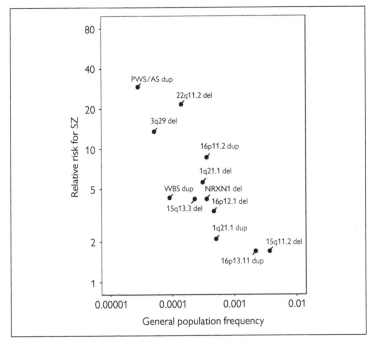

Figure 6.4 Frequencies and relative risks of SZ associated CNVs. CNV frequencies and relative risks for SZ were taken from Rees, Kendall, et al., 2016.

be eliminated from the population within a few generations if they were not replenished by new mutations.

As expected from genetic factors with such high ORs and penetrance for SZ and ID, the CNVs discussed here are very rare in the population (Figure 6.4). This is in contrast with the common SNPs identified in GWAS studies, which have very modest ORs.[28] Figure 6.4 shows the almost perfect relationship between the frequency of CNVs listed in Table 6.1 and their relative risk for SZ. It is very likely that many more genetic factors increase risk for SZ, but they are rare and/or of low ORs, so they cannot be identified with the available sample sizes.

Pathway Analyses

Despite numerous CNVs being identified as risk factors for neuropsychiatric disorders, inferring disease biology from these associations is often difficult, as they often overlap multiple genes. In addition to single CNV locus tests, a widely adopted analytical approach is to test sets of genes for CNV enrichment. These sets of genes are usually grouped by common biological functions or expression profiles, which allow physiological inferences to be made from significant associations. CNVs in patients diagnosed with SZ have been shown to be enriched for genes encoding members of the post-synaptic density protein complex. This association, first discovered through studies of de novo CNVs, is largely driven by genes belonging to N-methyl-D-aspartate receptor (NMDAR) and neuronal activity-regulated cytoskeleton-associated protein (ARC) complexes.[29] Independent support for the involvement of these post-synaptic gene-sets has come from case-control CNV studies[30,31,13] as well as exome sequencing studies of rare and de novo indel and point mutations.[32,33] These findings suggest that disruption of glutamatergic signaling is involved in SZ pathogenesis. Additional gene-sets associated with SZ CNVs include targets of the fragile X mental retardation protein (FMRP),[30,13] genes involved in neuronal calcium channel signaling,[30] and components of $GABA_a$ receptor complexes.[31] Moreover, associations with behavioral and neurodevelopmental gene-sets indicate that larger CNV analyses will implicate further biological systems in SZ pathophysiology.[31,13] There is also evidence that CNVs disrupting genes unrelated to brain function do not contribute to SZ risk.[31]

Conclusion

The last 10 years have witnessed the identification of a number of CNVs as strong risk factors for SZ and other neuro-psychiatric disorders. It now appears that the same genetic factors can lead to different disorders, while many carriers appear asymptomatic. SZ patients carrying known risk CNVs also have an excess of common risk alleles,[34] suggesting that a combination of common and rare risk factors influences disease risk. It is likely that larger studies will uncover additional neuropsychiatric risk CNVs, and the Psychaitric Genetics Consortium (PGC) CNV group is currently working on analyses of disorders that have been less well studied compared with SZ, such as BAD, ADHD, and post-traumatic stress disorder.[35] The contribution from smaller and complex structural variations, best discovered through whole-genome sequencing, to neuropsychiatric risk remains largely unexplored. As more samples are sequenced, future studies could reveal these mutations to be additional neuropsychiatric risk factors.

References

1. Lee, C., & Scherera, S. W. (2010). The clinical context of copy number variation in the human genome. *Expert Reviews in Molecular Medicine, 12*, e8. doi:10.1017/S1462399410001390

2. Iafrate, A. J., Feuk, L., Rivera, M. N., Listewnik, M. L., Donahoe, P. K., Qi, Y., . . . Lee, C. (2004). Detection of large-scale variation in the human genome. *Nature Genetics, 36*(9), 949–951.

3. Sebat, J., Lakshmi, B., Troge, J., Alexander, J., Young, J., Lundin, P., . . . Wigler, M. (2004). Large-scale copy number polymorphism in the human genome. *Science*, *305*(5683), 525–528.

4. Malhotra, D., & Sebat, J. (2012). CNVs: Harbingers of a rare variant revolution in psychiatric genetics. *Cell*, *148*(6), 1223–1241.

5. Lupski, J. R. (1998). Genomic disorders: structural features of the genome can lead to DNA rearrangements and human disease traits. *Trends in Genetics*, *14*(10), 417–422.

6. Lupski, J. R. (2007). Genomic rearrangements and sporadic disease. *Nature Genetics*, *14*, S43–S47.

7. Gu, W., Zhang, F., & Lupski, J. R. (2008). Mechanisms for human genomic rearrangements. *PathoGenetics 1*(4). doi:10.1186/1755-8417-1181-1184.

8. Walsh, T., McClellan, J. M., McCarthy, S. E., Addington, A. M., Pierce, S. B., Cooper, G. M., . . . Sebat, J. (2008). Rare structural variants disrupt multiple genes in neurodevelopmental pathways in schizophrenia. *Science*, *320*(5875), 539–543.

9. International Schizophrenia Consortium (ISC). (2008). Rare chromosomal deletions and duplications increase risk of schizophrenia. *Nature*, *455*(7210), 237–241.

10. Stefansson, H., Rujescu, D., Cichon, S., Pietilainen, O. P. H., Ingason, A., Steinberg, S., . . . Stefansson, K. (2008). Large recurrent microdeletions associated with schizophrenia. *Nature*, *455*(7210), 232–236.

11. Rees, E., Walters, J. T. R., Chambert, K. D., Isles, A. R., Chambert, K. D., C. O'Dushlaine, . . . Kirov, G. (2014a). CNV analysis in a large schizophrenia sample implicates deletions at 16p12.1 and *SLC1A1* and duplications at 1p36.33 and *CGNL1*. *Human Molecular Genetics*, *23*(6), 1669–1676.

12. Rees, E., Kendall, K., Pardiñas, A. F., Legge, S. E., Pocklington, A., Escott-Price, V., . . . Kirov, G. (2016). Analysis of intellectual disability copy number variants for association with schizophrenia. *JAMA Psychiatry*, *73*(9), 963–969.

13. CNV and Schizophrenia Working Groups of the Psychiatric Genomics, C. (2017). Contribution of copy number variants to schizophrenia from a genome-wide study of 41,321 subjects. *Nature Genetics*, *49*(1), 27–35.

14. Rees, E., Walters, J. T. R., Georgieva, L., Isles, A. R., Chambert, K. D., Richards, A. L., . . . Kirov, G. (2014b). Analysis of copy number variations at 15 schizophreniaassociated loci. *British Journal of Psychiatry*, *204*(2), 108–114.

15. Dittwald, P., Gambin, T., Szafranski, P., Li, J., Amato, S., Divon, M. Y., . . . Schaaf, C. P. (2013). NAHR-mediated copy-number variants in a clinical population: Mechanistic insights into both genomic disorders and Mendelizing traits. *Genome Research*, *23*(9), 1395–1409.

16. Coe, B. P., Witherspoon, K., Rosenfeld, J. A., van Bon, B. W. M., Vulto-van Silfhout, A. T., Bosco, P., . . . Eichler, E. E. (2014). Refining analyses of copy number variation identifies specific genes associated with developmental delay. *Nature Genetics*, *46*(10), 1063–1071.

17. Green, E. K., Rees, E., Walters, J. T. R., Smith, K. G., Forty, L., Grozeva, D., Moran, J. L., . . . Kirov, G. (2016). Copy number variation in bipolar disorder. *Molecular Psychiatry*, *21*(1), 89–93.

18. Girirajan, S., Rosenfeld, J. A., Coe, B. P., Parikh, S., Friedman, N., Goldstein, A., . . . Eichler, E. E. (2012). Phenotypic heterogeneity of genomic disorders and rare copy-number variants. *New England Journal of Medicine*, *367*(14), 1321–1331.

19. Sanders, S. J., He, X., Willsey, A. J., Ercan-Sencicek, A. G., Samocha, K. E., Cicek, A. E., . . . State, M. W. (2015). Insights into autism spectrum disorder genomic architecture and biology from 71 risk loci. *Neuron*, *87*(6), 1215–1233.

20. Rees, E., Kirov, G., Sanders, A., Walters, J. T. R., Chambert, K. D., Shi, J., . . . Owen, M. J. (2014). Evidence that duplications of 22q11.2 protect against schizophrenia. *Molecular Psychiatry*, *19*(1), 37–40.

21. Williams, N. M., Zaharieva, I., Martin, A., Langley, K., Mantripragada, K., Fossdal, R., . . . Thapar, A. (2010). Rare chromosomal deletions and duplications in attention-deficit hyperactivity disorder: A genome-wide analysis. *Lancet*, *376*(9750), 1401–1408.

22. McGrath, L. M., Yu, D., Marshall, C., Davis, L. K., Thiruvahindrapuram, B., Li, B., . . . Scharf, J. M. (2014). Copy number variation in obsessive-compulsive disorder and Tourette syndrome: A cross-disorder study. *Journal of the American Academy of Child & Adolescent Psychiatry*, *53*(8), 910–919.

23. Gazzellone, M. J., Zarrei, M., Burton, C. L., Walker, S., Uddin, M., Shaheen, S. M., . . . Scherer, S. W. (2016). Uncovering obsessive-compulsive disorder risk genes in a pediatric cohort by high-resolution analysis of copy number variation. *Journal of Neurodevelopmental Disorders*, *8*(1), 36.

24. Kirov, G., Rees, E., Walters, T. J., Escott-Price, V., Georgieva, L., Richards, A. L., . . . Owen, M. J. (2014). The penetrance of copy number variations for schizophrenia and developmental delay. *Biological Psychiatry*, *75*(5), 378–385.

25. Stefansson, H., Meyer-Lindenberg, A., Steinberg, S., Magnusdottir, B., Morgen, K., Arnarsdottir, S., . . . Doyle, O. M. (2014). CNVs conferring risk of autism or schizophrenia affect cognition in controls. *Nature*, *505*(7483), 361–366.

26. Kendall, K. M., Rees, E., Escott-Price, V., Einon, M., Thomas, R., Hewitt, J., . . . Kirov, G. (2017). Cognitive Performance Among Carriers of Pathogenic Copy Number Variants: Analysis of 152,000 UK Biobank Subjects. *Biological Psychiatry*, *82*(2), 103–110.

27. Rees, E., Moskvina, V., Owen, M. J., O'Donovan, M. C., & Kirov, G. (2011). De novo rates and selection of schizophrenia-associated copy number variants. *Biological Psychiatry*, *70*(12), 1109–1114.

28. Schizophrenia Working Group of the Psychiatric Genomics Consortium. (2014). Biological insights from 108 schizophrenia-associated genetic loci. *Nature*, *511*(7510), 421–427.

29. Kirov, G., Pocklington, A. J., Holmans, P., Ivanov, D., Ikeda, M., Ruderfer, D., . . . Owen, M. J. (2012). De novo CNV analysis implicates specific abnormalities of postsynaptic signalling complexes in the pathogenesis of schizophrenia. *Molecular Psychiatry*, *17*(2), 142–153.

30. Szatkiewicz, J. P., O'Dushlaine, C., Chen, G., Chambert, K., Moran, J. L., Neale, B. M., . . . Sullivan, P. F. (2014). Copy number variation in schizophrenia in Sweden. *Molecular Psychiatry*, *19*(7), 762–773.

31. Pocklington, A. J., Rees, E., Walters, J. T. R., Han, J., Kavanagh, D. H., Chambert, K. D., . . . Owen, M. J. (2015). Novel findings from CNVs implicate inhibitory and excitatory signaling complexes in schizophrenia. *Neuron*, *86*(5), 1203–1214.

32. Fromer, M., Pocklington, A. J., Kavanagh, D. H., Williams, H. J., Dwyer, S., Gormley, P., . . . O'Donovan, M. C. (2014). De novo mutations in schizophrenia implicate synaptic networks. *Nature*, *506*, 179–184.

33. Purcell, S. M., Moran, J. L., Fromer, M., Ruderfer, D., Solovieff, N., Roussos, P., . . . Sklar, P. (2014). A polygenic burden of rare disruptive mutations in schizophrenia. *Nature, 506*, 185–190.

34. Tansey, K. E., Rees, E., Linden, D. E., Ripke, S., Chambert, K. D., Moran, J. L., . . . O'Donovan, M. C. (2016). Common alleles contribute to schizophrenia in CNV carriers. *Molecular Psychiatry, 21*(8), 1085–1089.

35. Sullivan, P. F., Agrawal, A., Bulik, C., Andreassen, O. A., Borglum, A., Breen, G., . . . O'Donovan, M. (2017). Psychiatric genomics: An update and an agenda. *Am J Psychiatry*, appiajp201717030283. doi: 10.1176/appi.ajp.2017.17030283. [Epub ahead of print].

Table Reference

Isles, A. R., Ingason, A., Lowther, C., Walters, J., Gawlick, M., Stöber, G., . . . Kirov, G. (2016). Parental origin of interstitial duplications at 15q11.2-q13.3 in schizophrenia and neurodevelopmental disorders. *PLoS Genetics, 12*(5), e1005993.

Chapter 7

Pharmacogenomics and Precision Psychiatry

Julia C. Stingl and Gonzalo Laje

Take-Home Points

1. Pharmacogenomic tests in psychiatry are today of limited use.
2. Phenotype definition and limited understanding of pathophysiology constrain progress in personalized medicine in psychiatry.
3. Genetic variation in pharmacodynamic pathways so far has not been helpful at predicting outcomes.
4. Limited evidence-based dosing guidelines are available for actionable gene–drug pairs.

Introduction

Drug effects differ between individuals. Molecular medicine has opened a comprehensive understanding of molecular drug effects, and a developing shift is occurring in drug development towards drugs targeted to the molecular structure of the disease. However, variability between patients, including at the molecular level, may lead to variability in efficacy and safety of drug therapies.[1] Thus, pharmacogenetic diagnostics seeks to characterize patients' molecular profiles in order to better predict the individual benefit-to-risk ratio. Modern molecular technologies such as genomics, epigenomics, transcriptomics, or metabolomics have opened new possibilities of precision medicine approaches in drug therapy. A patient's individual molecular make-up can serve to explore the variability in benefit and/or risk in different vulnerable patient groups during a drug's life cycle.[2] Unpredicted variability in drug efficacy and tolerability causes enormous problems and costs, with 7–10% of hospital emergency admissions being due to severe side effects of drug therapy, and deaths from adverse drug reactions being among the most frequent causes of deaths according to the U.S. Vital Statistics report.[3] Especially in the field of psychiatric drug therapy, a huge burden of disease is caused by high rates of drug failure and inefficiency.[4] Hence, the prospect of individualized approaches aimed at tailoring the choice of the drug and/or dosage to the individual needs of the patient is of major clinical appeal. This appeal has propelled the use of pharmacogenomic diagnostics and the application of evidence-based pharmacogenetic guidelines to guide therapy.[5]

Slow Progress in Psychiatry

Despite great progress in GWAS analyses, progress in psychiatric pharmaco-genetics has been slow. There are numerous possible reasons behind the slow progression of findings, but two of the most salient are phenotype definition and limited understanding of mental illness's pathophysiology. The definition of a phenotype is basically how a "case" is characterized; genetic studies are very dependent on phenotype precision. Current psychiatric nosology has created definitions of illness that cluster symptoms where the presence of a certain number of these symptoms amounts to a diagnosis. These defini-tions are clearly outlined in the American Psychiatric Association's *Diagnostic and Statistical Manual of Mental Disorders, 5th Ed.* (DSM-5)[6] as well as in the *International Classification of Diseases, 10th Ed.* (ICD-10).[7] The definitions are designed to be reliable and relatively broad, consistent with the needs of clinicians.

However, genetic studies work best with phenotypes that are not just clini-cally reliable, but biologically based. The field of psychiatry has struggled with the biological characterization of its syndromes, despite significant progress in neuroscience research. Different symptoms, such as initial insomnia or psy-chomotor agitation, may be associated with different genes. Based on our cur-rent definition of depression, a patient may experience insomnia or agitation or both; thus, any signal in an association study using a depression phenotype may be influenced by the relative symptom frequency in the sample under study. The use of more stringent criteria to define phenotypes is likely to result in smaller samples that may be harder to collect, but they may improve power to detect genetic associations.

Pharmacogenetic studies face another layer of complexity: drug exposure. Hence, in pharmacogenetic studies, treatment outcome phenotypes should also include elements that are unique to the drug/s used such as pharmacoki-netics (what the body does to the drug), pharmacodynamics (what the drug does to the body), response, time to effect, tolerability, and drug adherence.[8]

Pharmacokinetic Tests

Pharmacokinetics comprise the absorption, distribution, metabolism, and elimination of a drug, each of which can often be quite well quantified in humans. Pharmacokinetics are important, since drugs have little chance at effi-cacy if their bioavailability is lower than needed or significantly higher than needed, where adverse effects may rapidly ensue. The pharmacogenetics of drug metabolism is known to affect many drugs commonly used in the treatment of depression and psychosis.[9] While the drugs most affected by polymorphic metabolizing enzymes tend to be old drugs that have been used for over 50 years, these drugs are still in common use in clinical practice, and dose tailoring can easily be done in these therapies because the dose range is broad, and the drug is often titrated to individual needs.

As an example, most antidepressant and antipsychotic drugs are metabolized by the polymorphic enzyme cytochrome P450 2D6 (CYP2D6). For this enzyme, enormous variability in enzyme activity exists that can be phenotyped in four groups of metabolizers: the ultrarapid (UM), rapid (EM), intermediate (IM), and poor metabolizer (PM) groups.[10] What group a patient belongs to can be determined by genotyping, where the bi-allelic genotype defines the activity score or phenotype group.[11] Genotyping or determination of the metabolizer group can be done with several validated methods. Non-genetic methods are also available. These methods directly determine metabolism of a probe drug that is a substrate for CYP2D6.[12] However, phenotyping demands the administration of a probe drug that is by itself a drug, and also may cause side effects; therefore, it is not commonly used in clinical practice, whereas genetic testing is easily applicable and getting less expensive.

Dose recommendations can be derived from the pharmacokinetic data on differences in drug clearance for these distinct metabolizer phenotypes.[13] As such, CYP2D6 dose adjustments have been developed with the aim to obtain similar drug exposure and bioequivalent plasma concentration time curves in patients with different genotype groups. These differences in oral clearance have been systematically analyzed and depicted as overview for the psychiatric drugs.[9]

Pharmacodynamic Testing

Markers associated with the pharmacodynamic aspect of a drug have been more elusive, as the exact mechanism of action of most psychiatric drugs is poorly understood. However, all this research on genetic variability of psychiatric drug targets, such as the serotonin transporter polymorphism as a target of antidepressants, has not resulted in any valid pharmacogenetics test that is available today on markers at the site of drug action, thus, at the present time, the value of a pharmacogenetics test that includes variation in pharmacodynamic genes is extremely limited. In current drug labels, psychiatric drugs include pharmacogenetics information on drug metabolism and safety (https://www.pharmgkb.org/view/drug-labels.do).

Clinical Guidelines and Recommendations

In clinical practice, stratified therapy approaches are in use that implement pharmacogenetic diagnostics, together with therapeutic drug monitoring as

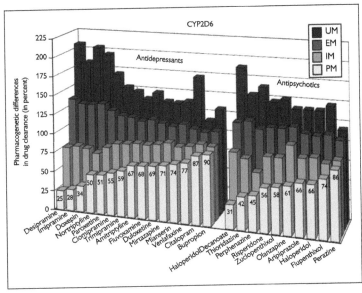

Figure 7.1 Dose adjustments according to the CYP2D6 phenotypes. Dose adjustments were based on differences in pharmacokinetic parameters (oral clearance, area under the concentration time curve, and concentration at steady state) observed between the phenotype groups. Stingl et al., *Molecular Psychiatry*, 2013; 18, 273–287.

therapy surveillance instrument or alone, but so far, there is little consensus as to when and if pharmacogenetic tests should be used in psychiatry.

Evidence-based dosing guidelines are available for actionable gene–drug pairs as issued by the Clinical Pharmacogenetics Implementation Consortium (CPIC) for tricyclic antidepressants and SSRIs for example.[14–16] In these guidelines, it is less the question who will be tested or at which opportunity, but rather, what happens if a patient with a known genotype or phenotype is asking for treatment adjustment or dose adjustment. Similar to these guidelines, the drug labels also contain mostly information on the risk for a patient with a distinctive genotype, and not information on the method that should be used or on the availability of genetic testing. On the website of PharmGKB, an overview on pharmacogenetics information in drug labels is provided and regularly updated (https://www.pharmgkb.org/view/drug-labels.do). And the type of information that is given is also characterized in different categories such as "mandatory" if testing is obligatory to determine the indication for a given drug, or "actionable" if the information has implications for drug therapy, such as, for example, for dose stratification. For psychiatric drugs, pharmacogenetic information in drug labels is either informative or actionable.

As can be seen, the listings of the various agencies differ in the number of drugs for which pharmacogenetic information is given. The U.S. Food and Drug Administration (FDA) was the first medical agency that developed a plan for providing pharmacogenetic information in drug labels. At present, the information given by the FDA seems to be the most elaborate, covering the largest number of substances, and also providing purely informative pharmacogenetic aspects on the labels. Gene–drug pairs for which evidence-based guidelines exist at the moment are listed on the CPIC website (https://cpicpgx.org/guidelines/), and these are currently used as the evidence base for the current and ongoing large implementation projects of pharmacogenetics diagnostics.[17] In Europe, the Ubiquitous Pharmacogenomics Consortium (UPGx) is implementing pharmacogenetic diagnostics in the hospital setting in different specializations. It is also developing a pharmacogenetic education program for the clinical and hospital staff, and a public movie on pharmacogenetics. The aim is to develop a ready-to-use and broad pharmacogenomics test system. Clinical implementation of this pharmacogenetics support system is tested enabling the individualizing of drug therapy. Implementation is tested in different fields of medicine, from transplantation medicine to psychiatry, in 16 European countries.[5]

Future Challenges

Future work in pharmacogenomics will have to elucidate the deeper genetic background, including rare genetic variants and epigenetics and their potential to explain individual patterns of therapy outcomes. This will allow better understanding of the molecular mechanisms of drug action, and its individual variability also in genes that are constributing to drug response. In psychiatry, these approaches may lead to a more biological understanding of psychiatric symptoms and disease, and finally provide the potential for new drug targets or individually tailored therapies.

References

1. Relling, M. V., & Evans, W. E. (2015). Pharmacogenomics in the clinic. *Nature*, *526*(7573), 343–350.

2. Eichler, H. G., Abadie, E., Breckenridge, A., Flamion, B., Gustafsson, L. L., Leufkens, H., Rowland, M., et al.(2011). Bridging the efficacy–effectiveness gap: A regulator's perspective on addressing variability of drug response. *Nature Reviews Drug Discovery*, *10*(7), 495–506.

3. Redelings, M. D., Sorvillo, F., & Simon, P. (2006). A comparison of underlying cause and multiple causes of death: U.S. Vital Statistics, 2000–2001. *Epidemiology, 17*(1), 100–103.

4. Crown, W. H., Finkelstein, S., Berndt, E. R., Ling, D., Poret, A. W., Rush, A. J., Russell, J. M., et al. (2002). The impact of treatment-resistant depression on health care utilization and costs. *Journal of Clinical Psychiatry, 63*(11), 963–971.

5. van der Wouden, C. H., Cambon-Thomsen, A., Cecchin, E., Cheung, K. C., Dávila-Fajardo, C. L., Deneer, V. H., Dolžan, V., et al. (2017). Implementing pharmacogenomics in Europe: Design and implementation strategy of the Ubiquitous Pharmacogenomics Consortium. *Clinical Pharmacology & Therapeutics, 101*(3), 341–358.

6. American Psychiatric Association. (2013). *Diagnostic and Statistical Manual of Mental Disorders (DSM-5®), Fifth Edition.* Arlington, VA: APA.

7. World Health Organisation. The ICD-10 classification of mental and behavioural disorders: diagnostic criteria for research. (1993). Available from: http://www.who.int/iris/handle/10665/37108.

8. Laje, G. (2013). Pharmacogenetics of mood disorders: What clinicians need to know. *CNS Spectrum, 18*(5), 272–284.

9. Kirchheiner, J., Nickchen, K., Bauer, M., Wong, M. L., Licinio, J., Roots, I., Brockmöller, J. (2004). Pharmacogenetics of antidepressants and antipsychotics: The contribution of allelic variations to the phenotype of drug response. *Molecular Psychiatry, 9*(5), 442–473.

10. Stingl, J. C., Brockmoller, J., & Viviani, R. (2013). Genetic variability of drug-metabolizing enzymes: The dual impact on psychiatric therapy and regulation of brain function. *Molecular Psychiatry, 18*(3), 273–287.

11. Gaedigk, A., Simon, S. D., Pearce, R. E., Bradford, L. D., Kennedy, M. J., & Leeder, J. S. (2008). The CYP2D6 activity score: Translating genotype information into a qualitative measure of phenotype. *Clinical Pharmacology & Therapeutics, 83*(2), 234–242.

12. Fuhr, U., Jetter, A., & Kirchheiner, J. (2007). Appropriate phenotyping procedures for drug metabolizing enzymes and transporters in humans and their simultaneous use in the "cocktail" approach. *Clinical Pharmacology & Therapeutics, 81*(2), 270–283.

13. Kirchheiner, J., Brosen, K., Dahl, M. L., Gram, L. F., Kasper, S., Roots, I., Sjöqvist, F., et al. (2001). CYP2D6 and CYP2C19 genotype-based dose recommendations for antidepressants: A first step towards subpopulation-specific dosages. *Acta Psychiatrica Scandinavica, 104*(3), 173–192.

14. Hicks, J. K., Sangkuhl, K., Swen, J. J., Ellingrod, V. L., Müller, D. J., Shimoda, K., Bishop, J. R., et al. (2016). Clinical Pharmacogenetics Implementation Consortium guideline (CPIC) for CYP2D6 and CYP2C19 genotypes and dosing of tricyclic antidepressants: 2016 update. 2016 Dec 20. *Clinical Pharmacology & Therapeutics.* doi: 10.1002/cpt.597.

15. Hicks, J. K., Bishop, J. R., Sangkuhl, K., Müller, D. J., Ji, Y., Leckband, S. G., Leeder, J. S., Graham, R. L., et al. (2015). Clinical Pharmacogenetics Implementation Consortium (CPIC) guideline for CYP2D6 and CYP2C19 genotypes and dosing of selective serotonin reuptake inhibitors. *Clinical Pharmacology & Therapeutics, 98*(2), 127–134.

16. Relling, M. V., & Klein, T. E. (2011). CPIC: Clinical Pharmacogenetics Implementation Consortium of the Pharmacogenomics Research Network. *Clinical Pharmacology & Therapeutics*, 89(3), 464–467.

17. Drew, L. (2016). Pharmacogenetics: The right drug for you. *Nature*, 537(7619), S60–S62.

Chapter 8

Endophenotypes

David C. Glahn, Laura Almasy, and John Blangero

Introduction

The dominant paradigm in psychiatric genetic research is to attempt to identify risk genes for mental illness by contrasting the allelic frequency of a variant between individuals diagnosed with a psychiatric disorder with unrelated comparison subjects at hundreds of thousands of points on the genome. A comparable, but less popular, experimental design utilizes related individuals and either association or genetic linkage analysis. In either case, the experimenter assumes that diagnostic entities represent coherent biological phenomena that map directly onto gene function. However, phenomenological psychotic diagnoses, like most complex disease entities, are relatively distant from gene action. Furthermore, there is growing evidence that individual genes do not directly code for current psychiatric diagnoses. Rather, it appears that genes influence some neurobiological processes that, when disrupted, confer risk for a disorder.

For example, Sekar and colleagues (2016) recently reported that the complement component 4 (*C4*) gene, located in the best-supported schizophrenia locus identified to date, influences synaptic pruning during adolescence in rodents.[1] Thus, it is possible that the *C4* gene, located within the major histocompatibility complex, increases risk for schizophrenia by influencing specific neurodevelopmental processes known to be altered in individuals with the illness.[2] In this context, synaptic pruning could be described as an intermediate phenotype or an endophenotype for schizophrenia. An intermediate phenotype is a measure indexing biological risk for a mental illness that is intermediate between gene expression and the disease.[3] An endophenotype is conceptually similar to an intermediate phenotype, except that the endophenotype concept is more carefully articulated and more closely approximates allied phenotypes used in other areas of human genetics, and endophenotypes must be heritable.[4] Thus, while both intermediate phenotypes and endophenotypes can be used to characterize the function of a risk gene, only endophenotypes can be used to query the genome for novel risk loci.[5] In this chapter, we define endophenotypes and describe different ways they have been applied to aid our understanding of the genetic architecture of psychiatric disorders.

What Are Endophenotypes?

The term "endophenotype" was first applied in psychiatric genetics by Gottesman and Shields (1972), who used the term to describe an internal phenotype discoverable by a "biochemical test or microscopic examination".[6] In an influential review nearly 30 years later, Gottesman and Gould (2003) clearly articulated testable criteria for endophenotypes. Specifcily, an endophenotype must: (1) be heritable; (2) be associated with the illness; (3) be independent of clinical state or require a challenge; (4) impairment must co-segregate with the illness within a family (that is, family members that do not meet diagnostic criteria show impairment relative to the general population); and (5) represent reproducible measurements.[4] In a follow-up paper, Gottesman and Gould noted that endophenotypes can best be conceptualized as the subset of biomarkers that are influenced by the same genetic factors that confer risk for the illness.[7] Thus, an endophenotype is a trait that is genetically related to the symptoms of an illness, but is not the illness per se.

Glahn and colleagues (2012) extend this assertion by suggesting that the joint genetic determination between the illness and endophenotype is fundamental to the concept. The primacy of pleiotropy led these investigators to develop a statistic, the Endophenotype Ranking Value, or *ERV*, for empirically ranking endophenotypes for an illness based upon their shared standardized genetic covariance.[8] The *ERV* is defined as the square root of the heritability of the endophenotype multiplied by the square root of the heritability of the illness, multiplied by the absolute value of their genetic correlation:

$$ERV = \sqrt{h_D^2 h_E^2}\,\left|\rho_G\right|$$

The advantage of this approach is that it allows one to select endophenotypes for an illness based upon evidence and strength of shared genetic etiology, which increases the likelihood that one could identify a gene that influences both the endophenotype and the illness. The *ERV* statistic also helps to focus the critical criteria for an endophenotype: it must be heritable and pleiotropic with the illness.

How Can Endophenotypes Advance Scientific Discovery?

As discussed, endophenotypes have two primary uses: gene discovery and gene characterization. Given that one of the requirements for an endophenotype is that it is heritable, it is entirely reasonable to use endophenotypes in gene discovery, either alone (univariate) or simultaneously with an indicator of affection status (bivariate or multivariate). In the univariate case, one would search the genome for loci that appear to influence the endophenotype. Assuming a genetic relationship between the endophenotype and illness was established, loci identified for the endophenotype are empirically nominated loci for the illness. Of course, the relationship between any particular locus and illness risk would necessarily need to be independently verified. A nice example of this approach is presented by Heck and colleagues (2014), who searched for loci influencing working memory performance in ~900 healthy subjects. While this analysis localized four genome-wide significant common variants, it also strongly implicated the "voltage-gated cation channel activity" (Gene Ontology ID [GO]:0022843) gene set in working memory performance.[9] These findings were replicated in an independent sample, extended to brain imaging, and intriguing, as variations in calcium channel genes appear to be associated with schizophrenia risk.[10] An alternate approach for gene discovery with endophenotypes is to directly test for loci influencing both the endophenotype and illness risk using a multivariate model.[5] This approach assumes that both the psychiatric disorder and the endophenotype are influenced by multiple genes, but only a subset of these genes influences both traits. Thus, by using a multivariate model, one improves statistical power to identify loci[11] and helps to characterize the biological process through which the gene/locus influences illness risk. An example of simultaneously modeling an endophenotype (right hippocampal volume) and illness risk (recurrent major depression) was provided by Mathias and colleagues (2015), who identified a pleiotropic locus at 18p11 in large extended pedigrees.[12] This suggests that a gene or genes in this region confers risk for major depression, potentially by also decreasing hippocampal volume. A conceptually similar analysis was conducted by Knowles and colleagues (2014), who identified a pleiotropic locus on 4q26 influencing both emotion recognition and amygdala volume.

   The commonly held conviction is that genes influence biological processes that in turn increase risk for psychiatric disorders.[3] If so, then the use of endophenotypes to characterize loci identified in more classical case-control or family-based analyses using only affection status is of paramount importance. Currently, there are no cellular markers for mental illness. This greatly complicates molecular biology experiments using functional genomic or proteomic techniques to investigate induced pluripotent stem cells (iPSC), an approach that could dramatically improve our understanding of illnesses like schizophrenia.[13] To the extent that endophenotypes provide clues about molecular processes or are themselves measureable within cells, then endophenotypes will help to fill this knowledge gap, furthering our understanding of pathobiology. This may be the ultimate utility of an endophenotype: a cellular-level measure of illness risk that can be used to help improve our understanding of mental illness.

References

1. Sekar, A., Bialas, A. R., de Rivera, H., Davis, A., Hammond, T. R., Kamitaki, N., . . . Schizophrenia Working Group of the Psychiatric Genomics Consortium. (2016). Schizophrenia risk from complex variation of complement component 4. *Nature*, *530*, 177–183.

2. Feinberg, I. (1982). Schizophrenia: Caused by a fault in programmed synaptic elimination during adolescence? *Journal of Psychiatric Research*, *17*, 319–334.

3. Meyer-Lindenberg, A., & Weinberger, D. R. (2006). Intermediate phenotypes and genetic mechanisms of psychiatric disorders. *Nature Reviews Neuroscience*, *7*, 818–827.

4. Gottesman, I. I., & Gould, T. D. (2003). The endophenotype concept in psychiatry: Etymology and strategic intentions. *American Journal of Psychiatry*, *160*, 636–645.

5. Glahn, D. C., Knowles, E. E., McKay, D. R., Sprooten, E., Raventos, H., Blangero, J., . . . Almasy, L. (2014). Arguments for the sake of endophenotypes: Examining common misconceptions about the use of endophenotypes in psychiatric genetics. *American Journal of Medical Genetics Part B: Neuropsychiatric Genetics*, *165*, 122–130.

6. Gottesman, I. I., & Shields, J. (1972). *Schizophrenia and Genetics: A Twin Study Vantage Point*. New York: Academic Press.

7. Gould, T., & Gottesman, I. (2006). Psychiatric endophenotypes and the development of valid animal models. *Genes, Brain & Behavior*, *5*, 113–119.

8. Glahn, D. C., Curran, J. E., Winkler, A. M., Carless, M. A., Kent, J. W. Jr., Charlesworth, J. C., . . . Blangero J. (2012). High dimensional endophenotype ranking in the search for major depression risk genes. *Biological Psychiatry*, *71*, 6–14.

9. Heck, A., Fastenrath, M., Ackermann, S., Auschra, B., Bickel, H., Coynel, D., . . . Papassotiropoulos, A. (2014). Converging genetic and functional brain imaging evidence links neuronal excitability to working memory, psychiatric disease, and brain activity. *Neuron*, *81*, 1203–1213.

10. Schizophrenia Working Group of the Psychiatric Genomics Consortium. (2014). Biological insights from 108 schizophrenia-associated genetic loci. *Nature*, *511*, 421–427.

11. Amos, C., de Andrade, M., & Zhu, D. (2001). Comparison of multivariate tests for genetic linkage. *Human Heredity*, *51*, 133–144.

12. Mathias, S. R., Knowles, E. E., Kent, J. W. Jr., McKay, D. R., Curran, J. E., de Almeida, M. A., . . . Glahn, D. C. (2016). Recurrent major depression and right hippocampal volume: A bivariate linkage and association study. *Human Brain Mapping*, *37*, 191–202.

13. Brennand, K. J., & Gage, F. H. (2012). Modeling psychiatric disorders through reprogramming. *Disease Models & Mechanisms*, *5*, 26–32.

Chapter 9

Imaging Genetics

Luanna Dixson, Heike Tost,
and Andreas Meyer-Lindenberg

Take-Home Points

1. The objective of an imaging genetic study is to identify genetic variants associated with inter-individual variation in different brain phenotypes.
2. Study of genetic contributions to heritable neural intermediate phenotypes has been a valuable approach for identifying novel psychiatric risk genes.
3. Candidate gene studies involve hypothesis-driven testing of genetic variants with prior links to the phenotype, while genome-wide association studies entail the rapid scanning of thousands of markers to detect genetic associations with quantitative traits or diagnoses.
4. Feed-back or feed-forward strategies may be used to facilitate gene discovery and exploration.
5. Establishment of multi-site consortia and the integration of metadata from bioinformatics resources has ushered in a new generation of analysis approaches using machine-learning algorithms.

Introduction: What Is Imaging Genetics?

It has long been known that various aspects of personality and behavior, as well as risk for neuropsychiatric illnesses, are influenced by inter-individual differences in a person's genetic makeup. Imaging genetics is a method to study how these features emerge at the level of brain structure, function, and wiring. In addition to investigating the role of genes in the healthy brain, imaging genetics approaches have been applied extensively to heritable psychiatric disorders and diseases, such as schizophrenia or autism.[1] Many of these illnesses are heterogeneous in presentation, possess environmental risk factors, and have behavioral and psychological features linked to observable changes in brain structure and function, such as the link between prefrontal cortex (PFC) activation and working memory function.[2] The decomposition of these complex features into brain phenotypes using neuroimaging techniques allows researchers to move beyond limited phenomenological definitions lacking biological validity. Identified brain phenotypes may furthermore represent more "intermediate" biological sub-processes and mechanisms, which in principle should be less genetically complex than the disease itself. This hypothesis has been partially borne out by meta-analysis studies demonstrating enhanced genetic penetrance for several neuroimaging phenotypes when compared to clinical measures.[3,4] A theoretical advantage of this approach is that increased gene effects on the level of brain phenotypes enable researchers to recruit smaller groups of individuals compared to formal genetic studies, reducing study costs and data acquisition time.[4] Finally, identifying mediatory neural circuitry is important for investigating underlying molecular mechanisms that can help target pharmacological and therapeutic interventions. In this chapter, we introduce the main neuroimaging modalities used in imaging genetic studies, outline some key trends, give some illustrative examples, and talk about future challenges for this exciting field.

The Intermediate Phenotype Concept

An important trend in imaging genetics is the study of intermediate phenotypes (also called "endophenotypes") that manifest risk on the level of neural phenotypes predicted to be closer to disease pathophysiology and gene effects. In order for an imaging-derived phenotype to be considered an intermediate phenotype, several criteria should be met.[5] First, the neuroimaging feature under investigation must segregate with illness in the population; i.e., it must more frequently occur with the disease. Second, the disease must have a heritable component linked to its genetic liability, meaning that relatives are more likely to be diagnosed than unrelated persons are meaning that relatives are more likely to be diagnosed with the disease than unrelated persons are. Third, the phenotype ought to be state-independent, which means it should be observable in individuals at higher genetic risk but without manifest disease. These could be healthy subjects carrying known risk alleles, or relatives with some shared genetic background. These individuals have the advantage of being enriched for genetic risk variants while being free from influential factors such as smoking or treatment. Lastly, it is important that the intermediate phenotype be reliable (i.e., sufficiently stable over time and can be replicated). In addition to elucidating mechanisms by which genes affect behavioral and clinical phenotypes, it is hoped that intermediate phenotypes will facilitate unbiased searches for psychiatric risk genes, and point towards mechanistically novel treatment targets.[6]

Genetic Association Studies

The first genetic studies of disease used linkage-based approaches in which chromosomal regions aggregating with disease were identified within an affected family. This approach has been successfully used to identify causative genes for brain-related diseases such as Huntington's chorea.[7] However, this strategy has been less successful for highly polygenic disorders such as schizophrenia, which arise from a complex interplay of environmental and genetic factors.[8] In order to study genetic contributions to these complex diseases, a frequentist approach (i.e., one that uses genotype frequencies for statistical inference) is often employed to estimate the probability of a genetic variant being associated with a quantitative phenotype or disease category. The basic idea behind these studies is that genetic variation that coincides more frequently with a disease category, or with higher or lower values of a continuous intermediate phenotype, may be linked to the disease susceptibility and warrant further investigation. The majority of imaging genetic studies have used this approach to study commonly occurring single-base pair changes in the genetic sequence, known as single nucleotide polymorphisms (SNPs). While the majority of SNPs do not have a known effect, SNPs which occur in regulatory or coding areas of DNA can alter the function and structure of associated proteins, and it is likely that a substantial part of the genome affects gene expression in multiple ways.[9] In this way, SNPs are thought to be the first links in a causal chain connecting molecular substrates to cellular physiology and higher level functioning. In the next few paragraphs, we discuss the major types of association studies conducted in imaging genetics.

Candidate Gene Studies

The first strategy used in imaging genetics was the "candidate gene" approach. In this method, a gene is selected on the basis of plausible molecular or cellular links to a disease or trait, and neuroimaging is used to study the effect of this gene on the brain (outlined in Figure 9.1A). Candidate gene strategies can be a powerful tool for prioritizing likely genes about which some neurobiological information is already known, or when specific pathways a gene affects are the focus of study (for example, it makes sense to investigate genes encoding enzymes and receptors in the dopaminergic system if this is the object of study). These studies have played an important role in focusing the initial research drive in imaging genetics by using information on molecular mechanisms, drug targets, gene expression, preclinical studies, and disease pathophysiology to select target genes to investigate. Unsurprisingly, the candidate gene approach greatly facilitates the biological interpretability of results. However, candidate gene studies are heavily reliant on extant knowledge about the neurobiology of the disease or phenotype under investigation, and have been famously likened to "packing your own lunchbox and then opening the lid to check to see what is in it" by S. Hyman.[10] Lastly, it is important that candidate genes studies be suitably powered with a reasonable sample size and that results can be replicated in an independent dataset.

Conducting an Imaging Genetic Study: The Basics

Most association studies in imaging genetics are relatively straightforward from a statistical point of view. Participants are split into three groups based on the autosomal SNP genotype they possess, and neuroimaging measures, for example, mean activity in a certain brain region, are compared and contrasted between genotype groups. This step involves making an assumption about the effect of the number of copies of the least frequently occurring (minor) allele on the phenotype. A common model is the additive genetic model, where the effect of an allele on the phenotype is believed to increase in a linear manner with each additional minor allele, so that for the "A" risk allele, the AG genotype confers an r-fold effect and the AA genotype confers a 2r-fold effect. For investigation of rarer common variants (i.e., <1% in a given population) other models may be pursued; for example, the "dominant model," which pools genotypes into two groups based on the risk allele (i.e., AA, AG vesus GG). The approach can be applied to variable numbers of SNPs and is well suited to the continuous intermediate phenotypes accessed by neuroimaging. In fMRI studies, significant allelic differences between groups can be demonstrated even with a small number of subjects[11]; however, a bare minimum of ~70–80 participants is required for investigation of those SNPs that do possess a sufficient minor allele frequency, with studies ideally featuring hundreds of subjects.[4,12] These data can then be entered into a regression model along with potential confounding factors, such as age and sex, to test if a SNP is statistically associated with the imaging phenotype. The respective candidate gene can then be followed up in further studies: for instance by knocking out the gene in rodents and testing for behavioral anomalies.

Two Canonical Candidate Gene Stories: COMT and SLC6A4

COMT

One of the most influential candidate gene stories in the neuroimaging genetic literature is that of the catechol-O-methyltransferase gene (COMT). This gene encodes a enzyme that degrades catecholamine neurotransmitters such as dopamine at synapses. Changes in dopamine have been strongly linked to the neurobiology of addiction, reward, and cognition.[13] It was postulated that this enzyme may play a particularly important role in modulating the dopamine levels in the prefrontal cortex where COMT expression is high and dopamine transporters (which attenuate the dopamine signal) are sparse.[14] A common base pair change in the 158th position of the coding sequence of the gene results in the substitution of an ancestral valine amino acid residue (Val) for methionine (Met) (COMT Val[158]Met). Insertion of Met at this point has a potent effect on the COMT protein, resulting in reduced enzymatic activity and subsequently increased dopamine concentrations in the PFC. Consequently, the question was posed whether gene effects in individuals possessing the *COMT* Val[158]Met polymorphism might be observed for dopamine-linked aspects of cognitive and behavioral function.

The very first study combining brain imaging and *COMT* Val[158]Met investigated working memory processes in patients with schizophrenia, their relatives, and healthy controls.[14] Working memory deficits are frequently seen in patients with schizophrenia and are dependent on prefrontal cortical brain regions. The study found that Val carriers, who should possess increased dopamine catabolism and thus lower dopamine levels in the PFC, showed a dose-dependent increase in prefrontal activation compared to methionine carriers when completing the task. The number of Val alleles was correlated with lower performance on the Wisconsin Card Sorting Test of executive function. The standard view is that these findings are due to a neural compensatory mechanism, termed *prefrontal inefficiency*, whereby more neural resources are recruited to perform a task in the setting of reduced dopamine metabolism.[15] Strikingly, the Val-mediated prefrontal inefficacy was starkest in the individuals with schizophrenia, but it could also be observed in unrelated healthy subjects who did not show impaired working memory performance. This gave rise to theory that the Val allele may mediate risk for schizophrenia via this neural mechanism, providing supportive evidence for the then-nascent concept of neuroimaging intermediate phenotypes.[16] A later study validated the effect of *COMT* genotype on dopamine availability using positron emission tomography (PET) imaging, providing quantitative evidence for a dosage-linked interaction between midbrain dopamine synthesis and prefrontal activity.[17] These findings contrast with the tenuous evidence of a role for *COMT* in schizophrenia from formal genetic studies, and bear testimony to the value of studying genetic variation on the level of neurobiological phenotypes purported to be closer to disease pathophysiology. Today *COMT* is one of the most well studied genes for schizophrenia, and it has inspired a host of neuroimaging genetic studies in its wake, especially in relation to catecholamine function. Moreover, in pharmacogenetic studies, the *COMT* Val[158]Met genotype has been linked to the efficacy of certain antidepressant medications, demonstrating how genetic findings can be related back to the clinic in the form of personalized medicine.[18,19] In sum, the *COMT* story shows the value of employing a candidate gene approach to validate existing theory, better understand risk circuitry, and guide patient-treatment strategies.

The Serotonin Transporter and the 5-HTTLPR Region

Another neurotransmitter of interest is serotonin. This neurotransmitter has been linked to known risk factors for several psychiatric disorders, such as the negative symptoms and increased stress responses seen in affective disorders.[20] A critical modulator of serotonergic neurotransmission is the serotonin transporter 5-HTT, encoded by the *SLC6A4* gene. 5-HTT attenuates serotonergic neurotransmission by transporting serotonin molecules from the synaptic cleft back to the presynaptic neuron, where they are metabolized. Drugs that target the serotonergic system (for example serotonin reuptake inhibitors) have shown efficacy in the treatment of depression.[21]

A "tandem repeat" variation at the promotor of the *SLC6A4* gene in the serotonin-transporter-linked polymorphic region (5-HTTLPR) leads to a long (L) and short (S) version of the 5-HTT transporter protein. The S-allele, which is associated with reduced 5-HTT transcription, has been linked to trait anxiety and risk for depression, with the strongest evidence found in individuals exposed to environmental adversity.[22] Evidence for an environmental interaction prompted investigation of the S-allele on amygdala activation, a brain region involved in the "fight or flight" response to threatening external stimuli.[11] In this study, the S-allele was associated with greater amygdala reactivity upon viewing of threatening faces. In animals, alterations of 5-HTT levels during neurodevelopment produces increased anxiety and alterations in wiring between the amygdala and anterior cingulate cortex (ACC).[23–25] This led to the hypothesis that the "S-allele" may impact amygdala-ACC neural pathway formation and functional interactions. Similar to depressed patients, healthy S-allele carriers show reduced gray matter volume in the amygdala and the ACC, which are two interconnected areas with strong links to serotonergic function.[25] The same study also reported decreased connectivity of the amygdala-ACC in S-allele carriers (particularly in the subgenual part) upon viewing aversive faces. In total, amygdala-subgenual ACC functional connectivity successfully accounted for a 30% variance in harm-avoidance scores. The 5-HTT transporter polymorphism is therefore an excellent example of how effects for "more penetrant" genes can be leveraged to dissect neural circuitry and complement imaging findings.

Genome-Wide Association Studies

The completion of the Human Genome Project and the advent of affordable microarray technology ushered in a second type of association study in neuroimaging genetics. In contrast to candidate gene studies, genome-wide association (GWA) studies use a data-driven approach to scan hundreds of thousands of genetic variants in parallel for association with a phenotype (see Figure 9.1C). In GWA studies, genetic markers from multiple individuals are quantified using microarray chips, which index blocks of common genetic variance in the population (i.e., variation in the genetic sequence that occurs in <5% individuals). It is important to note that a GWA SNP may not directly index the causal SNP itself, but rather be highly correlated with an untyped SNP in linkage disequilibrium with it. In regard to untyped SNPs, imputation techniques can be used to statistically infer missing SNP genotypes and extend the degree of genome-wide coverage. The first step in conducting a GWA study involves checking the quality of the genetics data and filtering on the basis of several factors. SNPs that deviate from Hardy Weinberg equilibrium or whose genotypes are not detectable within a certain proportion of the samples (typically <95%) are removed, along with individuals missing too many SNP genotypes overall. SNP genotypes that fall in too small a proportion of the study population to sufficiently reflect a minor allele frequency (MAF) of 10–20% are likewise filtered out. Lastly, outlier individuals, who share too much or too little genetic overlap after principal component or multi-dimensional scaling analysis, can be omitted or further examined. These may be family members or people of a different genetic ancestry who may mask true genetic effects. A well-known tool for performing these steps is the Plink software package developed by the Purcell Laboratory.[26] SNPs that meet a P < 5×10^{-8} are in accordance with a family-wise error rate of 5% (i.e., chance of false detection), and are considered good targets for replication and further investigation. It should be noted that multiple comparison correction for the testing of more than one phenotype for example, when voxel-wise comparisons are made must be performed before the genome-wide threshold is applied. Such multiple comparison correction was first developed for neuroimaging only, and it has been shown to be rather conservative for imaging genetics.[27] Meta and mega-analyses, which combine study results or perform analysis on pooled subject data, are increasingly being used to boost statistical power and summarize GWA study findings.[28–29]

Besides GWA-neuroimaging approaches, SNPs identified from GWA studies can make good candidate genes in light of their stronger genetic evidence for disease association. A well-known example is the investigation of the genome-wide significant risk SNP for psychosis, rs1344706 (*ZNF804A*), in healthy subjects performing a neurocognitive task associated with schizophrenia risk.[30] This study found an individual's risk-allele dosage was associated with altered correlations between the dorsal lateral prefrontal cortex (DLPFC) and hippocampus, similar to that seen in patients with schizophrenia completing the same task. A role for this SNP in brain function in schizophrenia has since received support from additional studies.[31–34]

While several studies have found associations of GWA-identified variants such as these with imaging phenotypes, the inverse is rarer, with few neuroimaging-based genome-wide SNP associations being identified so far. One of the first examples of this was the association of SNPs within the *ROBO1-ROBO2*, *TNIK*, and *CTXN3-SLC12A2* genes (P <10^{-6}) in a GWA study of DLPFC inefficiency in schizophrenia using the Sternberg item-recognition paradigm.[35]

One reason for this may be that GWA neuroimaging studies are simply underpowered to detect the thousands of small genetic variants predicted to contribute to disease risk.[8] There have been considerable efforts to deal with this issue by the formation of international imaging consortia that collate and share data for analysis. An example is the ENIGMA consortium, which combined data from multiple research groups to perform a huge genome-wide meta-analysis of genetic influences on hippocampal and intracranial volume in thousands of healthy individuals.[36] Other notable neuroimaging-GWA consortiums include IMAGEMEND and IMAGEN.[37–38]

Voxelwise GWA

In addition to candidate phenotype studies, whole-brain, voxelwise GWA (vGWA) involves a mass univariate search for associations of every SNP at *each* voxel *for* every voxel in the brain. This method was first employed to seek genome-wide associations with volumetric gray matter changes for 31,622 brain voxels in 740 elderly individuals who were healthy, or diagnosed with Alzheimer's disease or mild cognitive impairment.[39] This type of study demands extensive computational resources such as the use of computer clusters in order to obtain results in a timely manner. A later extension of this method discarded any SNPs not localized to genes to perform a voxelwise gene-wide association study.[40] However, the high dimensionality of the vGWA approach comes at a price, with few brain-wide–genome-wide SNPs surviving the strict multiple comparisons correction required.[41] Consequently, despite high hopes for this method, few studies to date have produced significant SNP associations. This is a potent issue in functional neuroimaging studies where temporal correlations between adjacent voxels in smoothed images reduce power to detect effects and potentially increase the type two error rate.[42] Issues of collinearity also extend to genomic data, which possesses a complex correlational structure linked to evolutionary influences and the non-random swapping of genetic material during chromosomal recombination. There has since been a drive to correct these issues by using dimensionality-reduction techniques that lessen the multiple testing burden. Examples include random field theory, lasso regression, kernel methods, and fast permutation procedures.[42] Researchers at Warwick University have also developed the Fast Voxelwise Genome Wide Association analysiS statistical toolbox (FVGWAS) for accelerating GWA in large search spaces.[43] In order for the multidisciplinary neuroimaging genetic community to make full use of these methods, it is important that software like this become more readily available.

Polygenic Risk Scores

In addition to GWA studies, the use of polygenic scores to study cumulative risk of SNPs with neuroimaging phenotypes has been implemented.[44] In its most basic form, a polygenic score may be constructed by summing up trait-associated alleles in individuals and computing a weighted score based on the strength of association with the neuroimaging phenotype. Polygenic risk scores of SNPs assembled from the largest schizophrenia GWA study to date, conducted by the Psychiatric Genomics Consortium, have produced mixed results with positive findings for altered brain activation during working memory, probabilistic learning, and executive processing, and negative findings for brain structural phenotypes.[45–49] Imagers who employ risk scores stand to benefit from reduced data dimensionality and the potential to use results as the basis of additional analyses.

Multivariate Methods

The growing size of imaging genetics datasets has ignited efforts to develop efficient analysis pipelines and computer algorithms able to handle complex multi-site studies. An emerging trend is the repurposing of multivariate statistics methods from bioinformatics to analyze imaging genetics data. One method that falls within this category is pathway-based analysis. Pathway-based analysis leverages *a priori* knowledge to gain insight into the biological functions of genes and pathways in genetic data.[50,51] The approach hinges on the finding that common genetic risk variants for psychiatric disorders and complex traits are not distributed randomly, but lie amongst sets of genes with overlapping functions.[52–55] There is a plethora of different methods, but the basic approach is to analyze sets of SNPs or genes grouped by common biological characteristics, such as a shared role in particular molecular functions or metabolic pathways.[56] The objective of such an analysis is to identify whether SNPs or genes more strongly associated with a phenotype of interest tend to significantly aggregate within specific "biological sets." In schizophrenia, pathway-based methods have identified gene sets related to memory processes and superior temporal gyrus thickness, yielding insight into plausible biological and molecular processes warranting further investigation.[57–59] A second type of exciting multivariate analysis method, uses machine-learning algorithms, such as random forests, which apply "decision trees" to distance metrics derived from the neuroimaging data in order to identify common predictive features.[60] Another interesting avenue is the development of methods to handle pleiotropic effects by teasing apart latent factors that jointly influence imaging and genetic variables. In many of these cases, the number of phenotypes outranks the number of predictors, presenting a challenging statistical problem. Methods adapted for this purpose include partial least squares, canonical correlation analysis, reduced rank regression, and independent component analysis.[41]

Future Directions

Epistasis
Epistasis is defined as the interaction between two genes that occurs when the effect of one locus on a phenotype is altered or masked by another locus.[61]

The study of epistasis is particularly important for complex traits where many SNPs are likely to have non-linear relationships. One method of studying epistasis is to select plausible genes on the basis of prior knowledge and test for multiway SNP-phenotype interactions using different genetic models (summarized in Figure 9.1B). A well-known epistasis study a well-known epistasis study investigated of SNPs in the schizophrenia risk gene *NRG1* and related partners, *ERBB* and *AKT*. In this study, subjects who bore a complete complement of risk genotypes from all three of these genes showed increased DLPFC activation during working memory.[62] No other genotype combination produced this result, leading researchers to conclude that these SNPs must confer a negative joint effect on DLPFC efficiency during working memory. Given that DLPFC inefficiency is one of the best-established intermediate phenotypes for schizophrenia, this phenotype has been fertile ground for interaction studies, with interaction of SNPs in *COMT-RSG4, GRM3-COMT,* and *DISC1-CIT-NDEL1,* with brain activation during working memory also being reported.[63-65] Many of these studies have been criticized for the biologically unrealistic investigation of two- or three-way SNP interactions. Recent efforts to address this issue have involved genome-wide assessment of epistasis with neuroimaging.[66]

Rare Variants

GWA studies were first designed to investigate commonly occurring genetic variants in a population (>5% of population). However, there is accumulating evidence that low-frequency, highly penetrant rare variants may account for some of the so-called missing heritability seen in complex traits.[67] In particular, large deletions, duplications, or inversions of DNA termed copy-number variants (CNVs) have provoked a lot of interest due to their aggregation in some psychiatric populations.[68–70] A recent MRI experiment showed that CNVs associated with schizophrenia and autism affected cognitive function and brain structure in healthy carriers in a dose-dependent fashion.[71] While studies of rare variants are sparse due to the difficulties in collecting a sufficient sample size, it is hoped that whole-genome and whole-exome sequencing will aid their discovery and help paint a more holistic picture of genetic disease architecture.

Bioinformatics

Many of the approaches discussed here can be viewed in light of an increasing interest in applying more functionally inspired approaches to the analysis of common genetic variants. This is seen in the increasing use of bioinformatics resources to categorize, annotate, and visualize genetic findings according to their expression level, protein interactions, and functional biochemistry. One novel approach is the use of post mortem brain expression banks, such as the Allen Brain Atlas or BrainCloud resources.[72,73] These resources have been used to investigate the spatial temporal gene expression patterns of genes disrupted by de novo genetic mutations seen in patients with schizophrenia.[74] Another study explored the relationship between gene-expression profiles

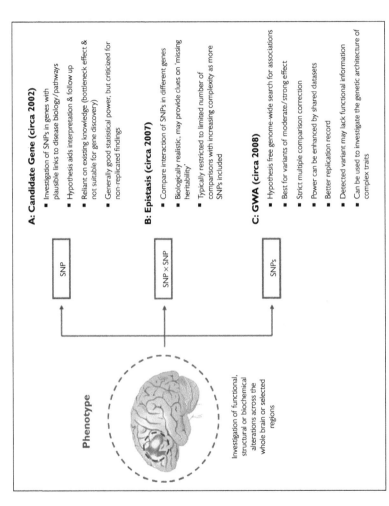

Phenotype

Investigation of functional, structural or biochemical alterations across the whole brain or selected regions

A: Candidate Gene (circa 2002)

SNP

- Investigation of SNPs in genes with plausible links to disease biology/pathways
- Hypothesis aids interpretation & follow up
- Reliant on existing knowledge (bottleneck effect & not suitable for gene discovery)
- Generally good statistical power, but criticized for non-replicated findings

B: Epistasis (circa 2007)

SNP × SNP

- Compare interaction of SNPs in different genes
- Biologically realistic, may provide clues on 'missing heritability'
- Typically restricted to limited number of comparisons with increasing complexity as more SNPs included

C: GWA (circa 2008)

SNPs

- Hypothesis free genome-wide search for associations
- Best for variants of moderate/strong effect
- Strict multiple comparison correction
- Power can be enhanced by shared datasets
- Better replication record
- Detected variant may lack functional information
- Can be used to investigate the genetic architecture of complex traits

Figure 9.1 An overview of three commonly used strategies to investigate genetic effects on brain images. Structural, functional, or biochemical investigations may be unconstrained (involve the whole search space) or involve a hypothesis-driven phenotype such as a region of interest. Genetic associations with these imaging phenotypes can then be investigated using several different analysis approaches, depending on the research question at hand.

and low frequency fluctuations from resting state fMRI.[75] While these methods are in their infancy, it can be expected that integration of these resources will be useful for facilitating novel analyses and post-hoc exploration of data.

Conclusion

Neuroimaging genetics is a highly dynamic and exciting field that has been rapidly expanding since its inception in the year 2000. In this chapter, we discussed the integration of neuroimaging and human genetics data in order to better understand risk mechanisms for psychiatric disease. While this endeavor is far from trivial, the potential rewards are considerable. Here we illustrated how imaging genetic strategies can be used to enable gene discovery, highlight neural risk circuitry, and inform treatment strategies. In addition to methodological advances, there is much to be learnt from new research frontiers focusing on gaining a better understanding of the joint effect of genes and environmental phenomena in the brain. Moreover, it is hoped that increased use of high powered collaborative data sets will produce novel genetic findings for further investigation. At present, researchers are increasingly integrating data with meaningful biological variables derived from databases and bioinformatics resources. It is hoped that these technological and methodological advances will lead to further insights into genetic influences on disease risk at the level of the brain.

References

1. Linden, D. E. (2012). The challenges and promise of neuroimaging in psychiatry. *Neuron*, 73(1), 8–22.

2. Callicott, J. H., Mattay, V. S., Bertolino, A., Finn, K., Coppola, R., Frank, J. A., . . . Weinberger, D. R. (1999). Physiological characteristics of capacity constraints in working memory as revealed by functional MRI. *Cerebral Cortex*, 9(1), 2026.

3. Munafo, M. R., Attwood, A. S., & Flint, J. (2004). Meta-analysis of genetic association studies. *Trends in Genetics*, 20, 439–444.

4. Mier, D., Kirsch, P., and Meyer-Lindenberg, A. (2010). Neural substrates of pleiotropic action of genetic variation in COMT: A meta-analysis. *Molecular Psychiatry*, 15(9), 918–927.

5. Gottesman, I. I., & Gould, T. D. (2003). The endophenotype concept in psychiatry: Etymology and strategic intentions. *American Journal of Psychiatry*, 160(4), 636–645.

6. Meyer-Lindenberg, A. (2010). From maps to mechanisms through neuroimaging of schizophrenia. *Nature*, 468 (7321), 194–202.

7. Dawn Teare, M., & Barrett, J. H. (2005). Genetic linkage studies. *Lancet*, 366 (9490), 1036–1044.

8. International Schizophrenia Consortium, Purcell, S. M., Wray, N. R., Stone, J. L., Visscher, P. M., O'Donovan, M. C., . . . Sklar, P. (2009). Common polygenic variation contributes to risk of schizophrenia and bipolar disorder. *Nature*, *460*(7256), 748–752. doi:10.1038/nature08185

9. ENCODE project consortium, Encode Project. (2012). An integrated encyclopedia of DNA elements in the human genome. *Nature*, *489*(7414), 57–74. doi:10.1038/nature11247

10. Abbott, A. (2008). Psychiatric genetics: The brains of the family. *Nature*, *454*(7201), 154–157.

11. Hariri, A. R., Mattay, V. S., Tessitore, A., Kolachana, B., Fera, F., Goldman, D., . . . Weinberger, D. R. (2002). Serotonin transporter genetic variation and the response of the human amygdala. *Science*, *297*(5580), 400–403.

12. Cao, H., Dixson, L., Meyer-Lindenberg, A., & Tost, H. (2015). Functional connectivity measures as schizophrenia intermediate phenotypes: Advances, limitations, and future directions. *Current Opinion in Neurobiology*, *36*, 7–14.

13. Iversen, L. L., Iversen, S. D., Dunnett, S. B., & Björklund, A. (2010). *Dopamine Handbook*. Oxford University Press, Oxford, Oxfordshire, UK

14. Egan, M. F., Goldberg, T. E., Kolachana, B. S., Callicott, J. H., Mazzanti, C. M., Straub, R. E., . . . Weinberger, D. R. (2001). Effect of COMT Val108/158 Met genotype on frontal lobe function and risk for schizophrenia. *Proceedings of the National Academy of Sciences USA*, *98*(12), 6917–6922.

15. Callicott, J. H., Mattay, V. S., Verchinski, B. A., Marenco, S., Egan, M. F., & Weinberger, D. R. (2003). Complexity of prefrontal cortical dysfunction in schizophrenia: More than up or down. *American Journal of Psychiatry*, *160*(12), 2209–2215. doi:10.1176/appi.ajp.160.12.2209

16. Meyer-Lindenberg, A., & Weinberger, D. R. (2006). Intermediate phenotypes and genetic mechanisms of psychiatric disorders. *Nature Reviews Neuroscience*, *7*(10), 818–827.

17. Meyer-Lindenberg, A. (2005). Midbrain dopamine and prefrontal function in humans: interaction and modulation by COMT genotype. *Nature Neuroscience*, *8*, 594–596.

18. Baune, B. T., Hohoff, C., Berger, K., Neumann, A., Mortensen, S., Roehrs, T., . . . Domschke, K. (2008). Association of the COMT val158met variant with antidepressant treatment response in major depression. *Neuropsychopharmacology*, *33*(4), 924–932.

19. Apud, J. A., Mattay, V., Chen, J., Kolachana, B. S., Callicott, J. H., Rasetti, R., . . . Weinberger, D. R. (2007). Tolcapone improves cognition and cortical information processing in normal human subjects. *Neuropsychopharmacology*, *32*(5), 1011–1020.

20. Goldman, N., Glei, D. A., Lin, Y. H., & Weinstein, M. (2010). The serotonin transporter polymorphism (5-HTTLPR): Allelic variation and links with depressive symptoms. *Depression and Anxiety*, *27*(3), 260–269.

21. Blier, P., & El Mansari, M. (2013). Serotonin and beyond: Therapeutics for major depression. *Philosophical Transactions of the Royal Society of London, B, Biological Sciences*, *368*(1615), 20120536.

22. Caspi, A., Sugden, K., Moffitt, T. E., Taylor, A., Craig, I. W., Harrington, H., . . . Poulton, R. (2003). Influence of life stress on depression: Moderation by a polymorphism in the 5-HTT gene. *Science*, *301*(5631), 386–389.

23. Kalueff, A. V., Jensen, C. L., & Murphy, D. L. (2007). Locomotory patterns, spatio-temporal organization of exploration and spatial memory in serotonin transporter knockout mice. *Brain Research*, *1169*, 87–97.

24. van der Marel, K., Homberg, J. R., Otte, W. M., & Dijkhuizen, R. M. (2013). Functional and structural neural network characterization of serotonin transporter knockout rats. *PLoS One*, *8*(2), e57780. doi:10.1371/journal.pone.0057780

25. Pezawas, L., Meyer-Lindenberg, A., Drabant, E. M., Verchinski, B. A., Munoz, K. E., Kolachana, B. S., . . . Weinberger, D. R. (2005). 5-HTTLPR polymorphism impacts human cingulate-amygdala interactions: A genetic susceptibility mechanism for depression. *Nature Neuroscience*, *8*(6), 828–834.

26. Purcell, S., Neale, B., Todd-Brown, K., Thomas, L., Ferreira, M. A., Bender, D., . . . Sham, P. C. (2007). PLINK: A tool set for whole-genome association and population-based linkage analyses. *American Journal of Human Genetics*, *81*(3), 559–575.

27. Meyer-Lindenberg, A., Nicodemus, K. K., Egan, M. F., Callicott, J. H., Mattay, V., & Weinberger, D. R. (2008). False positives in imaging genetics. *Neuroimage*, *40*(2), 655–661.

28. Major Depressive Disorder Working Group of the Psychiatric GWAS Consortium, Ripke, S., Wray, N. R., Lewis, C. M., Hamilton, S. P., Weissman, M. M., . . . Sullivan, P. F. (2013). A mega-analysis of genome-wide association studies for major depressive disorder. *Molecular Psychiatry*, *18*(4), 497–511.

29. Lee, Y. H. (2015). Meta-analysis of genetic association studies. *Annals of Laboratory Medicine*, *35*(3), 283–287.

30. Esslinger, C., Walter, H., Kirsch, P., Erk, S., Schnell, K., Arnold, C., . . . Meyer-Lindenberg, A. (2009). Neural mechanisms of a genome-wide supported psychosis variant. *Science*, *324*(5927), 605.

31. Rasetti, R., Sambataro, F., Chen, Q., Callicott, J. H., Mattay, V. S., & Weinberger, D. R. (2011). Altered cortical network dynamics: A potential intermediate phenotype for schizophrenia and association with ZNF804A. *Archives of General Psychiatry*, *68*(12), 1207–1217. doi:10.1001/archgenpsychiatry.2011.103

32. O'Donovan, M. C., Craddock, N., Norton, N., Williams, H., Peirce, T., Moskvina, V., . . . Molecular Genetics of Schizophrenia Collaboration. (2008). Identification of loci associated with schizophrenia by genome-wide association and follow-up. *Nature Genetics*, *40*(9), 1053–1055. doi:10.1038/ng.201

33. Riley, B., Thiselton, D., Maher, B. S., Bigdeli, T., Wormley, B., McMichael, G. O., . . . Kendler, K. S. (2010). Replication of association between schizophrenia and ZNF804A in the Irish Case-Control Study of Schizophrenia sample. *Molecular Psychiatry*, *15*(1), 29–37.

34. Donohoe, G., Morris, D. W., & Corvin, A. (2010). The psychosis susceptibility gene ZNF804A: Associations, functions, and phenotypes. *Schizophrenia Bulletin*, *36*(5), 904–909. doi:10.1093/schbul/sbq080

35. Potkin, S. G., Turner, J. A., Guffanti, G., Lakatos, A., Fallon, J. H., Nguyen, D. D., . . . Fbirn. (2009). A genome-wide association study of schizophrenia using brain activation as a quantitative phenotype. *Schizophrenia Bulletin*, *35*(1), 96–108.

36. Thompson, P. M., Andreassen, O. A., Arias-Vasquez, A., Bearden, C. E., Boedhoe, P. S., Brouwer, R. M., . . . Enigma Consortium. (2017). ENIGMA and the individual: Predicting factors that affect the brain in 35 countries worldwide. *Neuroimage*, *145*(Pt B), 389–408.

37. Frangou, S., Schwarz, E., Meyer-Lindenberg, A. (2016). Imaging Genetics for Mental Disorders (IMAGEMEND). *World Psychiatry 15*(2), 179–180.

38. Schumann, G., Loth, E., Banaschewski, T., Barbot, A., Barker, G., Buchel, C., . . . Imagen Consortium. (2010). The IMAGEN study: Reinforcement-related behaviour in normal brain function and psychopathology. *Molecular Psychiatry*, *15*(12), 1128–1139.

39. Stein, J. L., Hua, X., Lee, S., Ho, A. J., Leow, A. D., Toga, A. W., . . . Alzheimer's Disease Neuroimaging Initiative. (2010). Voxelwise genome-wide association study (vGWAS). *Neuroimage*, *53*(3), 1160–1174.

40. Hibar, D. P., Stein, J. L., Kohannim, O., Jahanshad, N., Saykin, A. J., Shen, L., . . . Initiative Alzheimer's Disease Neuroimaging. (2011). Voxelwise gene-wide association study (vGeneWAS): Multivariate gene-based association testing in 731 elderly subjects. *Neuroimage*, *56*(4), 1875–1891.

41. Liu, J., & Calhoun, V. D. (2014). A review of multivariate analyses in imaging genetics. *Frontiers in Neuroinformatics*, *8*, 29.

42. Ge, T., Feng, J., Hibar, D. P., Thompson, P. M., & Nichols, T. E. (2012). Increasing power for voxel-wise genome-wide association studies: The random field theory, least square kernel machines and fast permutation procedures. *Neuroimage*, *63*(2), 858–873.

43. Huang, M., Nichols, T., Huang, C., Yu, Y., Lu, Z., Knickmeyer, R. C., . . . Alzheimer's Disease Neuroimaging Initiative. (2015). FVGWAS: Fast voxelwise genome wide association analysis of large-scale imaging genetic data. *Neuroimage*, *118*, 613–627.

44. Dima, D., & Breen, G. (2015). Polygenic risk scores in imaging genetics: Usefulness and applications. *Journal of Psychopharmacology*, *29*(8), 867–871.

45. Kauppi, K., Westlye, L. T., Tesli, M., Bettella, F., Brandt, C. L., Mattingsdal, M., . . . Andreassen, O. A. (2015). Polygenic risk for schizophrenia associated with working memory-related prefrontal brain activation in patients with schizophrenia and healthy controls. *Schizophrenia Bulletin*, *41*(3), 736–743.

46. Lancaster, T. M., Ihssen, N., Brindley, L. M., Tansey, K. E., Mantripragada, K., O'Donovan, M. C., . . . Linden, D. E. (2015). Associations between polygenic risk for schizophrenia and brain function during probabilistic learning in healthy individuals. *Human Brain Mapping*,

47. Whalley, H. C., Papmeyer, M., Sprooten, E., Romaniuk, L., Blackwood, D. H., Glahn, D. C., . . . McIntosh, A. M. (2012). The influence of polygenic risk for bipolar disorder on neural activation assessed using fMRI. *Translational Psychiatry*, *2*, e130. doi:10.1038/tp.2012.60

48. Schizophrenia Working Group of the Psychiatric Genomics Consortium. (2014). Biological insights from 108 schizophrenia-associated genetic loci. *Nature*, *511*(7510), 421–427.

49. Voineskos, A. N., Felsky, D., Wheeler, A. L., Rotenberg, D. J., Levesque, M., Patel, S., . . . Malhotra, A. K. (2015). Limited evidence for association of genome-wide schizophrenia risk variants on cortical neuroimaging phenotypes. *Schizophrenia Bulletin*,

50. Mootha, V. K., Lindgren, C. M., Eriksson, K. F., Subramanian, A., Sihag, S., Lehar, J., . . . Groop, L. C. (2003). PGC-1alpha-responsive genes involved in oxidative phosphorylation are coordinately downregulated in human diabetes. *Nature Genetics*, *34*(3), 267–273.

51. Subramanian, A., Tamayo, P., Mootha, V. K., Mukherjee, S., Ebert, B. L., Gillette, M. A., . . . Mesirov, J. P. (2005). Gene set enrichment analysis: A knowledge-based approach for interpreting genome-wide expression profiles. *Proceedings of the National Academy of Sciences USA*, *102*(43), 15545–15550.

52. Jia, P., Wang, L., Meltzer, H. Y., & Zhao, Z. (2010). Common variants conferring risk of schizophrenia: A pathway analysis of GWAS data. *Schizophrenia Research*, *122*(1–3), 38–42.

53. Askland, K., Read, C., & Moore, J. (2009). Pathways-based analyses of whole-genome association study data in bipolar disorder reveal genes mediating ion channel activity and synaptic neurotransmission. *Human Genetics*, *125*(1), 63–79.

54. Holmans, P., Green, E. K., Pahwa, J. S., Ferreira, M. A., Purcell, S. M., Sklar, P., . . . Craddock, N. (2009). Gene ontology analysis of GWA study data sets provides insights into the biology of bipolar disorder. *American Journal of Human Genetics*, *85*(1), 13–24.

55. Lips, E. S., Cornelisse, L. N., Toonen, R. F., Min, J. L., Hultman, C. M., International Schizophrenia Consortium, . . . Posthuma, D. (2012). Functional gene group analysis identifies synaptic gene groups as risk factor for schizophrenia. *Molecular Psychiatry*, *17*(10), 996–1006.

56. Wang, K., Li, M., & Hakonarson, H. (2010). Analysing biological pathways in genome-wide association studies. *Nature Reviews Genetics*, *11*(12), 843–854.

57. Wolthusen, R. P., Hass, J., Walton, E., Turner, J. A., Rossner, V., Sponheim, S. R., . . . Ehrlich, S. (2015). Genetic underpinnings of left superior temporal gyrus thickness in patients with schizophrenia. *World Journal of Biological Psychiatry*, *6*,1–11.

58. Luksys, G., Fastenrath, M., Coynel, D., Freytag, V., Gschwind, L., Heck, A., . . . de Quervain, D. J. (2015). Computational dissection of human episodic memory reveals mental process-specific genetic profiles. *Proceedings of the National Academy of Sciences USA*, *112*(35), E4939–E4948. doi:10.1073/pnas.1500860112

59. Heck, A., Fastenrath, M., Ackermann, S., Auschra, B., Bickel, H., Coynel, D., . . . Papassotiropoulos, A. (2014). Converging genetic and functional brain imaging evidence links neuronal excitability to working memory, psychiatric disease, and brain activity. *Neuron*, *81*(5), 1203–1213. doi:10.1016/j.neuron.2014.01.010

60. Wang, Y., Goh, W., Wong, L., & Montana, G. (2013). Random forests on Hadoop for genome-wide association studies of multivariate neuroimaging phenotypes. *BMC Bioinformatics*, *14*(Suppl 16), S6.

61. Cordell, H. J. (2002). Epistasis: What it means, what it doesn't mean, and statistical methods to detect it in humans. *Human Molecular Genetics*, *11*(20), 2463–2468.

62. Nicodemus, K. K., Law, A. J., Radulescu, E., Luna, A., Kolachana, B., Vakkalanka, R., . . . Weinberger, D. R. (2010). Biological validation of increased schizophrenia risk with NRG1, ERBB4, and AKT1 epistasis via functional neuroimaging in healthy controls. *Archives of General Psychiatry*, *67*(10), 991–1001. doi:10.1001/archgenpsychiatry.2010.117

63. Buckholtz, J. W., Sust, S., Tan, H. Y., Mattay, V. S., Straub, R. E., Meyer-Lindenberg, A., . . . Callicott, J. H. (2007). fMRI evidence for functional epistasis between COMT and RGS4. *Molecular Psychiatry*, *12*(10), 893–5, 885.

64. Tan, H. Y., Chen, Q., Sust, S., Buckholtz, J. W., Meyers, J. D., Egan, M. F., . . . Callicott, J. H. (2007). Epistasis between catechol-O-methyltransferase and type II metabotropic glutamate receptor 3 genes on working memory brain function. *Proceedings of the National Academy of Sciences USA*, *104*(30), 12536–41.

65. Nicodemus, K. K., Callicott, J. H., Higier, R. G., Luna, A., Nixon, D. C., Lipska, B. K., . . . Weinberger, D. R. (2010). Evidence of statistical epistasis between DISC1, CIT and NDEL1 impacting risk for schizophrenia: Biological validation with functional neuroimaging. *Human Genetics*, *127*(4), 441–452.

66. Hibar, D. P., Stein, J. L., Jahanshad, N., Kohannim, O., Hua, X., Toga, A. W., . . . Thompson, P. M. (2015). Genome-wide interaction analysis reveals replicated epistatic effects on brain structure. *Neurobiology of Aging*, *36*(Suppl 1), S151–S158.

67. Gershon, E. S., Alliey-Rodriguez, N., & Liu, C. (2011). After GWAS: Searching for genetic risk for schizophrenia and bipolar disorder. *American Journal of Psychiatry*, *168*(3), 253–256.

68. Loohuis, L. M., Vorstman, J. A., Ori, A. P., Staats, K. A., Wang, T., Richards, A. L., . . . Ophoff, R. A. (2015). Genome-wide burden of deleterious coding variants increased in schizophrenia. *Nature Communications*, *6*, 7501.

69. Green, E. K., Rees, E., Walters, J. T., Smith, K. G., Forty, L., Grozeva, D., . . . Kirov, G. (2015). Copy number variation in bipolar disorder. *Molecular Psychiatry*, *21*, 89–93.

70. Marshall, C. R., & Scherer, S. W. (2012). Detection and characterization of copy number variation in autism spectrum disorder. *Nature Communications*, *838*, 115–135.

71. Stefansson, H., Meyer-Lindenberg, A., Steinberg, S., Magnusdottir, B., Morgen, K., Arnarsdottir, S., . . . Stefansson, K. (2014). CNVs conferring risk of autism or schizophrenia affect cognition in controls. *Nature*, *505*(7483), 361–366.

72. Hawrylycz, M. J., Lein, E. S., Guillozet-Bongaarts, A. L., Shen, E. H., Ng, L., Miller, J. A., . . . Jones, A. R. (2012). An anatomically comprehensive atlas of the adult human brain transcriptome. *Nature*, *489*(7416), 391–399. doi:10.1038/nature11405

73. Colantuoni, C., Lipska, B. K., Ye, T., Hyde, T. M., Tao, R., Leek, J. T., . . . Kleinman, J. E. (2011). Temporal dynamics and genetic control of transcription in the human prefrontal cortex. *Nature*, *478*(7370), 519–523.

74. Gulsuner, S., Walsh, T., Watts, A. C., Lee, M. K., Thornton, A. M., Casadei, S., . . . McClellan, J. M. (2013). Spatial and temporal mapping of de novo mutations in schizophrenia to a fetal prefrontal cortical network. *Cell*, *154*(3), 518–529.

75. Wang, G. Z., Belgard, T. G., Mao, D., Chen, L., Berto, S., Preuss, T. M., . . . Konopka, G. (2015). Correspondence between resting-state activity and brain gene expression. *Neuron*, *88*(4), 659–666.

Chapter 10

Bioinformatics in Psychiatric Genetics

Nikola S. Mueller, Ivan Kondofersky, Gökcen Eraslan, Karolina Worf, and Fabian J. Theis

Take-Home Points

1. Bioinformatic tools have been successfully used to identify links between genetic signals and psychiatric diseases.
2. Prioritization of SNPs plays an important role in GWAS studies, and we listed several techniques and trends on that topic.
3. Incorporation of network knowledge in analysis pipelines unravels even deeper understanding of the genetic architecture of a given disease.
4. An overview of available tools as well as corresponding biological databases storing existing literature findings was provided.

Introduction

The need for computational and statistical methods in psychiatric research was recognized as early as the 1980s.[1,2] This can be explained by the increasingly prominent examples of twins and relatives sharing the same psychiatric disorder and thus the associated logic that psychiatric disorders have a high degree of heritability,[3–5] which in turn led to the question of quantifying the genetic background statistically. Such approaches were complemented by animal models for the study of psychiatric disorders.[6] It was stated that for an animal model to be valid, it needs to be understood from the historical and evolutionary point of view, as these kind of models have been used for many decades to study psychiatric phenomena. The authors[6] conclude that to understand better the molecular mechanisms of a disease, genetics as a research field has to be included in psychiatric study. This claim is further supported by the realization that advances in genetics will make a large impact on clinical psychiatry[7]; the authors[7] point out that both genes and environment have an influence in psychiatric disorders and that genes have an impact on (brain) development. At the same time, many misconceptions in this research field are also stressed; for example, that high heritability would lead to ineffective clinical interventions, or genes that are associated with a certain disease are always "bad."[7]

These findings give a good view of how psychiatric genetics developed as a field, thus producing increasingly large phenotypical and molecular data sets. This has led to interest in development of tailored tools or data collection in online databases.[8–10] Bringing genetics into the equation, however, leads to a challenge that was previously unknown to this field: the problem of "big data."[11,12] In the age of big data, it is possible to perform studies in a way that was not possible due to, for instance, financial limitations of data generation a decade ago. For example, the cost for sequencing a whole human genome is currently estimated to be approximately US $1,000,[12] which means that it was reduced by more than 10,000 times in the space of only ten years. At the same time, technical advances allow the generated data to be of higher accuracy, and the process of data generation is speeded up enormously. With data generation improving at such a pace, many additional experimental designs can be performed realistically nowadays. These amounts of data also naturally limit the available analytical tools in psychiatric research, and at the same time create challenges for the development of new approaches. Here, psychiatric research fortunately can rely on many tools already developed in the research field of bioinformatics.[13]

One of the first promising approaches in bridging the gap between biological mechanisms and the actual psychiatric disorders was published in Schulze et al., 2005.[14] The authors performed a sophisticated genotype–phenotype association in bipolar disorder patients and were able to conclude that one specific locus on the human genome (DAOA/G30) was associated with persecutory delusions. This study was on a qualitatively high level, as the amount of data that was analyzed in a discovery cohort as well as a validation cohort was large and homogenous. However, the statistical analyses were mainly limited to a logistical regression approach, which for larger and more detailed data, clearly has its limits.

In the Psychiatric Genomics Consortium,[15] the authors provide a large comparison of five psychiatric disorders and associated genome-wide association studies. The data was collected within the Psychiatric Genomics Consortium and was one of the biggest studies, with well over 10,000 patients participating in the analysis. Here, the main findings consisted of considerable genetic correlation and thus a large amount of common single-nucleotide polymorphisms (SNPs) found (for example) in schizophrenia and bipolar disorder. The genetics data were found to be accountable for 17–29% of the variance in liability.

Other authors have already analyzed the role of bioinformatics and systems biology in the investigation of complex psychiatric disorders,[13] and have postulated that the real promise for better understanding psychiatric disorders is the study of the associated biology. The ultimate goal thereby is to use the available technology and ultimately create prognostic biomarkers that can be reliably translated into actual clinical treatment.

In this chapter, we aim to provide a review of multiple analysis techniques that have been successfully applied in some of the just-cited references in the genetic study of psychiatric disorders. We first describe some specific aspects of genome-wide association studies (GWAS). GWAS results are typically reported as variants representing an entire haplotype linkage disequilibrium (LD) block through a method called *clumping*. While this approach gives us genome-wide independent variants with the strongest association in the group of correlated variants (*clumps*), analyzing only such resulting lists of hits might lead us to miss putatively causal variants within the same block as the representative variant. One practice to deal with this problem is to extend the list of analyzed GWAS into a larger list that also includes variants in high LD with GWAS hits (*proxies*). There are many tools and web interfaces that allow us to perform such proxy searches via specifying the degree of dependence between variants such as r-squared.[16–19] In this context, we focus on prioritization of so-called GWAS hits or SNPs found to have a strong link to a psychiatric disorder. Furthermore, we consider some techniques that can be applied to the outcome of a GWAS study that enable us to put the results into an organized and structured context by combining single hits into networks. Therefore, we discuss the use and advantages of online databases and interaction networks and also focus on network-based stratification.

Prioritizing GWAS Hits

Genome-wide association studies (GWAS) have linked many loci associated with various psychiatric diseases such as schizophrenia and bipolar disorder. However, interpreting the biological relevance of GWAS hits—making sense of the GWAS findings in general—remains a challenging task. One important reason is the fact that the main unit of output in GWAS is a genomic region, where we typically observe many highly-correlated variants. This makes it difficult to pinpoint a putative functional variant. Therefore, effective prioritization techniques are needed in order to bridge the gap between several identified loci and the disease etiology.

The main goal of the prioritization of GWAS hits is to establish a reasonable link between an identified variant and the mechanisms underlying (or associated with) the disease by investigating possible effects of variants. Several ways have been proposed for handling this challenging task. In this section, we will review widely used methods.*

Overlap-Based Prioritization

The most widely used method to prioritize GWAS hits is to assess the overlap of the variants with the annotated regions in the genome. Depending

---

* Another technique, called the high-density, customized, genotyping-based fine mapping, is not covered in this chapter; see [20] for a nice review.

on whether a variant is protein-coding or non-coding, different types of annotations can be used for the prioritization. It ought to be noted that using different transcript sets might have severe effects on variant annotation.[21] The methods discussed in the following sections are summarized in Table 10.1.

Table 10.1 Overall View of Prioritization and Annotation Tools

Tool/Service	Annotations	Integrated Resources	Input	LD Search
HaploReg [47]	Regulatory elements, motifs, binding sites, eQTLs	GENCODE, dbSNP, NHGRI/ EBIGWAS hits, GRASP	dbSNP IDs or known GWAS hits	Yes
RegulomeDB [48]	Regulatory elements, motifs, binding sites, eQTLs	ROADMAP, ENCODE, ChromHMM	RSID, BED, VCF, GFF3, coordinates	No
GWAS3D [49]	Chromosome conformation, regulatory elements, conservation regions	ENCODE, ChromHMM	RSID, VCF, PLINK, coordinates	Yes
GEMINI [24]	Genes, pathways, TF binding, regulatory elements, conservation, clinical significance, custom annotations	dbSNP, UCSC, ClinVar, KEGG, ENSEMBL, PolyPhen, SIFT, CADD, ENCODE, 1000G, OMIM	VCF, PED	No
ANNOVAR/ wANNOVAR [22]	ChIP-seq, RNA-seq, DHS peaks, GWAS hits, TFBSs	RefSeq, UCSC, GENCODE, ENSEMBL, ENCODE	VCF, TSV, ANNOVAR, GFF3, disease/ phenotype terms	No
FunciSNP [50]	Chromatin features	1000G, ENCODE	dbSNP ids	Yes
DeepSEA [51]	TFBS, histone modifications, DHS	ENCODE, Roadmap	1kb sequence, VCF, BED	No
CADD [52]	Conservation, regulatory elements, genomic annotations	ENCODE, UCSC	VCF	No
GERP ++ [53]	Conservation	—	FASTA, genomic position	No
GenoWAP [54]	eQTL	—	GWAS results and p-values	No

Coding Variants

For the annotation of coding variants, ANNOVAR[22] and VEP (Ensembl's Variant Effect Predictor)[23] are widely used. These tools provide numerous filtering and annotation options and other convenient features. For example, ANNOVAR can detect and filter out transcripts with incomplete coding sequences, while VEP has wide range of plugins.[†] Another prominent algorithm in the field is GEMINI,[24] which integrates known annotations such as ENCODE, UCSC, and KEGG, user-defined annotations, as well as genotype and phenotype data. Its efficient storage and query framework facilitates downstream analysis. The main advantage of these tools is that they save researchers from making manual queries to various variant annotation and prediction sources using alternative set of transcripts; e.g., ENSEMBL, RefSeq.

SIFT[25] and PolyPhen[26] are popular tools that can predict whether amino acid changes will alter protein structure and function. Most variant annotation tools already include SIFT and PolyPhen scores in their outputs.

As functional units of the genome, genes are interpretable to some extent in the context of diseases, since they have been associated with specific phenotypes and diseases. Therefore, it is worth mentioning gene-based analysis methods. The Residual Variation Intolerance Score (RVIS) study aims for ranking genes based on how well they can tolerate mutations. The EXAC project is aiming for the consolidation of exome-sequencing data from many researchers in order to provide a comprehensive resource about coding variants. Annotations of rare variants in EXAC, together with the genic intolerance scores in RVIS, are useful resources that can be used to prioritize rare coding variants.

An alternative approach of variant prioritization is to assess the enrichment of group of variants. VEGAS[27] is such an example, in which gene-based enrichment tests are performed in order to identify disease-associated genes. It was successfully used to associate genes with anxiety disorder.[28] Other tools, such as DEPICT,[29] INRICH,[30] and GRAIL,[31] enable pathway-enrichment analysis of the genes related to GWAS hits. See endnotes 32 and 33 for applications to psychiatric disorders.

Non-Coding Variants and Epigenetics

Prioritization of non-coding variants is a more challenging task, since there is less evidence about the function of non-coding regions in general. A common approach is to check the enrichment of regulatory elements for identified GWAS variants, using sampling-based significance tests.[34,35]

ENCODE and Roadmap Epigenomics projects provide a comprehensive data source for epigenetic and regulatory annotations from numerous cell lines and tissues. PsychENCODE provides additional histone-modification data from brain. It has also been shown that allele-skewed DNA methylation

---

[†] For web interfaces, please check wannovar.usc.edu and ensembl.org/Tools/VEP.

is enriched in schizophrenia GWAS hits compared to other non-psychiatric disorders.[36] Gagliano et al. provided a great discussion about available brain-specific genomic annotations.[37] Interrogating non-coding variants putatively affecting the function of small non-coding RNAs is also used to shed light on the etiology of psychiatric disorders.[38] Haploreg, RegulomeDB, and FunciSNP are other integrative approaches that can be utilized to query the overlap of variant with regulatory elements. Machine-learning approaches such as GWAVA and CADD are trained with various variant features to predict the pathogenicity of variants and hence to prioritize them. FunSeq2 uses weighted scoring for a similar task.

One issue about analyzing GWAS hits and their proxies is that the variants that do not attain genome-wide significance might still have an impact on the disease through various biological mechanisms. Analysis of such *sub-threshold* variants has revealed new loci associated with cardiac traits where many variants are found to be enriched in enhancer regions.[39] In another approach, the authors used computational techniques to predict regulatory effects of variants and assess the disease association via multi-marker models where the variants altering the same regulatory element (such as a transcription factor [TF] binding site) in the same cell line are grouped together.[40] See endnotes 20, 41, and 42 for other examples of functional analysis and follow-up studies of GWAS.

Association-Based Prioritization

Gene expression readout is widely used in order to identify genetic variants leading to a variation in the expression levels. eQTL studies,[43] where expression is regarded as a quantitative trait and associated with variants, provide us with a more comprehensive view of genomic loci and therefore enable the identification of regulatory roles of the variants in question. The evidence provided by the expression data can also be utilized in GWAS so that the variants significantly altering expression of genes are prioritized. For example, Arloth et al.[44] identified that the transcriptional response of glucocorticoid receptor (GR) is altered by the SNPs in enhancer regions. Alternatively, the enrichment of risk loci for eQTLs can easily be examined using publicly available, tissue-specific data sources such as GTEx,[45] which has already been applied to psychiatric disorders.[34]

In another study, Tehranchi et al.[46] proposed a high-throughput sequencing-based method to identify variants, called *binding QTLs* (bQTLs), altering the binding affinity of transcription factors, using a pooled ChIP-seq approach. This powerful method enables researchers to directly interrogate the effect of risk variants on binding affinity and their regulatory impact, by comparing allele frequencies before and after chromatin immunoprecipitation, which in turn provides additional evidence about the disease etiology.

A serious challenge in exploring GWAS data is presented by the genetic heterogeneity in human diseases. This means that different causal variants can usually be found in different patients. Two distinct definitions of genetic heterogeneity exist: (1) patients harbor different variants causing changes in the same gene, or (2) the variants are mutating different genes, located in the same protein complex or pathway.[55] Most post-GWAS analyses are based on mutated genes and disregard the fact that variants led to their formation. Here, we focus on the discussion of the latter part.

Studies have already shown that rare mutations play an important role in neuropsychiatric diseases like autism or schizophrenia.[56–58] Genetic heterogeneity, however, makes analyses of these variants difficult, as many of them are not localized on the same genes and therefore do not overlap each other. Network-based methods have been developed to circumvent this problem. They are used for the identification of new causal genes or even whole interaction pathways in a given network, as well as for stratification of complex diseases. Valuable information is thereby extracted through the interaction partners of known causal genes. For the construction of such networks, the already available knowledge of biological databases is commonly used.

Biological Databases and Interaction Networks

Various biological databases, including different kinds of molecular interactions, are available nowadays. These can be divided into two types of molecular networks: (1) interactome networks containing metabolic, protein–protein, and/or gene regulatory interactions; and (2) functional networks containing phenotypic profiling, transcriptional profiling, and/or genetic interactions.[59] In network-based GWAS analyses, protein–protein interaction (PPI) networks are most commonly used. For their generation, high-throughput experiments, computational predictions, and literature curations are important sources.[60]

Usually, interaction networks are represented as graphs in form of $G = (V, E)$. Thereby, vertices (V) display genes or proteins and edges (E); i.e., tuples of two vertices, represent directed or undirected interactions between them. The most widely used PPI networks are BIND,[61] HPRD,[62] MIPS,[63] BioGRID,[64] DIP,[65] MINT,[66] IntAct,[67] and STRING.[68] MINT and IntAct are now combined into MIntAct.[69] Finally, some meta-databases like iRefIndex,[70] PINA2,[71] PathwayCommons,[72] and ConsensusPathDB[73] exist, which unite several databases in one.

Although most of these databases are updated regularly, it is recommended to utilize the available information with caution. Often the data in PPI networks are static and do not reflect the spatial and temporal dependence of protein interactions in real biological systems. Also, many PPIs are derived from high-throughput experiments in vitro and do not include tissue-specific information. Some are obtained through methods that do not reflect the real environment, like the yeast two-hybrid (Y2H) screen, where the interactions are measured in yeast cells. This can lead to interactions that do not occur in real cellular conditions. Another bias is generated by the fact that some protein interactions are more interesting and therefore more often studied than others. Thus the PPI data are far from complete, and the given databases change with every update.[60] Fortunately, nonstop exertion is the reason why computational approaches of disease genes are possible.[74] Functional (indirect) interactions like tissue-specific gene co-expression, literature co-citation, and genetic interactions could be biologically relevant to diseases and traits and thus meaningful for the discovery of enriched GWAS signals.[60] A newly generated database called the Integrated Interaction Database (IID)[75] includes tissue-specific interactions, and a tool called miT-ALOS[76] applicable for tissue-specific pathway analysis of miRNAs could be useful for current or future GWAS analysis. In the following sections, we show how the information stored in biological networks can be used for further downstream analysis by providing a comprehensive overview of available methods. The described methods and tools are summarized in Table 10.2 and Table 10.3.

Network-Based Disease Gene Prioritization

Prediction methods for disease gene prioritization rely on the observation that candidate genes of a given interaction network lie in proximity to known disease genes. A distinction is made between two scoring strategies: (1) local (parameter-free or connectivity-based) methods, using direct interactions and shortest path information between new identified genes and known disease genes; and (2) global (parameter-based or information flow–based) methods, using diffusion of the gene signal along the network to capture the overall interaction network structure. An overview of the most widely used prediction methods is given in Table 10.2.

One of the easiest and earliest methods for disease gene prioritization is to assess the information about direct interaction partners, which Endeavour[77] and CIPHER[78] both implement. CIPHER also compared this method to another approach, which calculates the shortest path length. In the Prioritizer[79] tool, this method was solely used. The first global predictions taking the whole network structure into account were GeneWanderer[80] and RWRH,[81] ranking the genes by the probability that starting from a known disease gene, each candidate gene will be reached by a random walk. Similar approaches were used in the network propagation of PRINCE[82] and the t-smoothed statistics of stSVM.[83]

A modification of the PageRank algorithm of Google is used in NIMMI[87] to add a weight for each protein. In this process, proteins with many interactions are scored higher than proteins with fewer connections. The association

Table 10.2 Modified Table of [74] Including the Different Scoring Strategies to Measure Proximities of PPI Network Elements

Strategy	Method	Function	Description	Reference
Local	Direct interactions	$N = \left\{ \begin{array}{l} 1, \text{if } \exists E \\ 0, \text{otherwise} \end{array} \right\}$	The direct neighbors get a count of 1 for N, if two nodes are directly interacting and 0 otherwise	Aerts et al. [77], Wu et al. [78]
	Shortest path length	$D = L$, where $L = L'$	The distance D between two proteins is the shortest path length L, whereas L' corresponds to any random path between them.	Franke et al. [79], Wu et al. [78]
Global	Diffusion kernel	$K = e^{-\beta L}$	The diffusion kernel K acts like a lazy random walk, where β controls the magnitude of diffusion. The Laplacian matrix L is defined as the adjacency matrix subtracted from the diagonal degree matrix.	Köhler et al. [80]
	Random walk with restart	$p^t = (1-r)Wp^{t-1} + rp^0$	The random walk with restarts begins at a source node, walks randomly from interacting node to node, and restarts at the source node with probability r. W is the normalized adjacency matrix, and p^t the probability vector of being at the nodes at iteration t.	Köhler et al. [80], Li & Patra [81]
	Propagation flow	$F^t = \alpha W'F^{t-1} + (1-\alpha)F^0$	In the network propagation function, each node propagates the information from the previous iteration to the next interacting node. F^0 is the prior information, α the diffusion parameter, and W' the degree normalized adjacency matrix.	Vanunu et al. [82]

Table 10.2 Continued

Strategy	Method	Function	Description	Reference
	P-step random walk kernel	$K = (\alpha I - L^{norm})^p$	The p-step random walk kernel results in a similarity matrix including the degree of topological relatedness of the network nodes. It needs a normalized Laplacian matrix, a constant value of α, and p random walk steps.	Cun and Fröhlich [83]

signals from the GWAS data are combined with the calculated weights to identify interesting sub-networks.

In dmGWAS,[88] a dense module searching (DMS) algorithm is used to identify candidate sub-networks or genes for complex diseases. It integrates the association signals of the GWAS data with a human PPI network. Then the DMS finds sub-networks enriched with genes that possess low p-values. The extension EW_dmGWAS[89] also integrates gene-expression profiles to generate edge weights. These are combined with the node weights derived from GWAS signals to identify modules with a maximum score. Another enhancement, called STAMS,[90] integrates the STRING database and uses the EW_dmGWAS search function with a new specific score normalization to find causal sub-networks.

In DAPPLE,[91] the authors used a permutation method to avoid any connectivity bias in the given PPI data. To each interaction a probability score was assigned, based on its neighboring interactions, the scale of the experiment, and the number of publications the interaction was found in.

The network-based analysis of genetic associations (NETBAG)[92] algorithm and its extension NETBAG+[93] were used to identify sub-networks affected by rare de novo variants in children with autism and in schizophrenia patients, respectively. In both methods, a background likelihood network, onto which all causal genes are mapped, is built, and then a "greedy search" algorithm is used to find high-scoring sub-networks (clusters) by iteratively adding those genes that increase the score.

Another approach for the identification of causal sub-networks is HotNet,[94] which was tested on somatic mutations of different cancer types. The algorithm uses a heat diffusion process to measure the influence between pairs of genes in a network. It assigns heat to each node (gene) in proportion to its mutation frequency and diffuses the heat through edges (interactions) of the network to the neighboring nodes. Afterwards, the network is divided into subnetworks by removing cold edges.

An additional method uses co-function networks to identify sets of mutually functionally related genes spanning multiple GWA loci. This PrixFixe[95] algorithm uses tagSNPs reported by GWAS, associated with different cancer types, to act as seeds for Linkage disequilibrium (LD) based query regions. Then a defined co-function network (CFN) is used to identify dense "prix fixe" (PF) subnetworks. Dense subnetworks are aggregated and genes are scored based on the frequency and strength of identifying such functional connections. High-scoring genes are then used to find causal pathways and new candidate genes.

Network-Based Stratification of Complex Diseases

Stratification of patients possessing complex diseases is a promising method to understand the underlying biology of the disease. It is also crucial to generating a better tailored clinical treatment. At the moment, this process is not in clinical practice, but is rather applied on a research level. Some approaches without using any network information were developed for common diseases, such as the identification of gene combinations for disease risk stratification in type 1 diabetes[96-98] and the discovery of a new loci for sporadic-Parkinson's disease by GWAS stratification.[99] Approaches using networks for the stratification can only be found for cancer patients by grouping them into their molecular subtypes. One of these methods is the "network-based stratification method" (NBS),[100] which maps the somatic tumor mutation profiles of the patients onto an interaction network. With network propagation,[82] the gene signal is smoothed along the edges of the network and the profiles are grouped into subtypes using non-negative matrix factorization (NMF)[101] and consensus clustering. Network-assisted co-clustering for the identification of cancer subtypes (NCIS)[102] is another clustering algorithm for cancer subtype identification incorporating molecular interaction networks with gene expression data. It uses a modified PageRank algorithm and semi-non-negative matrix tri-factorization (SNMTF) to group samples and genes synchronally into biologically meaningful clusters. NBS and NCIS are specifically built for cancer tumor mutations; new or adapted methods for non-somatic mutations will hopefully follow soon.

Conclusion

Altogether, in this chapter we provided an overview of common methods for SNP prioritization and further post-GWAS network-based analysis techniques in the context of psychiatric diseases. Suitable tools for the analysis of genetic influences on diseases are published on a regular basis, and databases are updated or created constantly to raise the available knowledge to a higher level.

Table 10.3 Overview of All Network-Based Methods, Including the Used Prediction Algorithm, Tool Name, Databases and Genetic Data

Algorithmic Approach	Tool name	Integrated Databases	Genetic Data
a) Disease gene identification			
Direct neighbor	Endeavour [77]	BIND	Causal genes
Shortest path length	Prioritizer [79]	BIND, HPRD, Reactome, KEGG	Causal genes
Direct neighbor/ shortest path length	CIPHER [78]	HPRD, OPHID, BIND, MINT	Causal genes + phenome
Random walk with restarts	RWRH [81]	HPRD	Causal genes
Random walk with restarts/Diffusion kernel	GeneWanderer [80]	HPRD, BIND, BioGRID, IntAct, DIP, STRING	Causal genes
Propagation flow	PRINCE [82]	HPRD + large scale experiments	Causal genes + phenotype similarity scores
P-step random walk kernel	stSVM [83]	PathwayCommons, KEGG pathways	Gene expression data (cancer tumors)
b) Disease pathway identification			
General approach using z-scores	jActiveModules [84]	iRefIndex	Gene expression data or GWAS SNPs
Random walk with restarts	PINBPA [86]	iRefIndex	GWAS SNPs
PageRank algorithm	NIMMI [87]	BioGRID	GWAS SNPs
Dense module searching (DMS) + greedy heuristic	dmGWAS [88]	PINA (MINT, IntAct, DIP, BioGRID, HPRD, MIPS)	GWAS SNPs
	EW_dmGWAS [89]	PINA (MINT, IntAct, DIP, BioGRID, HPRD, MIPS)	GWAS SNPs + gene expression data
	STAMS [90]	STRING, KEGG	GWAS SNPs
Multiple permutation approaches	DAPPLE [91]	InWeb	SNPs from different analyses
Greedy heuristic	NETBAG [92]	BIND, BioGRID, DIP, HPRD, InNetDB, IntAct, BiGG, MINT and MIPS	De novo CNVs
	NETBAG + [93]	BIND, BioGRID, DIP, HPRD, InNetDB, IntAct, BiGG, MINT and MIPS	De novo CNVs, de novo SNVs, GWAS SNPs

(continued)

Table 10.3 Continued

Algorithmic Approach	Tool name	Integrated Databases	Genetic Data
Heat diffusion	HotNet [94]	HPRD	Nonsynonymous somatic mutations
—	PrixFixe [95]	Two existing human co-function networks (CFNs)	GWAS SNPs
c) Stratification of complex diseases			
Propagation flow	NBS [100]	STRING, HumanNet, PathwayCommons	Somatic mutation profiles
Random walk	NCIS [102]	HPRD, Reactome, MSKCC, PID, KEGG	Gene expression profiles

One of the next steps for the scientific community analyzing genetic traits is to learn to utilize this additional information and no longer rely on possibly outdated resources. The collection of tools, databases, and methods in the present chapter suggest a comprehensive selection of available techniques that could be used for detailed investigation of genetic influences in psychiatric disorders.

As a promising outlook, we again turn to high-throughput experiments that enabled us to widely annotate the genome. Apart from the positional information of genomic annotations, which is extensively used in overlap-based prioritization methods, there are also machine-learning methods relying on manual extraction of features from the sequence.[103–105] However, thanks to the latest advances in the field of neural networks, methods that can learn features directly from the sequence have also been proposed. For example, DeepBind,[106] DeepSEA,[51] Basset,[107] and DANQ[108] are such tools that can harness the sequential features of such annotated regions and therefore enable us to predict regulatory regions and protein-binding sites. These new-generation methods can remarkably predict the key regulatory factors in the genome just from the sequence with exceptionally high accuracy in a tissue-specific fashion. More importantly, predicting the regulatory factors differentially between reference and alternative alleles provides new ways of variant prioritization based on the regulatory impact of the variant. Clinical application of the sequence model-based variant prioritization techniques, however, is yet to be established. To address this, a novel method called DeepWAS[40] has been proposed. It probes the disease association of groups of variants with a significant regulatory impact in the context of a specific cell line and transcription factor using a multi-marker association method. Considering the fact that the vast majority of GWAS hits are non-coding variants, the DeepWAS study places the regulatory variants at the center of the association studies. Furthermore, application of the method to major depressive disorder (MDD) demonstrates its value in the analysis of psychiatric disorders.

References

1. Nielsen, A. C. (1980). Choosing psychiatry: The importance of psychiatric education in medical school. *American Journal of Psychiatry, 137*, 428–431.

2. Cameron, P., & Persad, E. (1984). Recruitment into psychiatry: a study of the timing and process of choosing psychiatry as a career. *Canadian Journal of Psychiatry, 29*, 676–680.

3. Cardno, A. G., Marshall, E. J., Coid, B., Macdonald, A. M., Ribchester, T. R., . . . Davies, N. J. (1999). Heritability estimates for psychotic disorders: the Maudsley twin psychosis series. *Archives of General Psychiatry, 56*, 162–168.

4. McGuffin, P., Rijsdijk, F., Andrew, M., Sham, P., Katz, R., & Cardno, A. (2003). The heritability of bipolar affective disorder and the genetic relationship to unipolar depression. *Archives of General Psychiatry, 60*, 497–502.

5. McGuffin, P., Farmer, A. E., Gottesman, I. I., Murray, R. M., & Reveley, A. M. (1984). Twin concordance for operationally defined schizophrenia. Confirmation of familiality and heritability. *Archives of General Psychiatry, 41*, 541–545.

6. McKinney, W. T. (2001). Overview of the past contributions of animal models and their changing place in psychiatry. *Seminars in Clinical Neuropsychiatry, 6*, 68–78.

7. Rutter, M., & Plomin, R. (1997). Opportunities for psychiatry from genetic findings. *British Journal of Psychiatry, 171*, 209–219.

8. Purcell, S., Cherny, S. S., & Sham, P. C. (2003). Genetic Power Calculator: design of linkage and association genetic mapping studies of complex traits. *Bioinformatics, 19*, 149–150.

9. Konneker, T., Barnes, T., Furberg, H., Losh, M., Bulik, C. M., & Sullivan, P. F. (2008). A searchable database of genetic evidence for psychiatric disorders. *American Journal of Medical Genetics, B, Neuropsychiatric Genetics, 147B*, 671–675.

10. Abel, O., Powell, J. F., Andersen, P. M., Al-Chalabi, A. (2012). ALSoD: A user-friendly online bioinformatics tool for amyotrophic lateral sclerosis genetics. *Human Mutation, 33*, 1345–1351.

11. Marx, V. (2013). Biology: The big challenges of big data. *Nature, 498*, 255–260.

12. Stephens, Z. D., Lee, S. Y., Faghri, F., Campbell, R. H., Zhai, C., . . . Efron, M. J. (2015). Big data: Astronomical or genomical? *PLoS Biology, 13*, e1002195.

13. Alawieh, A., Zaraket, F. A., Li J-L, Mondello, S., Nokkari, A., . . . Razafsha, M. (2012). Systems biology, bioinformatics, and biomarkers in neuropsychiatry. *Frontiers in Neuroscience, 6*, 187.

14. Schulze, T. G., Ohlraun, S., Czerski, P. M., Schumacher, J., Kassem, L., . . . Deschner, M. (2005). Genotype-phenotype studies in bipolar disorder showing association between the DAOA/G30 locus and persecutory delusions: A first step toward a molecular genetic classification of psychiatric phenotypes. *American Journal of Psychiatry, 162*, 2101–2108.

15. Cross-Disorder Group of the Psychiatric Genomics Consortium, Lee, S. H., Ripke, S., Neale, B. M., Faraone, S. V., . . . Purcell, S. M. (2013). Genetic relationship between five psychiatric disorders estimated from genome-wide SNPs. *Nature Genetics, 45*, 984–994.

16. Johnson, A. D., Handsaker, R. E., Pulit, S. L., Nizzari, M. M., O'Donnell, C. J., & de Bakker, P. I. W. (2008). SNAP: a web-based tool for identification and annotation of proxy SNPs using HapMap. *Bioinformatics*, *24*, 2938–2939.

17. Arnold, M., Raffler, J., Pfeufer, A., Suhre, K., & Kastenmüller, G. (2015). SNiPA: an interactive, genetic variant-centered annotation browser. *Bioinformatics*, *31*, 1334–1336.

18. Machiela, M. J., & Chanock, S. J. (2015). LDlink: a web-based application for exploring population-specific haplotype structure and linking correlated alleles of possible functional variants. *Bioinformatics*, *31*, 3555–3557.

19. Chelala, C., Khan, A., & Lemoine, N. R. (2009). SNPnexus: a web database for functional annotation of newly discovered and public domain single nucleotide polymorphisms. *Bioinformatics*, *25*, 655–661.

20. Edwards, S. L., Beesley, J., French, J. D., & Dunning, A. M. (2013). Beyond GWASs: illuminating the dark road from association to function. *American Journal of Human Genetics*, *93*, 779–797.

21. McCarthy, D. J., Humburg, P., Kanapin, A., Rivas, M. A., Gaulton, K., . . . Cazier, J.-B. (2014). Choice of transcripts and software has a large effect on variant annotation. *Genome Medicine*, *6*, 26.

22. Wang, K., Li, M., & Hakonarson, H. (2010). ANNOVAR: functional annotation of genetic variants from high-throughput sequencing data. *Nucleic Acids Research*, *38*, e164.

23. McLaren, W., Gil, L., Hunt, S. E., Riat, H. S., Ritchie, G. R. S., . . . Thormann, A. (2016). The Ensembl Variant Effect Predictor. *Genome Biology*, *17*, 122.

24. Paila, U., Chapman, B. A., Kirchner, R., & Quinlan, A. R. (2013). GEMINI: integrative exploration of genetic variation and genome annotations. *PLoS Computational Biology*, *9*, e1003153.

25. Ng, P. C., & Henikoff, S. (2003). SIFT: Predicting amino acid changes that affect protein function. *Nucleic Acids Research*, *31*, 3812–3814.

26. Adzhubei, I. A., Schmidt, S., Peshkin, L., Ramensky, V. E., Gerasimova, A., . . . Bork, P. (2010). A method and server for predicting damaging missense mutations. *Nature Methods*, *7*, 248–249.

27. Liu, J. Z., McRae, A. F., Nyholt, D. R., Medland, S. E., Wray, N. R., . . . Brown, K. M. (2010). A versatile gene-based test for genome-wide association studies. *American Journal of Human Genetics*, *87*, 139–145.

28. Otowa, T., Maher, B. S., Aggen, S. H., McClay, J. L., van den Oord, E. J., & Hettema, J. M. (2014). Genome-wide and gene-based association studies of anxiety disorders in European and African American samples. *PLoS One*, *9*, e112559.

29. Pers, T. H., Karjalainen, J. M., Chan, Y., Westra H-J, Wood, A. R., . . . Yang, J. (2015). Biological interpretation of genome-wide association studies using predicted gene functions. *Nature Communications*, *6*, 5890.

30. Lee, P. H., O'Dushlaine, C., Thomas, B., & Purcell, S. M. (2012). INRICH: interval-based enrichment analysis for genome-wide association studies. *Bioinformatics*, *28*, 1797–1799.

31. Raychaudhuri, S., Plenge, R. M., Rossin, E. J., Ng, A. C. Y., International Schizophrenia Consortium, . . . Purcell, S. M. (2009). Identifying relationships among genomic disease regions: predicting genes at pathogenic SNP associations and rare deletions. *PLoS Genetics*, *5*, e1000534.

32. Lee, P. H., Perlis, R. H., Jung J-Y, Byrne, E. M., Rueckert, E., . . . Siburian, R. (2012). Multi-locus genome-wide association analysis supports the role of glutamatergic synaptic transmission in the etiology of major depressive disorder. *Translational Psychiatry, 2*, e184.

33. Cross-Disorder Group of the Psychiatric Genomics Consortium. (2013). Identification of risk loci with shared effects on five major psychiatric disorders: a genome-wide analysis. *Lancet, 381*, 1371–1379.

34. Schizophrenia Working Group of the Psychiatric Genomics Consortium. (2014). Biological insights from 108 schizophrenia-associated genetic loci. *Nature, 511*, 421–427.

35. Gjoneska, E., Pfenning, A. R., Mathys, H., Quon, G., Kundaje, A., . . . Tsai, L.-H. (2015). Conserved epigenomic signals in mice and humans reveal immune basis of Alzheimer's disease. *Nature, 518*, 365–369.

36. Gagliano, S. A., Ptak, C., Mak, D. Y. F., Shamsi, M., Oh, G., . . . Knight, J. (2016). Allele-skewed DNA modification in the brain: Relevance to a schizophrenia GWAS. *American Journal of Human Genetics, 98*, 956–962.

37. Gagliano, S. A. (2016). It's all in the brain: A review of available functional genomic annotations. *Biological Psychiatry [Internet]*. Available from: http://dx.doi.org/10.1016/j.biopsych.2016.08.011.

38. Hauberg, M. E., Holm-Nielsen, M. H., Mattheisen, M., Askou, A. L., Grove, J., . . . Børglum, A. D. (2016). Schizophrenia risk variants affecting microRNA function and site-specific regulation of NT5C2 by miR-206. *European Neuropsychopharmacology, 26*, 1522–1526.

39. Wang, X., Tucker, N. R., Rizki, G., Mills, R., Krijger, P. H., de . . . Wit, E. (2016). Discovery and validation of sub-threshold genome-wide association study loci using epigenomic signatures. *eLife, 5*, e10557. doi:10.7554/eLife.10557. Available from: https://elifesciences.org/articles/10557.

40. Eraslan, G., Arloth, J., Martins, J., Iurato, S., Czamara, D., . . . Binder, E. B. (2016). DeepWAS: Directly integrating regulatory information into GWAS using deep learning supports master regulator MEF2C as risk factor for major depressive disorder [Internet]. *BioRxiv*. Available from: http://dx.doi.org/10.1101/069096.

41. Hou, L., & Zhao, H. (2013). A review of post-GWAS prioritization approaches. *Frontiers in Genetics, 4*, 280.

42. Tak, Y. G., & Farnham, P. J. (2015). Making sense of GWAS: using epigenomics and genome engineering to understand the functional relevance of SNPs in non-coding regions of the human genome. *Epigenetics & Chromatin, 8*, 57.

43. Gilad, Y., Rifkin, S. A., & Pritchard, J. K. (2008). Revealing the architecture of gene regulation: the promise of eQTL studies. *Trends in Genetics, 24*, 408–415.

44. Arloth, J., Bogdan, R., Weber, P., Frishman, G., Menke, A., . . . Wagner, K. V. (2015). Genetic differences in the immediate transcriptome response to stress predict risk-related brain function and psychiatric disorders. *Neuron, 86*, 1189–1202.

45. Melé, M., Ferreira, P. G., Reverter, F., DeLuca, D. S., Monlong, J., . . . Sammeth, M. (2015). Human genomics. The human transcriptome across tissues and individuals. *Science, 348*, 660–665.

46. Tehranchi, A. K., Myrthil, M., Martin, T., Hie, B. L., Golan, D., & Fraser, H. B. (2016). Pooled ChIP-Seq links variation in transcription factor binding to complex disease risk. *Cell, 165*, 730–741.

47. Ward, L. D., & Kellis, M. (2016). HaploReg v4: systematic mining of putative causal variants, cell types, regulators and target genes for human complex traits and disease. *Nucleic Acids Research*, *44*, D877–D881.

48. Boyle, A. P., Hong, E. L., Hariharan, M., Cheng, Y., Schaub, M. A., . . . Kasowski, M. (2012). Annotation of functional variation in personal genomes using RegulomeDB. *Genome Research*, *22*, 1790–1797.

49. Li, M. J., Wang, L. Y., Xia, Z., Sham, P. C., & Wang, J. (2013). GWAS3D: Detecting human regulatory variants by integrative analysis of genome-wide associations, chromosome interactions and histone modifications. *Nucleic Acids Research*, *41*, W150–W158.

50. Coetzee, S. G., Rhie, S. K., Berman, B. P., Coetzee, G. A., & Noushmehr, H. (2012). FunciSNP: an R/bioconductor tool integrating functional non-coding data sets with genetic association studies to identify candidate regulatory SNPs. *Nucleic Acids Research*, *40*, e139.

51. Zhou, J., & Troyanskaya, O. G. (2015). Predicting effects of noncoding variants with deep learning–based sequence model. *Nature Methods*, *12*, 931–934.

52. Kircher, M., Witten, D. M., Jain, P., O'Roak, B. J., Cooper, G. M., & Shendure, J. (2014). A general framework for estimating the relative pathogenicity of human genetic variants. *Nature Genetics*, *46*, 310–315.

53. Davydov, E. V., Goode, D. L., Sirota, M., Cooper, G. M., Sidow, A., & Batzoglou, S. (2010). Identifying a high fraction of the human genome to be under selective constraint using GERP ++. *PLoS Computational Biology*, *6*, e1001025.

54. Lu, Q., Yao, X., Hu, Y., & Zhao, H. (2016). GenoWAP: GWAS signal prioritization through integrated analysis of genomic functional annotation. *Bioinformatics*, *32*, 542–548.

55. Leiserson, M. D. M., Eldridge, J. V., Ramachandran, S., & Raphael, B. J. (2013). Network analysis of GWAS data. *Current Opinion in Genetics & Development*, *23*, 602–610.

56. Bucan, M., Abrahams, B. S., Wang, K., Glessner, J. T., Herman, E. I., . . . Sonnenblick, L. I. (2009). Genome-wide analyses of exonic copy number variants in a family-based study point to novel autism susceptibility genes. *PLoS Genetics*, *5*, e1000536.

57. Walsh, T., McClellan, J. M., McCarthy, S. E., Addington, A. M., Pierce, S. B., . . . Cooper, G. M. (2008). Rare structural variants disrupt multiple genes in neurodevelopmental pathways in schizophrenia. *Science*, *320*, 539–543.

58. McClellan, J., & King, M.-C. (2010). Genetic heterogeneity in human disease. *Cell*, *141*, 210–217.

59. Vidal, M., Cusick, M. E., & Barabási A-L. (2011). Interactome networks and human disease. *Cell*, *144*, 986–998.

60. Jia, P., & Zhao, Z. (2014). Network-assisted analysis to prioritize GWAS results: principles, methods and perspectives. *Human Genetics*, *133*, 125–138.

61. Bader, G. D. (2003). BIND: the Biomolecular Interaction Network Database. *Nucleic Acids Research*, *31*, 248–250.

62. Mishra, G. R. (2006). Human protein reference database—2006 update. *Nucleic Acids Research*, *34*, D411–4.

63. Pagel, P., Kovac, S., Oesterheld, M., Brauner, B., Dunger-Kaltenbach, I., . . . Frishman, G. (2004). The MIPS mammalian protein-protein interaction database. *Bioinformatics*, *21*, 832–834.

64. Stark, C., Breitkreutz B-J, Reguly, T., Boucher, L., Breitkreutz, A., & Tyers, M. (2006). BioGRID: a general repository for interaction datasets. *Nucleic Acids Research, 34,* D535–D539.

65. Salwinski, L. (2004). The Database of Interacting Proteins: 2004 update. *Nucleic Acids Research, 32,* 449D–451.

66. Licata, L., Briganti, L., Peluso, D., Perfetto, L., Iannuccelli, M., . . . Galeota, E. (2012). MINT, the molecular interaction database: 2012 update. *Nucleic Acids Research, 40,* D857–861.

67. Kerrien, S., Aranda, B., Breuza, L., Bridge, A., Broackes-Carter, F., . . . Chen, C. (2012). The IntAct molecular interaction database in 2012. *Nucleic Acids Research, 40,* D841–6.

68. Szklarczyk, D., Franceschini, A., Wyder, S., Forslund, K., Heller, D., Huerta- . . . Cepas, J. (2015). STRING v10: protein-protein interaction networks, integrated over the tree of life. *Nucleic Acids Research, 43,* D447–452.

69. Licata, L., & Orchard, S. (2016). The MIntAct Project and Molecular Interaction databases. *Methods in Molecular Biology, 1415,* 55–69.

70. Razick, S., Magklaras, G., & Donaldson, I. M. (2008). iRefIndex: a consolidated protein interaction database with provenance. *BMC Bioinformatics, 9,* 405.

71. Cowley, M. J., Pinese, M., Kassahn, K. S., Waddell, N., Pearson, J. V., . . . Grimmond, S. M. (2011). PINA v2.0: mining interactome modules. *Nucleic Acids Research, 40,* D862–5.

72. Cerami, E. G., Gross, B. E., Demir, E., Rodchenkov, I., Babur, O., . . . Anwar, N. (2010). Pathway Commons, a web resource for biological pathway data. *Nucleic Acids Research, 39,* D685–690.

73. Kamburov, A., Stelzl, U., Lehrach, H., & Herwig, R. (2013). The ConsensusPathDB interaction database: 2013 update. *Nucleic Acids Research, 41,* D793–800.

74. Wang, X., Gulbahce, N., & Yu, H. (2011). Network-based methods for human disease gene prediction. Brief. Funct. *Genomics.*10:280–293.

75. Kotlyar, M., Pastrello, C., Sheahan, N., & Jurisica, I. (2016). Integrated interactions database: tissue-specific view of the human and model organism interactomes. *Nucleic Acids Research, 44,* D536–541.

76. Preusse, M., Theis, F. J., & Mueller, N. S. (2016). miTALOS v2: Analyzing tissue specific microRNA function. *PLoS One, 11,* e0151771.

77. Aerts, S., Lambrechts, D., Maity, S., Van Loo, P., Coessens, B., De . . . Smet, F. (2006). Gene prioritization through genomic data fusion. *Nature Biotechnology, 24,* 537–544.

78. Wu, X., Jiang, R., Zhang, M. Q., & Li, S. (2008). Network-based global inference of human disease genes. *Molecular Systems Biology, 4,* 189.

79. Franke, L., van Bakel, H., Fokkens, L., de Jong, E. D., Egmont-Petersen, M., & Wijmenga, C. (2006). Reconstruction of a functional human gene network, with an application for prioritizing positional candidate genes. *American Journal of Human Genetics, 78,* 1011–1025.

80. Köhler, S., Bauer, S., Horn, D., & Robinson, P. N. (2008). Walking the interactome for prioritization of candidate disease genes. *American Journal of Human Genetics, 82,* 949–958.

81. Li, Y., & Patra, J. C. (2010). Genome-wide inferring gene-phenotype relationship by walking on the heterogeneous network. *Bioinformatics, 26,* 1219–1224.

82. Vanunu, O., Magger, O., Ruppin, E., Shlomi, T., & Sharan, R. (2010). Associating genes and protein complexes with disease via network propagation. *PLoS Computational Biology, 6*, e1000641.

83. Cun, Y., & Fröhlich, H. (2013). Network and data integration for biomarker signature discovery via network smoothed T-statistics. *PLoS One, 8*, e73074.

84. Ideker, T., Ozier, O., Schwikowski, B., & Siegel, A. F. (2002). Discovering regulatory and signalling circuits in molecular interaction networks. *Bioinformatics, 18*(Suppl 1), S233–240.

85. Cline, M. S., Smoot, M., Cerami, E., Kuchinsky, A., Landys, N., . . . Workman, C. (2007). Integration of biological networks and gene expression data using Cytoscape. *Nature Protocols, 2*, 2366–2382.

86. Wang, L., Matsushita, T., Madireddy, L., Mousavi, P., & Baranzini, S. E. (2015). PINBPA: cytoscape app for network analysis of GWAS data. *Bioinformatics, 31*, 262–264.

87. Akula, N., Baranova, A., Seto, D., Solka, J., Nalls, M. A., . . . Singleton, A. (2011). A network-based approach to prioritize results from genome-wide association studies. *PLoS One, 6*, e24220.

88. Jia, P., Zheng, S., Long, J., Zheng, W., & Zhao, Z. (2011). dmGWAS: dense module searching for genome-wide association studies in protein-protein interaction networks. *Bioinformatics, 27*, 95–102.

89. Wang, Q., Yu, H., Zhao, Z., & Jia, P. (2015). EW_dmGWAS: edge-weighted dense module search for genome-wide association studies and gene expression profiles. *Bioinformatics, 31*, 2591–2594.

90. Hillenmeyer, S., Davis, L. K., Gamazon, E. R., Cook, E. H., Cox, N. J., & Altman, R. B. (2016). STAMS: STRING-assisted module search for genome wide association studies and application to autism. *Bioinformatics [Internet]*, Available from: http://dx.doi.org/10.1093/bioinformatics/btw530

91. Rossin, E. J., Lage, K., Raychaudhuri, S., Xavier, R. J., Tatar, D., . . . Benita, Y. (2011). Proteins encoded in genomic regions associated with immune-mediated disease physically interact and suggest underlying biology. *PLoS Genetics, 7*, e1001273.

92. Gilman, S. R., Iossifov, I., Levy, D., Ronemus, M., Wigler, M., & Vitkup, D. (2011). Rare de novo variants associated with autism implicate a large functional network of genes involved in formation and function of synapses. *Neuron, 70*, 898–907.

93. Gilman, S. R., Chang, J., Xu, B., Bawa, T. S., Gogos, J. A., . . . Karayiorgou, M. (2012). Diverse types of genetic variation converge on functional gene networks involved in schizophrenia. *Nature Neuroscience, 15*, 1723–1728.

94. Vandin, F., Upfal, E., & Raphael, B. J. (2011). Algorithms for detecting significantly mutated pathways in cancer. *Journal of Computational Biology, 18*, 507–522.

95. Taşan, M., Musso, G., Hao, T., Vidal, M., MacRae, C. A., & Roth, F. P. (2015). Selecting causal genes from genome-wide association studies via functionally coherent subnetworks. *Nature Methods, 12*, 154–159.

96. Winkler, C., Krumsiek, J., Lempainen, J., Achenbach, P., Grallert, H., . . . Giannopoulou, E. (2012). A strategy for combining minor genetic susceptibility genes to improve prediction of disease in type 1 diabetes. *Genes & Immunity, 13*, 549–555.

97. Winkler, C., Krumsiek, J., Buettner, F., Angermüller, C., Giannopoulou, E. Z., . . . Theis, F. J. (2014). Feature ranking of type 1 diabetes susceptibility genes improves prediction of type 1 diabetes. *Diabetologia*, *57*, 2521–2529.

98. Winkler, C., Krumsiek, J., Buettner, F., Angermüller, C., Giannopoulou, E. Z., . . . Theis, F. J. (2015). Erratum to: Feature ranking of type 1 diabetes susceptibility genes improves prediction of type 1 diabetes. *Diabetologia*,58:206.

99. Hill-Burns, E. M., Wissemann, W. T., Hamza, T. H., Factor, S. A., Zabetian, C. P., & Payami, H. (2014). Identification of a novel Parkinson's disease locus via stratified genome-wide association study. *BMC Genomics*, *15*, 118.

100. Hofree, M., Shen, J. P., Carter, H., Gross, A., & Ideker, T. (2013). Network-based stratification of tumor mutations. *Nature Methods*, *10*, 1108–1115.

101. Hartsperger, M. L., Blöchl, F., Stümpflen, V., & Theis, F. J. (2010). Structuring heterogeneous biological information using fuzzy clustering of k-partite graphs. *BMC Bioinformatics*, *11*, 522.

102. Liu, Y., Gu, Q., Hou, J. P., Han, J., & Ma, J. (2014). A network-assisted co-clustering algorithm to discover cancer subtypes based on gene expression. *BMC Bioinformatics*, *15*, 37.

103. Ghandi, M., Lee, D., Mohammad-Noori, M., & Beer, M. A. (2014). Enhanced regulatory sequence prediction using gapped k-mer features. *PLoS Computational Biology*, *10*, e1003711.

104. Ghandi, M., Mohammad-Noori, M., Ghareghani, N., Lee, D., Garraway, L., & Beer, M. A. (2016). gkmSVM: an R package for gapped-kmer SVM. *Bioinformatics*, *32*, 2205–2207.

105. Lee, D. (2016). LS-GKM: a new gkm-SVM for large-scale datasets. *Bioinformatics*, *32*, 2196–2198.

106. Alipanahi, B., Delong, A., Weirauch, M. T., & Frey, B. J. (2015). Predicting the sequence specificities of DNA- and RNA-binding proteins by deep learning. *Nature Biotechnology*, *33*, 831–838.

107. Kelley, D. R., Snoek, J., & Rinn, J. L. (2016). Basset: learning the regulatory code of the accessible genome with deep convolutional neural networks. *Genome Research*, *26*, 990–999.

108. Quang, D., & Xie, X. (2016). DanQ: a hybrid convolutional and recurrent deep neural network for quantifying the function of DNA sequences. *Nucleic Acids Research*, *44*, e107.

Chapter 11

Epigenomic Exploration of the Human Brain

Tobias B. Halene, Gregor Hasler, Amanda Mitchell, and Schahram Akbarian

Take-Home Points

1. Epigenetic landscapes in human brain cells remain plastic throughout the human lifespan.
2. Ongoing dynamic regulation occurs even in neurons and other post-mitotic cells.
3. Defective chromatin structure is responsible for a range of neurological disorders and a subset of cases with psychosis, dementia, and other degenerative conditions.
4. DNA sequence analysis alone will not uncover the functional impact of disease-relevant mutations without epigenetic exploration.
5. Chromatin-modifying drugs could improve treatment for neurological and psychiatric disease.

Introduction

Even today, most psychiatric disorders lack an explanatory molecular or cellular pathology. In most cases, they are likely to be the consequence of a multifactorial etiology with numerous environmental and genetic components.

Despite significant overlap, clinicians and researcher still classify these disorders into distinct (*Diagnostic and Statistical Manual* [DSM]) categories. Considering that conventional medications elicit a sufficient therapeutic response in only 50% or less of patients diagnosed with schizophrenia,[1] or depression and anxiety,[2,3] we are left with the formidable challenge of understanding the pathophysiology of unique human diseases and developing safe and efficient therapies that actually work for the majority of patients.

Although serendipity played a major role in the discovery of every major psychiatric drug class that was discovered in the last century (lithium, chlorpromazine, iproniazid, etc.), the way we practice medicine has changed: we can no longer expect discoveries resulting from careful months-long observation of institutionalized patients because length of stay continues to decrease.

144

Instead, we strive to take the knowledge gained from basic science research from bench to bedside.

One promising direction in neuroscience research is epigenetics,[4] which has—for at least 15 years—piqued the interest of neuroscientists and psychiatrists, so that even popular scientific literature has caught on to the trend. Epigenetics is the tempting proposition that environment and experience can leave a lasting mark in our bodies, a welcome alternative to the rather dull prospect of genetic determinism.

On a more concrete level, this is because human and animal brain studies have shown that many epigenetic markings, including DNA methylation and various histone modifications, remain "plastic" throughout the human lifespan, with ongoing dynamic regulation even in neurons and other differentiated cells once believed to be set in stone after birth. Changing neuronal activity, learning and memory, and numerous other processes all have been shown to be associated with DNA methylation and histone modification and histone variant changes at specific genomic sequences in brain chromatin.[5–7]

Clinical genetic findings from genetic syndromes with a single causative mutation show that the disrupted protein often regulates chromatin structure and function,[8] an indication that the brain indeed is sensitive to dysregulation of the epigenetic machinery. Such types of mutations even have been linked to cases of adult-onset psychosis or dementia,[8] so that neurological and psychiatric conditions could conceivably arise from more widespread chromatin defects affecting the immature brain.

By mapping and superimposing epigenomic landscapes of brain cells with the genetic risk architecture of common psychiatric disease such as schizophrenia, we are starting to decipher the disease-relevant function for a growing number of non-coding sequences that do not code for proteins but harbor mutations for psychiatric disorders. New insight into structure and function of the genome in brain disorders will probably also come from the description of chromosomal loopings and other features of the three-dimensional genome.[9,10] In this chapter, we will touch upon each point after a concise introduction into the various markings and molecules that make the epigenome.

The Epigenome—General Principles

The medley of covalent DNA and histone modifications and variant histones provides the major building blocks for the "epigenome" and forms the epigenetic landscapes that define the functional architecture of the genome, including its organization into many tens of thousands of transcriptional units, clusters of condensed chromatin, and other features that are differentially regulated in different cell types and developmental stages of the organism.[11–13] Several reviews provide excellent starting points for the reader interested to learn more.[14–17]

Common Technical Terms Used in Chromatin Studies

(i) *Nucleosomes:* the elementary unit of chromatin, 146 base pairs of genomic DNA wrapped around an octamer of core histones like a thread wrapped around a spool. Nucleosomes are connected by linker DNA and linker histones. Transcription start sites are often located in a nucleosome-free interval DNA, thought to ease access of the transcriptional initiation complex and other regulators of gene expression.

(ii) *Euchromatin:* lightly packed chromatin, typically at sites of actively transcribed genes and units poised for transcription.

(iii) *Heterochromatin*: tightly packed chromatin. Constitutive heterochromatin (e.g., pericentric and telomeric repeat DNA or the inactivated X-chromosome of female somatic cells and other chromosomal structures often found in close proximity to the nuclear envelope and also around the nucleolus). Facultative heterochromatin includes silenced genes that can switch to a state of active transcription upon differentiation or other stimuli (see Figure 11.1).

Key Players of the Epigenetic Landscape

(i) *DNA methylation*: One of several epigenetic mechanisms to control gene expression. The major forms of DNA methylation in the human brain are DNA cytosine C5 modifications, primarily the methylation (m) and hydroxymethylation (hm) of cytosines in CpG dinucleotides. Both provide the bulk of epigenetic modifications in vertebrate DNA.[18] While both methylation and hydroxymethylation are most frequently encountered at the site of CpG dinucleotides, there are many methylated sites of non-CpG cytosine dinucleotides methylated in brain tissue.[19] Interestingly, many studies report promoter DNA methylation changes in preclinical models of psychosis, depression, and addiction, as well as in brain tissue from human subjects diagnosed with one of these conditions. For recent overviews on DNA methylation and hydroxymethylation in the context of human brain development and disease, see references 20 and 21. Other recently discovered or yet incompletely understood modifications are DNA N(6) adenine methylation[22] and N(6)methyladenosine.[23]

(ii) *Histone modifications:* Chemical histone modification is much more complex than DNA methylation. It is now thought that there are far more than 100 amino acid residue-specific post-translational modifications (PTMs) in a typical vertebrate cell.[24,25] For an overview on the principle, see Figure 11.1. It is important to emphasize that histone PTM rarely occur in isolation; instead, multiple histone PTM appear to be co-regulated and, as a group, define chromatin states,[26] adding further complexity to an already high number of epigenetic regulators. Many active promoters, for example, are defined by high levels of histone H3 lysine 4 methylation and various histone lysine acetylation markings.[14]

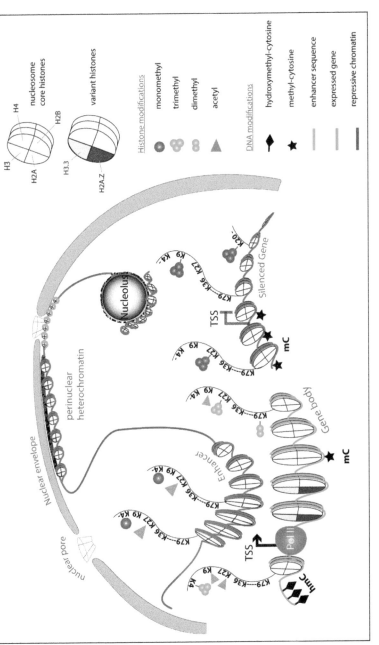

Figure 11.1 The epigenome from nucleus to nucleosome: Schematic illustration of (green) gene poised for transcription by polymerase II (Pol II) initiation complex, with nucleosome free interval at transcription start site (TSS). Distal enhancer sequence (blue) which in loop-like structure moves in close proximity to active gene. Red marks a small subset of heterochromatic portions of the genome, including silenced gene and heterochromatic structures bordering the nuclear envelope and pore complex, and also the nucleolar periphery. A small subset of representative histone variants and histone H3 site-specific lysine (K) residues at N-terminal tail and H4K20 residue are shown as indicated, together with panel of mono- and trimethyl-, or acetyl modifications that differentiate between active promoters, transcribed gene bodies, and repressive chromatin, as indicated. DNA cytosines that are hydroxyl-methylated at the C5 position are mostly found at active promoters, while methylated cytosines are positioned within the body of actively transcribed genes and around repressed promoters and in constitutive heterochromatin.

(iii) *Histone variants*: In addition to the core histones H2A/H2B/H3/H4, histone variants exist (see Figure 11.1). The role of these variant histones—which differ from the canonical histone only at a very few amino acid positions—is often discussed in the context of replication-independent expression and assembly,[27] and several histone variants robustly affect nucleosome stability and compaction.[28] Recent studies have shown that replication-independent turnover of nucleosomes provides a highly dynamic regulatory mechanism throughout the brain's entire lifespan, with two specific histone variants H3.3 and H2A.Z assigned with an essential role in learning and synaptic plasticity.[7,29,30]

(iv) *The epigenome is packaged into higher order chromatin structures*: The epigenetic decorations described here would fall short of adequately describing the chromatin architecture at a given genomic locus, let alone the entire epigenome. This is because organizing DNA into nucleosomes only increases packaging density sevenfold compared to naked DNA, whereas the actual packaging density in the interphase nucleus is about three orders of magnitude higher.[31] Chromosomal arrangements in the interphase nucleus are not random. Loci of active gene expression are more likely to be clustered together and positioned towards a central position within the nucleus, while heterochromatin and silenced loci can be found towards the nuclear periphery.[32,33] Chromatin forms loopings that are highly structured and associated with transcriptional regulation. Surprisingly, distal regulatory elements such as enhancers or silencers, hundreds of kilobases apart from a gene promoter on the linear genome, interact directly with that specific promoter by forming a loop.[34,35] Three-dimensional chromatin architectures are commonly mapped using derivatives of chromosome conformation capture (3C).[36] Importantly, 3C and other techniques that measure interaction and spatial proximity of non-contiguous DNA elements in brain cells are feasible techniques with postmortem brain tissue[37,38] and are therefore attractive approaches to studying dynamic changes of the 3D genome in the context of brain development and psychiatric disease. Indeed, chromosomal loop-bound regulatory elements appear to link non-coding DNA and the genetic risk architecture of schizophrenia.[99]

Lifelong Plasticity of Brain Epigenomes

Most, or perhaps all, epigenetic markings are likely to be reversible even in post-mitotic cells, and subject to bidirectional regulation. There is no *a priori* reason for a specific epigenetic mark to only accumulate while the brain is maturing and aging.[39–44] Instead, chromatin markings appear to remain plastic throughout the lifespan of the human brain, with implications for the neurobiology of psychiatric disease. Human cerebral cortex, for example, shows complex and gene-specific changes in the amount of methylcytosine (mC5 = cytosine methylated at the carbon 5 position). There is a fast rise in mC5 at many promoters during the transition from peri- to postnatal age that then continues at a slower pace into old age in conjunction with subtle changes in expression of transcripts originating from these promoters.[45–48] Such age-related epigenetic drifts could contribute to vulnerability to neuropsychiatric disease, including schizophrenia.[48]

The epigenetic landscapes of histone modifications also undergo substantial reorganization across the lifespan of the human brain. For example, histone methylation markings that differentiate between open and repressive chromatin surrounding N-methyl-D-aspartate receptor gene promoters show highly dynamic changes in cerebellar cortex during the transition from perinatal stages and infancy to adulthood[49] that reflect, in part, development changes in the corresponding gene transcripts.[50] Furthermore, hundreds of loci undergo histone methylation changes in cortical neurons during the first few years of life,[44] and there is strong and steady accumulation of variant histones such as H3.3 during childhood years, while levels essentially plateau around adolescence.[7]

Post-traumatic stress disorder (PTSD) can illustrate the explanatory appeal of epigenetics for the pathophysiology of psychiatric disease. Epigenetic markers inside the nuclei of neurons and glia serving memory function could convey lasting alterations in a subject's emotional and physical health and resilience toward an "environmental" stimulus (e.g., trauma).[51] For example, a recent study on peripheral cells collected pre- and post-deployment from U.S. military service members identified global DNA methylation levels in repetitive DNA sequences, including LINE-1 and Alu repeat elements, as biomarkers that were significantly associated with resilience or, conversely, vulnerability to PTSD.[52] Similarly, studies in civilian/urban populations discovered that changes in blood DNA methylation signatures in PTSD subjects selectively affected cytokine and steroid signaling, immune defense, and inflammation-related genes, which is consistent with several lines of evidence implicating peripheral immune dysregulation in this disorder.[53,54] Based on the aforementioned studies in blood, one would predict that brain chromatin is also involved in the neurobiology of PTSD. Human postmortem brain does show distinct DNA and histone methylation changes in amygdala and hippocampus, ventral striatum, and other anatomical structures with a critical role for emotion, affect, and memory.[51] Indeed, there is excessive methylation of the glucocorticoid receptor gene promoter NR3C1 and ribosomal DNA repeats in the hippocampus of adult suicide victims who also suffered childhood abuse.[55,56] In peripheral tissue of Holocaust survivors, methylation of the stress-sensitive gene FK506 binding protein was altered, with potential for intergenerational transmission to offspring after the preconception trauma of the survivor.[57] Potentially long-lasting epigenetic changes have also been reported at hundreds of loci in blood cells of subjects who suffered from severe malnutrition in early childhood.[58]

While postmortem brain samples of psychiatric disease cases are notoriously hampered by the fact that most subjects received psychoactive medication prior to death, evidence from animal studies suggests that at least a subset of the chromatin changes in diseased brain are not mere epiphenomena due to medication or postmortem confounds such as tissue autolysis, but have close associations with the disease process. To mention just two examples, the hippocampal glucocorticoid receptor gene *Nr3c1* shows excessive methylation not only in patients,[55] but also in adults rats brought up with suboptimal maternal[59] and other types of early life stress.[60] Similarly, chronic social defeat stress in mice and rats elicits histone acetylation changes in ventral striatum and hippocampus akin to those encountered in depressed human subjects.[61–63]

Monogenetic Etiologies of Neuropsychiatric Disease Include Mutations in Proteins Involved in Reading, Writing, or Erasure of Epigenetic Markings

Hundreds of genes encode proteins that either write, erase, or read the molecular marks of the epigenome[64,65]; however, we want to stress that some experts feel this type of terminology can be misleading, especially because the regulation of many epigenetic markings could turn out to be only a "cog" in the chromatin remodeling machinery and not a key driver.[66] The genome encodes three DNA methyltransferases, *DNMT1, DNMT3a, DNMT3b*, that establish and maintain DNA methylation markings. The collective set of reader, writer, and eraser proteins includes at least 15 genes associated with monogenetic forms of neurodevelopmental or adult-onset neuropsychiatric disease.[8] While an exhaustive discussion would be beyond the scope of this chapter, it is important to note that until recently, chromatin defects in the brain were considered static, early developmental lesions in the context of rare genetic syndromes. It is now clear that mutations and maladaptation of the epigenetic machinery cover a much wider continuum, including adult-onset neurodegenerative disease. For example, while partial loss-of-function mutations in the DNA methyltransferase *DNMT3B* were already known to cause a multi-organ syndrome called ICF 1 (Immunodeficiency, Centromere instability, Facial anomalies), which includes mental retardation and defective brain development,[67,68] it was only recently discovered that select mutations in DNA methyltransferase coding regions, including *DNMT1*, are responsible for some cases of hereditary sensory and autonomic neuropathy, type 1 (HSAN1),[69] a rare neurodegenerative condition characterized by various neuropathies and early onset. In other pedigrees, *DNMT1* mutations were linked to narcolepsy and late-onset deafness and cerebellar ataxia.[70] Likewise, structural variants in the X-linked gene *MECP2*, encoding the methyl-CpG-binding protein 2, not only cause Rett syndrome (RTT), a disorder of early childhood associated with cognitive deficits and a broad range of neurological symptoms,[71,72] but are thought to be responsible for some cases of autism and schizophrenia as well.[73] Furthermore, DNA variants and mutations encompassing the

KMT1D gene (9q34.3), encoding a histone H3-lysine 9 specific methyltransferase were initially recognized as the causative genes responsible for a distinct neurodevelopmental and multi-organ syndrome (Kleefstra mental retardation syndrome).[74] Meanwhile, *KMT1D* mutations are also responsible for some cases with schizophrenia,[75] various nonspecific psychiatric phenotypes, and even neurodegenerative disease in the post-adolescence period.[76] Mutations within the coding sequence can affect expression levels of a set of regulatory proteins involved in DNA or histone methylation and could cause neuropsychiatric disease even after brain development has largely been completed, including some cases diagnosed with psychosis or early-onset dementia. One could speculate that *DNMT1, MECP2, KMT1D, KMT2F,* and other monogenetic causes of neuropsychiatric disease[8] could then also play a wider role in the pathophysiology of autism, schizophrenia, and other illnesses, outside of the previously discussed and among the overall population of psychiatric patients cases with mutations and deletions of these chromatin regulatory proteins.

Epigenomic Studies in Diseased Postmortem Brain

Researchers currently invest considerable effort and resources in exploring the molecular pathology of common psychiatric disorders for which postmortem brain collections exist, including autism, schizophrenia, and depression. All lack a unifying neuropathology, but dysregulated gene expression in cerebral cortex and other brain regions is likely to play a role. For schizophrenia, comparison of tissue from diseased cases and controls led to a large number of studies that collectively suggested altered expression of a distinct set of gene transcripts in at least a subset of disease cases. For schizophrenia and mood disorders, well-known examples involve transcripts for GABA-ergic inhibitory signaling, or myelination and other oligodendrocyte-specific function; more generalized metabolic pathways, as well as many markers of pre- and postsynaptic neurotransmission.[77-91] Again, the vast majority of these transcriptional alterations are subtle and not uniformly encountered. Furthermore, most postmortem brain studies are conducted with small sample sizes of often far fewer than 100 brains, which is not ideal, given the heterogeneity of molecular pathologies. For other disorders, including autism, the available number of postmortem brains for research is very limited. To overcome some of these limitations, research initiatives such as "PsychENCODE" bundle resources and share data to map cortical transcriptomes and epigenomes of hundreds of brains diagnosed with schizophrenia and other common psychiatric disease, and controls.[92] Interestingly, exome-sequencing studies involving more than 600 cases with schizophrenia are beginning to identify groups of genes, including, for example, regulators of postsynaptic glutamatergic signaling, that show increased mutational burden in disease cases.[93]

Epigenomic Profiling to Assign Potential Function to Disease-Associated DNA Structural Variants and Polymorphisms Outside of Protein Coding Sequences

A significant portion of disease-associated mutations and polymorphisms is thought to affect sequences that code for "function" rather than a protein. The challenge here is that the analysis of DNA sequence gives little information about "normal" function, and that single-nucleotide polymorphisms (SNPs) identified by genome-wide association are usually a block of sequence harboring multiple SNPs without clear information about which one contributes to disease risk. The promise of epigenetic studies is to identify active regulation (e.g., DNA methylation, histone modifications, non-coding transcript, transcription factor binding site, etc.) or specific spatial conformations (e.g., promoter-enhancer loopings) at the site of non-coding DNA within a risk haplotype, which could assign chromatin-regulatory function.

An early example was *GAD1* encoding glutamic acid decarboxylase (67KDa) GABA synthesis enzyme: *GAD1* haplotypes and polymorphisms, positioned within few Kb from the gene transcription start site, confer genetic risk for accelerated loss of frontal lobe gray matter[94,95] and, via epistatic interaction with catechol-o-methyltransferase (*COMT*) alleles, regulate synaptic dopamine and modulate overall GABA tissue levels in the prefrontal cortex.[96] Such types of genetic variants surrounding the *GAD1* promoter appear to contribute to the disease-related decline in *GAD67* transcript and affect epigenetic regulation of the proximal *GAD1* promoter in subjects with schizophrenia postmortem brain, including the balance between "open" and "repressive" histone methylation markings histone H3 trimethyl-lysines, K4me3 and K27me3.[97] Moreover, chromosomal conformations at the *GAD1* locus include 50kb loop formations that carry enhancer elements enriched with transcription factor motifs into physical proximity of the *GAD1* gene promoter, and these loops could be disrupted in the prefrontal cortex of some subjects with schizophrenia,[98] where they would contribute to decreased gene expression and deficits in open chromatin-associated histone H3-lysine 4 methylation.[97,98] It is thought that proper *GAD1* expression is important for cortical inhibitory circuitry and synchronization of cortical networks.[99,100] Therefore, the reported epigenomic alterations at the *GAD1* promoter and the concurrent changes in local chromosomal promoter-enhancer loopings[98] speak to the disease-relevant role of epigenomic dysregulation in brains of subjects diagnosed with psychosis.

Another recent insightful example concerns the *CACNA1C* calcium channel gene body. Risk alleles were associated with decreased reporter gene activity.[37] A third, recent example is the NMDA receptor subunit gene *GRIN2B* that is broadly implicated in schizophrenia.[101–104] At the *GRIN2B* locus, a chromosomal conformation bypassing 450kb of linear genome harbors sequence polymorphisms that may contribute to risk for schizophrenia and personality traits associated with schizophrenia[9] (see Figure 11.2). These early examples highlight the enormous potential of epigenomic studies, conducted in human brain tissue, to illuminate the molecular pathology of psychiatric disease cases, including a deeper understanding for the underlying genetic architecture.

Epigenomic Drug Targets in Brain

Drugs that interfere with transcriptional regulation hold promise for novel psychopharmacological treatments. Interestingly, sodium valproate, a frequently prescribed anti-epileptic drug and mood stabilizer, is a weak but broad-acting inhibitor of histone deacetylase (HDAC) enzymes.[105] Histone acetylation appears to facilitate transcription while HDAC is commonly associated with repressive chromation remodeling as it cleaves off the acetyl-groups from the histone lysine residues.[106] While the therapeutic range of valproate in clinical populations appears to be below HDAC inhibition levels.[107] HDAC inhibitors (HDACi) are thought to upregulate gene expression at some loci by shifting the balance toward acetylation (of promoter-bound histones). In the pre-clinical model, HDACi improve learning and memory function in a variety of paradigms[108] and may exert therapeutic effects in psychiatric and neurodegenerative disease.[61,109,110,111–114]

Similar to HDACi, there is some evidence for the therapeutic potential of drugs affecting histone methylation. Of interest are small molecules such as BIX-01294, which inhibit a select set of histone methyltransferases (HMTs).[115] Behavioral changes after BIX-01294 treatment include altered reward and addiction behavior in the context of cocaine and other stimulant exposure.[116] The drug's mechanism of action could, at least in part, involve the inhibition of repressive chromatin remodeling at several gene promoters including brain-derived neurotrophic factor (BDNF), *Cdk5*, *Arc*, and others, resulting in increased spine density and synaptic connectivity.[116]

Lastly, several DNA methylation inhibitors alter synaptic plasticity and hippocampal learning and memory in mice and rats, which could be used to modulate reward and addiction-related behavior.[42,117–121] We predict that the therapeutic potential of chromatin-modifying drugs will soon be tested on a broader basis, given these promising findings currently emerging from preclinical and translational research.

Can the Epigenetics of Peripheral Tissue Inform Psychiatric Research?

Our reliance on postmortem tissue for neuro-epigenetic research has major limitations. Age influences the regulation of gene expression in a profound,

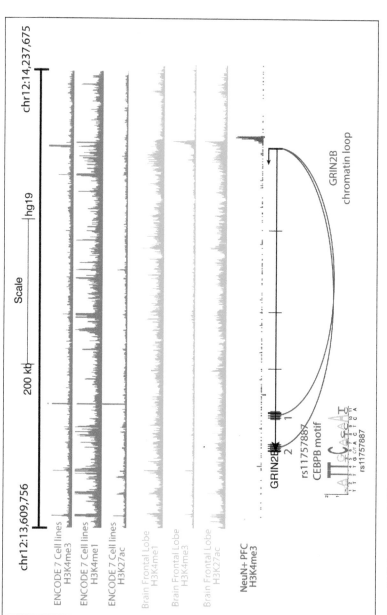

Figure 11.2 Linear map of 600kb genome sequence centered on the *GRIN2B* gene (chromosome 12): The browser tracks on top show histone H3-lysine 4 tri- and mono-methylation (H3K4me3/H3K4me1) and histone H3-lysine 27 acetylation for (blue) ENCODE cell lines[134] and (light green) human postmortem frontal lobe tissue, and H3K4me3 track from sorted neuronal nuclei (prefrontal cortex).[135] Notice that histone modification landscapes, specifically H3K4me1 and H3K27ac with localized "peaks," are not limited to transcription start site or exons but also involve intronic and intragenic sequences. At the bottom, two-long range chromosomal loop formations that interconnect sequences surrounding the *GRIN2B* transcription start site with sequences surrounding the 3' end of the gene. This includes a promoter-enhancer interaction at the site of a CCAAT/Enhancer Binding

non-linear fashion,[122] and our knowledge of how death and the postmortem interval affect the epigenetic landscape remains limited.[123] There is no standardized method to evaluate the psychiatric history of the sample donor postmortem.[124] What is available in brain banks and clinical records might not suffice for less than severe psychiatric conditions, including personality and stress-related disorders. As a result, a large proportion of mental disorders, in particular anxiety disorders, are not well represented in brain banks. Stem cell–derived neuronal cultures may offer an alternative approach in the future, but most studies to date have utilized peripheral tissues (blood and buccal cells) for neuro-epigenetic research in clinical populations. For DNA methylation, some inter-individual variation related to psychiatric symptoms was found to be consistent across tissues.[125,126] For histone marks, however, a recent study suggests that the cell type-specific signature may be more prominent than the subject-specific signature.[127] But the same study also demonstrates that there are similarities across tissues that open up the potential for identifying epigenetic risk for mental illness in peripheral tissues. Therefore, peripheral tissues may be a useful option to study psychiatric illnesses where sufficient numbers of postmortem brains are not available.

Synopsis and Outlook

"Neuroepigenetics" is an emerging field of psychiatric research. Epigenetic landscapes in human brain cells remain plastic throughout the human lifespan, and ongoing dynamic regulation occurs even in neurons and other post-mitotic cells.[44–47]

The range of neurological conditions due to a primary chromatin defect extends far beyond the early developmental period and is likely to be responsible for a subset of cases with psychosis, dementia, and other neurodegenerative disease.[69,128,129]

The exploration of chromatin structure will uncover the impact of disease-relevant mutations,[130] a task difficult to accomplish with DNA sequence analysis alone. Chromatin-modifying drugs could lead to novel treatments for neurological and psychiatric disease.[131,132]

Finally, it is worth mentioning that, based on next-generation sequencing of epigenetic markings in sperm, 4% of the human genome could maintain nucleosomal organization and many types of epigenetic decoration when transmitted through the germ line. This includes many loci considered of critical importance for early pre- and post-implantation development, imprinted gene clusters, microRNA clusters, homeobox (HOX) gene clusters, and the promoters of many stand-alone developmental transcription and signaling factors.[133] These and related findings will further stimulate research aimed at uncovering evidence for the epigenetic heritability of psychiatric disease.

Conflict of Interest

The authors declare no conflict of interest.

Acknowledgments

Work conducted in the Schahram Akbarian's laboratory is sponsored by grants from the National Institutes of Health.

References

1. Lehman, A. F., Lieberman, J. A., Dixon, L. B., et al. (2004). Practice guideline for the treatment of patients with schizophrenia, second edition. *American Journal of Psychiatry, 161*(2 Suppl), 1–56.

2. Krishnan, V., & Nestler, E. J. (2011). Linking molecules to mood: new insight into the biology of depression. *American Journal of Psychiatry, 167*(11), 1305–1320.

3. Cipriani, A., Furukawa, T. A., Salanti, G., et al. (2000). Comparative efficacy and acceptability of 12 new-generation antidepressants: a multiple-treatments meta-analysis. *Lancet, 373*(9665), 746–758.

4. Labrie, V., Pai, S., & Petronis, A. (2012). Epigenetics of major psychosis: progress, problems and perspectives. *Trends in Genetics, 28*(9), 427–435.

5. Robison, A. J., & Nestler, E. J. (2011). Transcriptional and epigenetic mechanisms of addiction. *Nature Reviews Neuroscience, 12*(11), 623–637.

6. Day, J. J., & Sweatt, J. D. (2011). Epigenetic mechanisms in cognition. *Neuron, 70*(5), 813–829.

7. Maze, I., Wenderski, W., Noh, K. M., et al. (2011). Critical role of histone turnover in neuronal transcription and plasticity. *Neuron, 87*(1), 77–94.

8. Jakocevski, M., & Akbarian, S. (2012). Epigenetic mechanisms in neurodevelopmental and neurodegenerative disease. *Nature Medicine, 18*(8), 1194–1204.

9. Bharadwaj, R., Peter, C. J., Jiang, Y., et al. (2011). Conserved higher-order chromatin regulates NMDA receptor gene expression and cognition. *Neuron, 84*(5), 997–1008.

10. Roussos, P., Mitchell, A. C., Voloudakis, G., et al. (2011). A role for noncoding variation in schizophrenia. *Cell Reports, 9*(4), 1417–1429.

11. Rodriguez-Paredes, M., & Esteller, M. (2011). Cancer epigenetics reaches mainstream oncology. *Nature Medicine, 17*(3), 330–339.

12. Li, G., & Reinberg, D. (2011). Chromatin higher-order structures and gene regulation. *Current Opinion in Genetics & Development, 21*(2), 175–186.

13. Allis, C. D., & Jenuwein, T. (2016). The molecular hallmarks of epigenetic control. *Nature Reviews Genetics, 17*(8), 487–500.

14. Zhou, V. W., Goren, A., & Bernstein, B. E. (2011). Charting histone modifications and the functional organization of mammalian genomes. *Nature Reviews Genetics, 12*(1), 7–18.

15. Ederveen, T. H., Mandemaker, I. K., & Logie, C. (2011). The human histone H3 complement anno 2011. *Biochimica Biophysica Acta, 1809*(10), 577–586.

16. Kinney, S. M., Chin, H. G., Vaisvila, R., et al. (2011). Tissue-specific distribution and dynamic changes of 5-hydroxymethylcytosine in mammalian genomes. *Journal of Biological Chemistry, 286*(28), 24685–93.

17. Soshnev, A. A., Josefowicz, S. Z., & Allis, C. D. (2011). Greater than the sum of parts: Complexity of the dynamic epigenome. *Molecular Cell, 62*(5), 681–694.

18. Kriaucionis, S., & Heintz, N. (2000). The nuclear DNA base 5-hydroxymethylcytosine is present in Purkinje neurons and the brain. *Science, 324*(5929), 929–930.

19. Xie, W., Barr, C. L., Kim, A., et al. (2011). Base-resolution analyses of sequence and parent-of-origin dependent DNA methylation in the mouse genome. *Cell, 148*(4), 816–831.

20. Kinde, B., Gabel, H. W., Gilbert, C. S., Griffith, E. C., & Greenberg, M. E. (2011). Reading the unique DNA methylation landscape of the brain: Non-CpG methylation, hydroxymethylation, and MeCP2. *Proceedings of the National Academy of Sciences USA, 112*(22), 6800–6806.

21. Kato, T., & Iwamoto, K. (2011). Comprehensive DNA methylation and hydroxymethylation analysis in the human brain and its implication in mental disorders. *Neuropharmacology, 80*, 133–139.

22. Koziol, M. J., Bradshaw, C. R., Allen, G. E., Costa, A. S., Frezza, C., & Gurdon, J. B. (2011). Identification of methylated deoxyadenosines in vertebrates reveals diversity in DNA modifications. *Nature Structural & Molecular Biology, 23*(1), 24–30.

23. Chen, T., Hao, Y. J., Zhang, Y., et al. (2011). m(6)A RNA methylation is regulated by microRNAs and promotes reprogramming to pluripotency. *Cell Stem Cell, 16*(3), 289–301.

24. Tan, M., Luo, H., Lee, S., et al. (2011). Identification of 67 histone marks and histone lysine crotonylation as a new type of histone modification. *Cell, 146*(6), 1016–1028.

25. Baumann, K. (2011). Post-translational modifications: Crotonylation versus acetylation. *Nature Reviews Molecular Cell Biology, 16*(5), 265.

26. Berger, S. L. (2000). The complex language of chromatin regulation during transcription. *Nature, 447*(7143), 407–412.

27. Woodcock, C. L. Chromatin architecture. *Current Opinion in Structural Biology.* 2006;16(2), 213–220.

28. Jin, C., & Felsenfeld, G. (2000). Nucleosome stability mediated by histone variants H3.3 and H2A.Z. *Genes & Development, 21*(12), 1519–1529.

29. Wenderski, W., & Maze, I. (2011). Histone turnover and chromatin accessibility: Critical mediators of neurological development, plasticity, and disease. *Bioessays, 38*(5), 410–419.

30. Zovkic, I. B., Paulukaitis, B. S., Day, J. J., Etikala, D. M., & Sweatt, J. D. (2011). Histone H2A.Z subunit exchange controls consolidation of recent and remote memory. *Nature, 515*(7528), 582–586.

31. Belmont, A. S. Mitotic chromosome structure and condensation. *Current Opinion in Cell Biology.* 2006;18(6), 632–638.

32. Cremer, T., & Cremer, C. (2000). Chromosome territories, nuclear architecture and gene regulation in mammalian cells. *Nature Reviews Genetics, 2*(4), 292–301.

33. Duan, Z., Andronescu, M., Schutz, K., et al. (2011). A three-dimensional model of the yeast genome. *Nature*, *465*(7296), 363–367.

34. Wood, A. J., Severson, A. F., & Meyer, B. J. (2011). Condensin and cohesin complexity: the expanding repertoire of functions. *Nature Reviews Genetics*, *11*(6), 391–404.

35. Gaszner, M., & Felsenfeld, G. (2000). Insulators: exploiting transcriptional and epigenetic mechanisms. *Nature Reviews Genetics*, *7*(9), 703–713.

36. Dekker, J., Rippe, K., Dekker, M., & Kleckner, N. (2000). Capturing chromosome conformation. *Science*, *295*(5558), 1306–1311.

37. Mitchell, A., Roussos, P., Peter, C., Tsankova, N., & Akbarian, S. (2011). The future of neuroepigenetics in the human brain. *Progress in Molecular Biology and Translational Science*, *128*, 199–228.

38. Mitchell, A. C., Bharadwaj, R., Whittle, C., et al. (2011). The genome in three dimensions: a new frontier in human brain research. *Biological Psychiatry*, *75*(12), 961–969.

39. Ooi, S. K., & Bestor, T. H. (2000). The colorful history of active DNA demethylation. *Cell*, *133*(7), 1145–1148.

40. Klose, R. J., & Zhang, Y. (2000). Regulation of histone methylation by demethylimination and demethylation. *Nature Reviews Molecular Cell Biology*, *8*(4), 307–318.

41. Loenarz, C., & Schofield, C. J. (2011). Physiological and biochemical aspects of hydroxylations and demethylations catalyzed by human 2-oxoglutarate oxygenases. *Trends in Biochemical Science*, *36*(1), 7–18.

42. Miller, C. A., & Sweatt, J. D. (2000). Covalent modification of DNA regulates memory formation. *Neuron*, *53*(6), 857–869.

43. Guo, J. U., Su, Y., Zhong, C., Ming, G. L., & Song, H. (2011). Hydroxylation of 5-methylcytosine by TET1 promotes active DNA demethylation in the adult brain. *Cell*, *145*(3), 423–434.

44. Cheung, I., Shulha, H. P., Jiang, Y., et al. (2011). Developmental regulation and individual differences of neuronal H3K4me3 epigenomes in the prefrontal cortex. *Proceedings of the National Academy of Sciences USA*, *107*(19), 8824–8829.

45. Siegmund, K. D., Connor, C. M., Campan, M., et al. (2000). DNA methylation in the human cerebral cortex is dynamically regulated throughout the life span and involves differentiated neurons. *PLoS One*, *2*(9), e895.

46. Hernandez, D. G., Nalls, M. A., Gibbs, J. R., et al. (2011). Distinct DNA methylation changes highly correlated with chronological age in the human brain. *Human Molecular Genetics*, *20*(6), 1164–1172.

47. Numata, S., Ye, T., Hyde, T. M., et al. (2011). DNA methylation signatures in development and aging of the human prefrontal cortex. *American Journal of Human Genetics*, *90*(2), 260–272.

48. Jaffe, A. E., Gao, Y., Deep-Soboslay, A., et al. (2011). Mapping DNA methylation across development, genotype and schizophrenia in the human frontal cortex. *Nature Neuroscience*, *19*(1), 40–47.

49. Stadler, F., Kolb, G., Rubusch, L., Baker, S. P., Jones, E. G., & Akbarian, S. (2000). Histone methylation at gene promoters is associated with developmental regulation and region-specific expression of ionotropic and metabotropic glutamate receptors in human brain. *Journal of Neurochemistry*, *94*(2), 324–336.

50. Akbarian, S., Sucher, N. J., Bradley, D., et al. (1999). Selective alterations in gene expression for NMDA receptor subunits in prefrontal cortex of schizophrenics. *Journal of Neuroscience, 16*(1), 19–30.

51. Zovkic, I. B., & Sweatt, J. D. (2013). Epigenetic mechanisms in learned fear: Implications for PTSD. *Neuropsychopharmacology, 38*(1), 77–93.

52. Rusiecki, J. A., Chen, L., Srikantan, V., et al. (2011). DNA methylation in repetitive elements and post-traumatic stress disorder: a case-control study of US military service members. *Epigenomics, 4*(1), 29–40.

53. Uddin, M., Aiello, A. E., Wildman, D. E., et al. (2011). Epigenetic and immune function profiles associated with posttraumatic stress disorder. *Proceedings of the National Academy of Sciences USA, 107*(20), 9470–9475.

54. Smith, A. K., Conneely, K. N., Kilaru, V., et al. (2011). Differential immune system DNA methylation and cytokine regulation in post-traumatic stress disorder. *American Journal of Medical Genetics B, Neuropsychiatric Genetics, 156B*(6), 700–708.

55. McGowan, P. O., Sasaki, A., D'Alessio, A. C., et al. (2000). Epigenetic regulation of the glucocorticoid receptor in human brain associates with childhood abuse. *Nature Neuroscience, 12*(3), 342–348.

56. McGowan, P. O., Sasaki, A., Huang, T. C., et al. (2000). Promoter-wide hypermethylation of the ribosomal RNA gene promoter in the suicide brain. *PLoS One, 3*(5), e2085.

57. Yehuda, R., Daskalakis, N. P., Bierer, L. M., et al. (2015). Holocaust exposure induced intergenerational effects on FKBP5 methylation. *Biological Psychiatry, 80*(5), 372–380.

58. Peter, C. J., Fischer, L. K., Kundakovic, M., et al. (2016). DNA methylation signatures of early childhood malnutrition associated with impairments in attention and cognition. *Biological Psychiatry, 80*(10), 765–774.

59. Weaver, I. C., Cervoni, N., Champagne, F. A., et al. (2000). Epigenetic programming by maternal behavior. *Nature Neuroscience, 7*(8), 847–854.

60. Bockmuhl, Y., Patchev, A. V., Madejska, A., et al. (2011). Methylation at the CpG island shore region upregulates Nr3c1 promoter activity after early-life stress. *Epigenetics, 10*(3), 247–257.

61. Covington, H. E., 3rd, Maze, I., LaPlant, Q. C., et al. (2000). Antidepressant actions of histone deacetylase inhibitors. *Journal of Neuroscience, 29*(37), 11451–11460.

62. Hollis, F., Wang, H., Dietz, D., Gunjan, A., & Kabbaj, M. (2011). The effects of repeated social defeat on long-term depressive-like behavior and short-term histone modifications in the hippocampus in male Sprague-Dawley rats. *Psychopharmacology (Berlin), 211*(1), 69–77.

63. Sun, H., Kennedy, P. J., & Nestler, E. J. (2011). Epigenetics of the depressed brain: role of histone acetylation and methylation. *Neuropsychopharmacology, 38*(1), 124–137.

64. Filippakopoulos, P., Qi, J., Picaud, S., et al. (2011). Selective inhibition of BET bromodomains. *Nature, 468*(7327), 1067–1073.

65. Janzen, W. P., Wigle, T. J., Jin, J., & Frye, S. V. (2011). Epigenetics: Tools and technologies. *Drug Discovery Today: Technologies, 7*(1), e59–e65.

66. Henikoff, S., & Shilatifard, A. (2011). Histone modification: cause or cog? *Trends in Genetics, 27*(10), 389–396.

67. Hansen, R. S., Wijmenga, C., Luo, P., et al. (1999). The DNMT3B DNA methyl-transferase gene is mutated in the ICF immunodeficiency syndrome. *Proceedings of the National Academy of Sciences USA, 96*(25), 14412–14417.

68. Okano, M., Bell, D. W., Haber, D. A., & Li, E. (1999). DNA methyltransferases Dnmt3a and Dnmt3b are essential for de novo methylation and mammalian development. *Cell, 99*(3), 247–257.

69. Klein, C. J., Botuyan, M. V., Wu, Y., et al. (2011). Mutations in DNMT1 cause hereditary sensory neuropathy with dementia and hearing loss. *Nature Genetics, 43*(6), 595–600.

70. Winkelmann, J., Lin, L., Schormair, B., et al. (2011). Mutations in DNMT1 cause autosomal dominant cerebellar ataxia, deafness and narcolepsy. *Human Molecular Genetics, 21*(10), 2205–2210.

71. Amir, R. E., Van den Veyver, I. B., Wan, M., Tran, C. Q., Francke, U., & Zoghbi, H. Y. (1999). Rett syndrome is caused by mutations in X-linked MECP2, encoding methyl-CpG-binding protein 2. *Nature Genetics, 23*(2), 185–188.

72. Chouery, E., Ghoch, J. A., Corbani, S., et al. (2011). A novel deletion in ZBTB24 in a Lebanese family with immunodeficiency, centromeric instability, and facial anomalies syndrome type 2. *Clinical Genetics, 82*(5), 489–493.

73. Piton, A., Gauthier, J., Hamdan, F. F., et al. (2011). Systematic resequencing of X-chromosome synaptic genes in autism spectrum disorder and schizophrenia. *Molecular Psychiatry, 16*(8), 867–880.

74. Kleefstra, T., van Zelst-Stams, W. A., Nillesen, W. M., et al. (2000). Further clinical and molecular delineation of the 9q subtelomeric deletion syndrome supports a major contribution of EHMT1 haploinsufficiency to the core phenotype. *Journal of Medical Genetics, 46*(9), 598–606.

75. Kirov, G., Pocklington, A. J., Holmans, P., et al. (2011). De novo CNV analysis implicates specific abnormalities of postsynaptic signalling complexes in the pathogenesis of schizophrenia. *Molecular Psychiatry, 17*(2), 142–153.

76. Verhoeven, W. M., Egger, J. I., Vermeulen, K., van de Warrenburg, B. P., & Kleefstra, T. (2011). Kleefstra syndrome in three adult patients: further delineation of the behavioral and neurological phenotype shows aspects of a neurodegenerative course. *American Journal of Medical Genetics A, 155A*(10), 2409–2415.

77. Martins-de-Souza, D., Gattaz, W. F., Schmitt, A., et al. (2000). Alterations in oligodendrocyte proteins, calcium homeostasis and new potential markers in schizophrenia anterior temporal lobe are revealed by shotgun proteome analysis. *Journal of Neural Transmitters, 116*(3), 275–289.

78. Regenold, W. T., Phatak, P., Marano, C. M., Gearhart, L., Viens, C. H., & Hisley, K. C. (2000). Myelin staining of deep white matter in the dorsolateral prefrontal cortex in schizophrenia, bipolar disorder, and unipolar major depression. *Psychiatry Research, 151*(3), 179–188.

79. Katsel, P., Davis, K. L., & Haroutunian, V. (2000). Variations in myelin and oligodendrocyte-related gene expression across multiple brain regions in schizophrenia: a gene ontology study. *Schizophrenia Research, 79*(2–3), 157–173.

80. Aston, C., Jiang, L., & Sokolov, B. P. (2000). Microarray analysis of postmortem temporal cortex from patients with schizophrenia. *Journal of Neuroscience Research, 77*(6), 858–866.

81. Hakak, Y., Walker, J. R., Li, C., et al. (2000). Genome-wide expression analysis reveals dysregulation of myelination-related genes in chronic schizophrenia. *Proceedings of the National Academy of Sciences USA, 98*(8), 4746–4751.

82. Tkachev, D., Mimmack, M. L., Ryan, M. M., et al. (2000). Oligodendrocyte dysfunction in schizophrenia and bipolar disorder. *Lancet*, *362*(9386), 798–805.

83. Duncan, C. E., Webster, M. J., Rothmond, D. A., Bahn, S., Elashoff, M., Shannon & Weickert, C. (2010). Prefrontal GABA(A) receptor alpha-subunit expression in normal postnatal human development and schizophrenia. *Journal of Psychiatric Research*, *44*(10), 673–681.

84. Charych, E. I., Liu, F., Moss, S. J., & Brandon, N. J. (2000). GABA(A) receptors and their associated proteins: implications in the etiology and treatment of schizophrenia and related disorders. *Neuropharmacology*, *57*(5–6), 481–495.

85. Woo, T. U., Kim, A. M., & Viscidi, E. (2000). Disease-specific alterations in glutamatergic neurotransmission on inhibitory interneurons in the prefrontal cortex in schizophrenia. *Brain Research*, *1218*, 267–277.

86. Akbarian, S., & Huang, H. S. (2000). Molecular and cellular mechanisms of altered GAD1/GAD67 expression in schizophrenia and related disorders. *Brain Research Review*, *52*(2), 293–304.

87. Guidotti, A., Auta, J., Davis, J. M., et al. (2000). GABAergic dysfunction in schizophrenia: new treatment strategies on the horizon. *Psychopharmacology (Berlin)*, *180*(2), 191–205.

88. Dracheva, S., Elhakem, S. L., McGurk, S. R., Davis, K. L., & Haroutunian, V. (2000). GAD67 and GAD65 mRNA and protein expression in cerebrocortical regions of elderly patients with schizophrenia. *Journal of Neuroscience Research*, *76*(4), 581–592.

89. Hashimoto, T., Bazmi, H. H., Mirnics, K., Wu, Q., Sampson, A. R., & Lewis, D. A. (2000). Conserved regional patterns of GABA-related transcript expression in the neocortex of subjects with schizophrenia. *American Journal of Psychiatry*, *165*(4), 479–489.

90. Benes, F. M. (2011). Amygdalocortical circuitry in schizophrenia: from circuits to molecules. *Neuropsychopharmacology*, *35*(1), 239–257.

91. Sibille, E., Wang, Y., Joeyen-Waldorf, J., et al. (2000). A molecular signature of depression in the amygdala. *American Journal of Psychiatry*, *166*(9), 1011–1024.

92. Psych, E. C., Akbarian, S., Liu, C., et al. (2011). The PsychENCODE project. *Nature Neuroscience*, *18*(12), 1707–1712.

93. Fromer, M., Pocklington, A. J., Kavanagh, D. H., et al. (2011). De novo mutations in schizophrenia implicate synaptic networks. *Nature*, *506*(7487), 179–184.

94. Addington, A. M., Gornick, M., Duckworth, J., et al. (2000). GAD1 (2q31.1), which encodes glutamic acid decarboxylase (GAD67), is associated with childhood-onset schizophrenia and cortical gray matter volume loss. *Molecular Psychiatry*, *10*(6), 581–588.

95. Straub, R. E., Lipska, B. K., Egan, M. F., Goldberg, T. E., Kleinman, J. E., & Weinberger, D. R. (2007). Allelic variation in GAD1 (GAD67) is associated with schizophrenia and influences cortical function and gene expression. *Molecular Psychiatry*, *12*(9), 854–869.

96. Marenco, S., Savostyanova, A. A., van der Veen, J. W., et al. (2011). Genetic modulation of GABA levels in the anterior cingulate cortex by GAD1 and COMT. *Neuropsychopharmacology*, *35*(8), 1708–1717.

97. Huang, H. S., Matevossian, A., Whittle, C., et al. (2000). Prefrontal dysfunction in schizophrenia involves mixed-lineage leukemia 1-regulated histone methylation at GABAergic gene promoters. *Journal of Neuroscience*, *27*(42), 11254–62.

98. Bharadwaj, R., Jiang, Y., Mao, W., et al. (2011). Conserved chromosome 2q31 conformations are associated with transcriptional regulation of GAD1 GABA synthesis enzyme and altered in prefrontal cortex of subjects with schizophrenia. *Journal of Neuroscience, 33*(29), 11839–51.

99. Rocco, B. R., Lewis, D. A., & Fish, K. N. (2015). Markedly lower glutamic acid decarboxylase 67 protein levels in a subset of boutons in schizophrenia. *Biological Psychiatry, 79*(12), 1006–1015.

100. Lewis, D. A. (2011). Inhibitory neurons in human cortical circuits: substrate for cognitive dysfunction in schizophrenia. *Current Opinion in Neurobiology, 26*, 22–26.

101. Talkowski, M. E., Rosenfeld, J. A., Blumenthal, I., et al. (2011). Sequencing chromosomal abnormalities reveals neurodevelopmental loci that confer risk across diagnostic boundaries. *Cell, 149*(3), 525–537.

102. Epi, K. C., Epilepsy Phenome/Genome, P., Allen, A. S., et al. (2011). De novo mutations in epileptic encephalopathies. *Nature, 501*(7466), 217–221.

103. Hamdan, F. F., Srour, M., Capo-Chichi, J. M., et al. (2011). De novo mutations in moderate or severe intellectual disability. *PLoS Genetics, 10*(10), e1004772.

104. O'Roak, B. J., Deriziotis, P., Lee, C., et al. (2011). Exome sequencing in sporadic autism spectrum disorders identifies severe de novo mutations. *Nature Genetics, 43*(6), 585–589.

105. Guidotti, A., Auta, J., Chen, Y., et al. (2011). Epigenetic GABAergic targets in schizophrenia and bipolar disorder. *Neuropharmacology, 60*(7–8), 1007–1016.

106. Sharma, R. P., Rosen, C., Kartan, S., et al. (2000). Valproic acid and chromatin remodeling in schizophrenia and bipolar disorder: preliminary results from a clinical population. *Schizophrenia Research, 88*(1–3), 227–231.

107. Hasan, A., Mitchell, A., Schneider, A., Halene, T., & Akbarian, S. (2011). Epigenetic dysregulation in schizophrenia: molecular and clinical aspects of histone deacetylase inhibitors. *European Archives of Psychiatry Clinical Neuroscience, 263*(4), 273–284.

108. Lopez-Atalaya, J. P., Valor, L. M., & Barco, A. (2011). Epigenetic factors in intellectual disability: the Rubinstein-Taybi syndrome as a paradigm of neurodevelopmental disorder with epigenetic origin. *Progress in Molecular Biology & Translational Science, 128*, 139–176.

109. Morris, M. J., Karra, A. S., & Monteggia, L. M. (2011). Histone deacetylases govern cellular mechanisms underlying behavioral and synaptic plasticity in the developing and adult brain. *Behavioral Pharmacology, 21*(5–6), 409–419.

110. Schroeder, F. A., Lin, C. L., Crusio, W. E., & Akbarian, S. (2000). Antidepressant-like effects of the histone deacetylase inhibitor, sodium butyrate, in the mouse. *Biological Psychiatry, 62*(1), 55–64.

111. Chuang, D. M., Leng, Y., Marinova, Z., Kim, H. J., & Chiu, C. T. (2000). Multiple roles of HDAC inhibition in neurodegenerative conditions. *Trends in Neuroscience, 32*(11), 591–601.

112. Baltan, S., Murphy, S. P., Danilov, C. A., Bachleda, A., & Morrison, R. S. (2011). Histone deacetylase inhibitors preserve white matter structure and function during ischemia by conserving ATP and reducing excitotoxicity. *Journal of Neuroscience, 31*(11), 3990–3999.

113. Fischer, A., Sananbenesi, F., Mungenast, A., & Tsai, L. H. (2011). Targeting the correct HDAC(s) to treat cognitive disorders. *Trends in Pharmacological Science, 31*(12), 605–617.

114. Tsou, A. Y., Friedman, L. S., Wilson, R. B., & Lynch, D. R. (2000). Pharmacotherapy for Friedreich ataxia. *CNS Drugs, 23*(3), 213–223.

115. Kubicek, S., O'Sullivan, R. J., August, E. M., et al. (2000). Reversal of H3K9me2 by a small-molecule inhibitor for the G9a histone methyltransferase. *Molecular Cell, 25*(3), 473–481.

116. Maze, I., Covington, H. E., 3rd, Dietz, D. M., et al. (2011). Essential role of the histone methyltransferase G9a in cocaine-induced plasticity. *Science, 327*(5962), 213–216.

117. Levenson, J. M., Roth, T. L., Lubin, F. D., et al. (2000). Evidence that DNA (cytosine-5) methyltransferase regulates synaptic plasticity in the hippocampus. *Journal of Biological Chemistry, 281*(23), 15763–73.

118. Han, J., Li, Y., Wang, D., Wei, C., Yang, X., & Sui, N. (2011). Effect of 5-aza-2-deoxycytidine microinjecting into hippocampus and prelimbic cortex on acquisition and retrieval of cocaine-induced place preference in C57BL/6 mice. *European Journal of Pharmacology, 642*(1–3), 93–98.

119. LaPlant, Q., Vialou, V., Covington, H. E. 3rd, et al. (2011). Dnmt3a regulates emotional behavior and spine plasticity in the nucleus accumbens. *Nature Neuroscience, 13*(9), 1137–1143.

120. Lubin, F. D., Roth, T. L., & Sweatt, J. D. (2000). Epigenetic regulation of BDNF gene transcription in the consolidation of fear memory. *Journal of Neuroscience, 28*(42), 10576–86.

121. Miller, C. A., Gavin, C. F., White, J. A., et al. (2011). Cortical DNA methylation maintains remote memory. *Nature Neuroscience, 13*(6), 664–666.

122. Colantuoni, C., Lipska, B. K., Ye, T., et al. (2011). Temporal dynamics and genetic control of transcription in the human prefrontal cortex. *Nature, 478*(7370), 519–523.

123. Ferrer, I., Martinez, A., Boluda, S., Parchi, P., & Barrachina, M. (2000). Brain banks: benefits, limitations and cautions concerning the use of post-mortem brain tissue for molecular studies. *Cell Tissue Bank, 9*(3), 181–194.

124. McCullumsmith, R. E., Hammond, J. H., Shan, D., & Meador-Woodruff, J. H. (2011). Postmortem brain: an underutilized substrate for studying severe mental illness. *Neuropsychopharmacology, 39*(1), 65–87.

125. Davies, M. N., Volta, M., Pidsley, R., et al. (2011). Functional annotation of the human brain methylome identifies tissue-specific epigenetic variation across brain and blood. *Genome Biology, 13*(6), R43.

126. Stenz, L., Zewdie, S., Laforge-Escarra, T., et al. (2011). BDNF promoter I methylation correlates between post-mortem human peripheral and brain tissues. *Neuroscience Research, 91*, 1–7.

127. Dincer, A., Gavin, D. P., Xu, K., et al. (2011). Deciphering H3K4me3 broad domains associated with gene-regulatory networks and conserved epigenomic landscapes in the human brain. *Translational Psychiatry, 5*, e679.

128. Winkelmann, J., Lin, L., Schormair, B., et al. (2012). Mutations in DNMT1 cause autosomal dominant cerebellar ataia, deafness and narcolepsy. *Human Molecular Genetics, 21*(10), 2205–2210.

129. Jakovcevski, M., & Akbarian, S. (2011). Epigenetic mechanisms in neurological disease. *Nature Medicine, 18*(8), 1194–204.

130. Fullard, J. F., Halene, T. B., Giambartolomei, C., Haroutunian, V., Akbarian, S., & Roussos, P. (2016). Understanding the genetic liability to schizophrenia through the neuroepigenome. *Schizophrenia Research, 177*(1–3), 115–124.

131. Jakovcevski, M., Akbarian, S., & Di Benedetto, B. (2011). Pharmacological modulation of astrocytes and the role of cell type-specific histone modifications for the treatment of mood disorders. *Current Opinion in Pharmacology*, 26, 61–66.

132. Tremolizzo, L., Rodriguez-Menendez, V., Conti, E., Zoia, C. P., Cavaletti, G., & Ferrarese, C. (2011). Novel therapeutic targets in neuropsychiatric disorders: the neuroepigenome. *Current Pharmaceutical Design*, 20(11), 1831–1839.

133. Hammoud, S. S., Purwar, J., Pflueger, C., Cairns, B. R., & Carrell, D. T. (2011). Alterations in sperm DNA methylation patterns at imprinted loci in two classes of infertility. *Fertility & Sterility*, 94(5), 1728–1733.

Chapter 12

Epigenetics in Psychiatry

Subha Subramanian and James B. Potash

Take-Home Points

1. Epigenetics is of great interest in psychiatry because it has the potential to provide mechanistic links between genetic variation that increases susceptibility to mental disorders, and environmental exposures that influence risk.
2. The most heavily studied epigenetic marks in the context of psychiatric illness are DNA methylation, and histone acetylation and methylation. While the field is still young, some evidence has implicated variation in these marks in response to stressors and to substance use, as well as in psychiatric illnesses such as PTSD and schizophrenia.
3. Fundamental challenges in this area of research include the inability to access brain tissue from live patients, and the heterogeneity of epigenetic marks across tissues and across cell types.
4. A great deal of epigenetic variation has yet to be assayed, as, for example, genome-wide approaches to the recently discovered 5-hydroxymethylcytosine and non-CpG methylation marks have not yet been employed in the context of psychiatric illness.

Introduction

The term "epigenetics" originates from the work of Conrad Waddington, a developmental biologist who was interested in the factors that influence the course an organism takes from genetic potential to maturity. These factors include environmental insults such as childhood trauma and life stressors that contribute to the etiology of mental disorders; therefore, psychiatric researchers have been intrigued by the potential of epigenetics to elucidate the interaction between nature and nurture in these conditions.

Investigators first focused on the methylation of DNA (DNAm), an epigenetic modification on cytosine nucleotides adjacent to guanine. Methylated cytosines were discovered in 1925,[1] yet their biological role was only noted 40 years later by Griffith and Mahler, who noted that DNAm and demethylation influence protein synthesis in neurons and might play a role in memory.[2] In 1975, Holliday and others posited that DNAm might influence gene expression,[3,4] and data supporting this concept followed soon after.[5] Holliday additionally proposed that changes in DNAm might be the basis for carcinogenesis, after which hypomethylation and hypermethylation were described in cancer biology.[6–8]

Biochemical modifications of histones also influence gene expression, a concept David Allis referred to as the *histone code*.[9] Histones are protein subunits that spool the genomic sequence, forming chromatin. The pattern of modifications on these histone subunits determines if chromatin is uncondensed (euchromatin) and open for active transcription, or condensed (heterochromatin) and closed, preventing transcription. Other variations of interest in psychiatric epigenetics occur in non-coding RNAs, such as micro RNAs (miRNAs), which also regulate gene expression.

Overtime, the term "epigenetics" has evolved to broadly describe the study of any DNA- or chromatin-related factor that influences gene expression. The narrow definition involves persistence through cell division, and the narrowest definition requires inheritance of the relevant marks. Like the genome, the epigenome may be heritable, though this is not yet entirely clear. There are a few studies suggesting intergenerational inheritance of DNA methylation, with potential examples in animal models and in humans.[10–12]

Much of the allure within the field of epigenetics stems from the reversibility of epigenetic marks. The potential to identify early stages of psychiatric disorders through epigenetic biomarkers, and subsequently interrupt the progress of pathogenesis through altering the epigenetic landscape, holds enormous promise. Similarly, the potential to treat existing disease through reversing epigenetic marks is exciting. Recent work has demonstrated the potential to use the Cas9 DNA-editing enzyme as the basis for a system that can edit DNA methylation in post-mitotic neurons in a highly targeted fashion.[13]

Relevance to Psychiatry

There is ample reason to believe that epigenetic mechanisms might play a role in psychiatric disorders. First, while the heritability of some psychiatric disorders is quite high, it is not 100% for any disorder, and it is less than 50% for some (e.g., the heritability of schizophrenia [SCZ], bipolar disorder [BD], and major depressive disorder [MDD] are 81%, 75%, and 38%, respectively).[14] This suggests that other factors influence disease etiology. Second, the interplay between genetic susceptibility and environmental factors is particularly plausible for some disorders, such as MDD and post-traumatic stress disorder (PTSD). For example, mothers experiencing stress and depression during pregnancy and the post-partum show an increased risk of psychiatric disorders in their children.[15,16] Likewise, rodents exposed to stressful stimuli *in utero* deliver pups with anxiety-like and depression-like behaviors, decreased social interaction, and increased corticosterone levels.[17,18] Third, many psychiatric illnesses begin in adolescence or later in life, suggesting that it is not simply genetic variations present at birth that are causative. Many illnesses like depression and BD are also episodic. The fluctuating and variable nature of such disorders is consistent with epigenetic mechanisms that are reversible. Fourth, mood stabilizers and antidepressants alter epigenetic marks to influence gene function. Valproic acid is a BD medication that inhibits histone deacetylases (HDACs). Imipramine is a tricyclic antidepressant that also inhibits the histone deacetylase, *HDAC5*. However, we do not know whether these changes play a role in the mechanism of action of these medications. Finally, neuronal plasticity, the construction and pruning of synapses between neurons, plays a role in addiction biology, and epigenetics provides a potential mechanistic explanation for the changes that have been observed, as discussed further in this chapter.

Epigenetic Mechanisms

DNA Methylation

DNA methyltransferases catalyze DNAm by transferring a methyl group from 5-adenosylmethionine to position 5 of the cytosine ring, producing 5-methylcytosine (5mC). Methylation predominantly occurs on cytosine-guanine dinucleotides (CpGs), though in embryonic stem cells, 5mCs have recently been found to sometimes occur adjacent to adenosines, cytosines, or thymines (non-CpGs).[19,20]

Highly methylated regions typically lead to decreased transcription of genes downstream. This occurs via several mechanisms: methylated cytosines block transcription factors from binding to the gene; methylated cytosines also recruit methyl-CpG binding proteins, which then condense chromatin structure. This "closed" state of chromatin inhibits active transcription. In contrast, unmethylated regions are generally associated with increased transcription.

While methylation can be reversible, population studies suggest that methylation plays a role in some stable modifications. For example, the nutrition deficiency in pregnant women during the Dutch Famine of 1944–1945 led to a twofold increase in SCZ risk in their offspring;[21] the famine was associated with long-term DNAm changes, including decreased DNAm of insulin-like growth factor 2 and differential methylation in metabolic syndrome pathways.[22,23]

Some methylation changes parallel neuronal development and are dynamic through time. Jaffe et al. identified an association between increased DNAm and decreased neuronal progenitor and embryonic cells during the second fetal trimester; decreased DNAm is subsequently associated with an increased number of adult neurons. Their study further demonstrated that many SCZ risk-associated loci were near the regions that showed methylation changes between prenatal and postnatal periods.[24]

Histone Acetylation and Methylation

Histones are the basic units of chromatin. About 147 nucleotides wrap around histone octamers, forming nucleosomes. Each octamer consists of two copies of histones H2A, H2B, H3, and H4. Nucleosome arrangement regulates the dynamic state of chromatin, such that genes within condensed chromatin are not transcribed, while those within open chromatin are transcribed.

Post-translational modifications on the N-terminals of histone amino acids orchestrate the fluidity of chromatin conformation. Acetyl-, methyl-, ubiquitin-, and SUMO-, groups may be tagged onto lysine residues; methyl- groups can also be added to arginine; and phosphate groups may be attached to serine or threonine. Further, lysine side chains may hold up to three methyl groups. The enzymes responsible for deacetylation and acetylation of lysine residues are HDACs and histone acetyl transferases (HATs), respectively.

Non-Coding RNA

The majority of transcripts are not translated into proteins, but many transcripts do have functions within neurons. These non-coding RNAs can be short (<200 nt) or long (<200 nt) and are further classified by genomic origin and mechanism of action. Many of these interact with histone modifying complexes or DNA methyltransferases to regulate gene expression. Thus, non-coding RNAs play a role in the epigenetic landscape.

Though research on RNA interference (RNAi) is still in its infancy, evidence pinpoints miRNAs—21–23 nucleotides of non-protein coding DNA sequences—as modulators of brain development and structural plasticity. Large-scale genome-wide studies have identified disease-associated single-nucleotide polymorphisms (SNPs) within and near miRNA genes, such as miR-137, which is discussed further in this chapter.

Methods and Models

Detection

The exploration of epigenetic profiles may begin globally or regionally. Methods that detect global methylation—i.e., the total level of DNAm across the genome—include: high-performance liquid chromatography (HPLC), liquid chromatography coupled with mass spectrometry (LC-MS), and enzyme-linked immunosorbent assay (ELISA). These methods allow for rapid, quantifiable, reproducible data. ELISA requires DNA inputs of 10 ng; HPLC or LC-MS requires DNA inputs from 1 ng to 1 ug.

Global methylation platforms are advantageous if only broad patterns are being sought or if resources are limited. If higher resolution is needed to characterize particular 5mC sites, DNA is treated with bisulfite or restriction enzymes. These reactions often require 500 ng of DNA. Bisulfite conversion deaminates cytosine to uracil; 5mC is not converted. Polymerase chain reaction (PCR) amplification thereafter will transcribe uracil as thymine and 5mC sites as cytosines. This distinction allows for the identification of methylated sites upon subsequent hybridization or sequencing.

For histone studies, targeted antibodies are used in chromatin immunoprecipitation (ChIP) studies. To assay individual genes, ChIP is combined with quantitative PCR of the gene fragment in question. ChIP–seq, which combines chromatin immunoprecipitation with DNA sequencing, has aided in deciphering the histone code on a large-scale level. Limitations include the number of antibodies that can be used per platform and the steady-state view of chromatin structure ChIP provides.

Tissue-Specificity

The ideal place to look for epigenetic changes relevant to psychiatric disorders is live brain tissue. But we cannot get at this tissue in living patients. One alternative is to examine postmortem brain samples from patients. However, these are limited in number, and there are concerns about the potential for artifact.

Another approach to this challenge is to examine epigenetic profiles of human peripheral blood or saliva. Both tissues allow investigators to analyze larger populations over a period of time, which is an advantage for cohort-based studies or biomarker discovery. The challenge here is that tissue-type and cell-type specificity is well known for DNAm, at least for some loci.[25,26] It is this very specificity that helps confer some of the unique features of each tissue and cell type. Within the brain itself, there are region-specific differences, as shown by Ladd-Acosta et al.[27] Nonetheless, across the genome, there are many regions where DNAm does correlate substantially across tissues. Studies have found correlations of DNAm in blood and postmortem brain tissues to range from r = 0.61–0.91.[28,29] Correlation studies have also compared brain to saliva, which consists of ~70% lymphocytes and ~30% epithelial cells. One study compared DNAm from both saliva and blood to postmortem brain, and reported that saliva may show more similar DNAm patterns to brain than does blood.[30]

Another area of investigation tests whether saliva DNAm correlates more strongly with neuronal DNAm or glial cell DNAm. Glial cell pathology has been an area of recent interest and has been implicated in SCZ.[31] Differences in DNAm between neurons and glial cells have been observed,[32] suggesting that examination of these cell types separately could be illuminating. A further implication of these differences is that there is a need, when making comparisons across samples, to adjust for potential differences between neuron and glial proportions. Methods for doing so have been recently developed.[33] The same issue arises in blood and saliva studies, as these two are composed on disparate cell types. A method for this kind of adjustment, proposed by Houseman et al., has become widely used.[34]

Additional approaches to the selection of tissues for the study of psychiatric illnesses include using live brain tissues from animal models, surrogate central nervous system (CNS) tissues in live patients, and induced neurons derived from patients through the use of stem cell technology.

Animal Models

Rodent models offer multiple advantages in epigenetics, including the ability to test a single isolated exposure, introduce drugs in the prenatal period, obtain brain tissue, and observe multiple developmental stages in a relatively brief period.

Stress, a well-known risk factor for psychiatric disorders, has been explored using a variety of paradigms.[35] Studies have capitalized on the ability to analyze methylation patterns in rodent brain tissue, specifically particular brain regions, after exposure to these kinds of stress paradigms.[36–38]

Data Analytic Considerations

Many new statistical packages and approaches have been developed to analyze genome-wide DNAm data. At least five comprehensive packages make use of Illumina methylation array data: methylumi, minfi, wateRmelon, ChAMP, and RnBeads. All five are available through Bioconductor, which utilizes the R statistical programming language, and allows for the import of raw files or of methylation values.[39] Similarly, a variety of tools have been created to analyze the results derived from sequencing bisulfite-treated DNA. These include Bismark, BSMAP, and BS-seeker2,[40] ERNE 2,[41] and WALT.[42] One new method, methyLiftover, allows for the integration of DNAm data between sequencing and array-based approaches.[43]

Findings

DNA Methylation in Psychiatric Phenotypes

Studies have been conducted to test the relationship of DNAm to psychiatric disorders, both at the level of one or several candidate genes and at the genome-wide level. A brief overview of these is provided in Table 12.1.

Table 12.1 DNA Methylation

Disease	Type of Study	Genes Implicated	Citation
SCZ	Genome-wide	BDNF, ST6GALNAC1, FAM63B	Mill et al. 2008, Dempster et al. 2011, Aberg et al. 2014, Dempster et al. 2014
	Candidate gene	COMT, RELN, BNDF, OXTR	Costa et al. 2002, Grayson et al. 2005, Abdolmaleky et al. 2006, Tamura et al. 2007, Kundakovic et al. 2015, Rubin et al. 2016, Ursini et al. 2016
BD	Genome-wide	GP2R4, CTNNA2,	Mill 2008, Dempster 2011
	Candidate gene	COMT, HTR2A, NR3C1, HCG9, 5-HTTLPR	Abdolmaleky 2006, Ghadirivasfi 2011, Sugawara 2011, Kaminsky 2012
MDD	Genome-wide	PRIMA1, STK32C, DGKH, GSK3B, SGK1	Sabunciyan et al. 2012, Dempster et al. 2014, Cordova-Palomera et al. 2015, Numata 2015
	Candidate gene	CRF, BDNF	Elliott et al. 2010, Sterrenburg et al. 2011
PTSD	Genome-wide	NPFFR2	Smith et al. 2011
	Candidate gene	NR3C1, FKBP5, PACAP, ADCYAP1R1	Ressler et al. 2011, Klengal et al. 2013
Addiction	Genome-wide	PPM1G	Ruggeri et al. 2015
	Candidate gene	TET1, MeCP2, DNMT	Deng et al. 2010, Im et al. 2010, Kaas et al. 2013

An early example of an intriguing result implicating DNAm variation in psychiatric illness came from Grayson et al.,[44] who compared DNA from postmortem brains of people with SCZ and controls. They observed increased DNAm in cases within the promoter region of *RELN*, a gene whose protein product had previously been found to be downregulated in SCZ in GABA-ergic neurons.

The Petronis laboratory published the earliest epigenome-wide study of SCZ and BD in 2008. They used a CpG island microarray approach covering 7,834 regions and interrogated genomic DNA samples from postmortem frontal cortices of SCZ and BD and matched controls. Methylation changes were identified at ~100 sites across the genome, with glutamate receptor-related and GABA-signaling genes (*GRIA2* and *MARLIN-1*) among the strongest results.[45]

Recent epigenome studies of SCZ have expanded coverage to over 450,000 CpG loci. Montano et al. examined a discovery set of ~650 SCZ cases and controls, and a replication set totaling ~500. There were 923 CpGs found to be differentially methylated, of which 172 replicated in the second sample. Genes involved in neuronal function (such as *NCOR2* and *SULT4A1*) and T-cell development (*ZC3H12D, TCF3*) were highlighted.[46]

The first genome-wide DNA methylation study of MDD examined 39 postmortem frontal cortex MDD samples and 26 controls using the Comprehensive High-throughput Arrays for Relative Methylation (CHARM) platform, covering 3.5 million CpGs. There were 224 candidate regions identified having DNAm differences >10%, and these were enriched in genes relevant for neuronal growth and development. Further experimental validation showed the greatest differences in *PRIMA1*, with 12–15% increased DNAm in MDD.[47] However, these were not replicated in an independent sample. Another study compared unmedicated MDD subjects to controls using blood samples and the Illumina methylation array. Significant differences in DNAm were observed at 363 CpG sites in the discovery set. Eighty-four genes were replicated in an independent sample, such as *DGKH, GSK3B*, and *SGK1*.[48]

In PTSD, there have largely been studies that assessed peripheral blood and examined candidate genes. One important study identified *ADCYAP1R1* as a gene for which DNAm varies with PTSD status.[49] The first genome-wide DNAm study examined 110 people with and without PTSD, using an Illumina microarray. They reported one result that met criteria for experiment-wide significance, in the gene *NPFFR2*.[50]

DNA Methylation in Stress Paradigms

Among the seminal early studies examining an epigenetic role in the impact of the environment on behavioral phenotypes was one from Michael Meany's group at McGill University using an animal model. In 2004, they reported that in the postnatal period, decreased maternal bonding behavior in rats—as measured by low frequencies of arched-back nursing and licking and grooming—reduced expression of glucocorticoid receptors and increased levels of stress hormones such as adrenocorticotropic hormone (ACTH) and corticosterone in their offspring. Decreased levels of glucocorticoid receptors (GR) in the hippocampus were associated with increased DNAm in the exon 1_7 GR promoter. The team found that this outcome led to diminished negative hypothalamic-pituitary-adrenal (HPA) axis feedback and increased reactivity to stress throughout the lifetime of the offspring.[51]

The same group later compared the homologous promoter in human postmortem hippocampus from suicide victims, with and without a history of childhood abuse, with controls. They found increased methylation of the promoter in abused subjects, consistent with the findings in the offspring of the poorly mothered rats.[52]

A review of 40 subsequent studies in animals and humans following up these results (most of them focused on the GR exon variant 1_F in humans or the $GR1_7$ in rats) found that 89% of human studies and 70% of animal studies of early-life adversity reported increased methylation at this exon variant.[53]

Another important stress-related gene for which there is ample evidence for epigenetics playing a mediating role in psychiatric disease is *FKBP5*. The protein product of this gene is a co-chaperone protein that regulates the activity of the glucocorticoid receptor. Glucocorticoid hormones can elevate *FKBP5* expression by altering DNAm patterns at the *FKBP5* locus.[38] Childhood adversity has been observed to decrease DNAm at a regulatory element in intron 7 of *FKBP5*, increasing its expression in response to glucocorticoid receptor signaling, thus dampening the negative feedback mechanism of the HPA axis.[54]

Histone Modifications

A number of studies have examined how variation in modifications of histones correlates with psychiatric disorder, using both candidate gene and genome-wide approaches. An overview of these results is provided in Table 12.2.

Acetylation and methylation are the two heavily studied modifications of histone complexes. These typically occur on lysine residues, which are designated by the letter "K." For example, hypo-acetylation on lysines 9 and 14 on H3 (H3K9K14) was associated with decreased expression of glutamic acid decarboxylase 1,[55] a gene encoding an enzyme for GABA-synthesis that is deregulated in SCZ and BD.[56] Enzymes that modify acetylation, the HDAC family, have been implicated in disease. Postmortem samples showed increased *HDAC1*, *3*, and *4* levels in SCZ patients.[57] *HDAC2* levels were increased in the nucleus accumbens in postmortem MDD samples, and in chronic-stress rodent models of the disorder.[58]

One early observation was that administration of HDAC inhibitors improved depression in animal models.[59–61] Recent studies have demonstrated that histone modifications are seen in the setting of using additional psychiatric medications. For example, histone H3 changes were noted around the leptin receptor gene after administration of valproate, and also lithium.[62]

Histone acetylation has been well studied in the realm of drug addiction. HDAC4 attenuates H3K9/K14 acetylation levels and inhibits place preference and cocaine self-administration in mice; however, chronic cocaine exposure decreases *HDAC4* activity. Because *HDAC4* regulates synaptic development and plasticity, one hypothesis is that cocaine exposure leads to epigenetic

Table 12.2 Histone Modifications

Disease	Type of Study	Histone Mechanisms Assessed	Citation
SCZ	Genome-wide	H3K4 trimethylation	Shi et al. 2009, Cheung et al. 2010, Bharadwaj et al. 2014
	Site-based	H3K9K14 acetylation	Tang, Dean, & Thomas 2011
BD	Genome-wide	—	—
	Site-based	H3K9K14 acetylation	Tang, Dean, & Thomas 2011
MDD	Genome-wide	—	—
	Site-based	ACF (ATP-utilizing chromatin assembly and remodeling factor) H3K14 acetylation	Sun et al. 2015
PTSD	Genome-wide	—	—
	Site-based	H3 and H4 acetylation	Levenson et al. 2004, Matsumoto et al. 2013
Addiction	Genome-wide	H3K9me3	Maze et al. 2010
	Gene-based	HDAC4, HDAC5, H3K9, H3K14ac, H3K9me2, H3K9me3	Kumar et al. 2005, Renthal et al. 2007, Maze et al. 2010, Sando et al. 2012

changes and addiction via this enzyme.[63] Similarly, repeated cocaine exposure downregulates *G9a* and *GLP* (G9a-like protein) which methylate lysine 9 of histone 3. G9a opposes ΔFosB, a transcription factor associated with increased dendritic spine density in chronic cocaine exposure.[61,64]

The results of pathway analysis based on genome-wide association study (GWAS) data from over 60,000 participants from the Psychiatric Genomics Consortium (PGC) implicated *H3K4* methylation across MDD, BD, and SCZ.[65] Interestingly, the antipsychotic drug clozapine increases the tri-methylation pattern of *H3K4* in mouse models.[66]

Non-Coding RNAs

Researchers looking at SCZ were the first to implicate miRNA expression variation in psychiatric illness. Beveridge et al. assayed postmortem brain from dorsolateral prefrontal cortex and noted 16 differentially expressed miRNAs that were significantly associated with SCZ. Among their results, miRNA miR-107 and members of the miR-15 family have repeatedly been identified by other investigators.[67] Some miRNAs, like miR-29c, miR-106, and miR-132, show evidence across SCZ, BD, and MDD.[68] An overview of results in this domain is provided in Table 12.3.

SNPs in miRNA genes have also been associated with psychiatric disorders. The Psychiatric Genetics Consortium analyzed 17,836 cases and 33,859 controls and found that rs1625579 was within the miRNA-137 transcript and associated with SCZ. Through a GWAS meta-analysis including 52 studies, the Psychiatric Genetics Consortium also found that SCZ risk genes were more likely to be regulated by miRNAs, and that miR-9-5-p was the top miRNA associated with SCZ.[69]

Challenges

Investigators examining epigenetic variation in relation to psychiatric disorders face a number of obstacles to defining associations and mechanisms. We

Table 12.3 Small Non-Coding RNA

Disease	Type of Study	miRNA	Gene Targets	Citation
SCZ	Genome-wide	miRNA-132, miR-137, miR-9-5-p, miRNA-181b, miR-485-5p	GRIA2, VSNL1, BDNF, DRD1, NRG1, DNMT3A, GATA2, DPYSL3	Beveridge et al. 2008, Santarelli et al. 2011, Miller et al. 2012, Hauberg et al. 2016
	Site-specific	miRNA-137	M1R137HG, GPLX1, NSF, SYT1	Van Erp et al. 2014, Siegert et al. 2015, Wright et al. 2016
BD	Genome-wide	miR-499	CACNB2	Forstner et al. 2015
	Site-specific	mi-RNA-34	ANK3, CACNB3	Bavamian et al. 2015
MDD	Genome-wide			
	Site-specific	miR-335	GRM4	Li et al. 2015
PTSD	Genome-wide	—	—	—
	Site-specific	miR-608	AChE	Wingo et al. 2015, Lin et al. 2016
Addiction	Genome-wide	miR-181a, MiR-124, MiR-212, let-7d	—	Chandrasekar & Dreyer 2009, Hollander et al. 2010
	Site-specific	—	—	—

have spoken already of the challenging tissue issue. Beyond tissues, there is the problem that particular cell types within a tissue may vary epigenetically. Further, given the uniquely high level of neuronal differentiation in the brain, there could be a level of cell-specificity in epigenetic marks not seen elsewhere in the body. Another concern is that epigenetic marks show developmental stage-specific variation. Epigenetic signatures crucial to the understanding of psychiatric disease are likely to exist at early stages of development (such as the fetus); yet, we are typically limited to postnatal samples. It is possible that new approaches using 3-D human brain organoids might allow insight into epigenetic programs at these earlier stages.

Disentangling disease effects from treatment effects is often complicated, as most study participants included in analyses are taking medications. Accessing unmedicated individuals is one way of circumventing this problem; other potential solutions include determining medication effects in animal models, human induced pluripotent stem cells, or human brain organoids.

Finally, the issue of causation is more problematic in epigenetic than in genetic studies. Whereas a mutation or genetic variation can always be presumed to have preceded the disease, the temporal relationship between an epigenetic mark and a disease cannot easily be established. Did the epigenetic mark precede illness and was it a cause of the illness, or did the variation follow the illness as a compensatory reaction? Did it precede a stressor, or was it induced by a stressor? Longitudinal studies of cohorts provide the best way to establish temporality, but these are time-consuming, costly, and suffer from loss to follow-up.

New Horizons

Several new approaches are becoming available. First, stress has been recently found to induce changes to a novel epigenetic mark, 5-hydroxymethylcytosine (5hmC) that might affect behavior. 5hmC is thought to be an intermediate metabolic product of oxidized methylated cytosine and has been observed to alleviate transcriptional repression mediated by 5-methylcytosines.[70] Although whether 5hmC is involved in psychiatric illness is currently unknown, 5hmC is implicated in regulating mammalian brain development, neurogenesis, and gene expression.[71,72] Future studies might incorporate methods to distinguish 5mC from 5hmC, such as Tet-assisted bisulfite sequencing (TAB-seq) or oxidative bisulfite-sequencing (oxBS-seq).[73,74]

A second future direction involves the study of non-CpG methylation in the stressed brain. Gou et al. provided direct molecular evidence showing that non-CpG methylation affects gene expression and discovered that non-CpG methylation in adult mouse neurons was conserved in the adult human brain.[75] Methods such as whole-genome bisulfite sequencing may aid in accessing such novel epigenetic marks.

Studies are now emerging to examine DNAm in very large patient samples. For example, the Psychiatric Genetic Consortium PTSD group has an Epigenome-Wide Association Study (EWAS) component coupled with its GWAS. Integration across the two study types could prove a powerful approach for the detection of PTSD-implicated genes. A similar strategy might be of value for disorders like MDD and addiction.

References

1. Johnson, T. B., & Coghill, R. (1925). The discovery of 5-methyl-cytosine in tuberculinic acid, the nucleic acid of the tubercle bacillus. *The American Chemical Society, 47*, 2838–2844.

2. Griffith, J. S., & Mahler, H. R. (1969). DNA ticketing theory of memory. *Nature, 223*(5206), 580–582.

3. Holliday, R., & Pugh, J. E. (1975). DNA modification mechanisms and gene activity during development. *Science, 187*(4173), 226–232.

4. Riggs, A. D. (1975). X inactivation, differentiation, and DNA methylation. *Cytogenetics & Cell Genetics, 14*(1), 9–25.

5. McGhee, J. D., & Ginder, G. D. (1979). Specific DNA methylation sites in the vicinity of the chicken beta-globin genes. *Nature, 280*(5721), 419–420.

6. Holliday, R. (1979). A new theory of carcinogenesis. *British Journal of Cancer, 40*(4), 513–522.

7. Feinberg, A. P., & Vogelstein, B. (1983). Hypomethylation distinguishes genes of some human cancers from their normal counterparts. *Nature, 301*(5895), 89–92.

8. Baylin, S. B., Hoppener, J. W., de Bustros, A., Steenbergh, P. H., Lips, C. J., & Nelkin, B. D. (1986). DNA methylation patterns of the calcitonin gene in human lung cancers and lymphomas. *Cancer Research, 46*(6), 2917–2922.

9. Strahl, B. D., & Allis, C. D. (2000). The language of covalent histone modifications. *Nature, 403*(6765), 41–45.

10. Franklin, T. B., Russig, H., Weiss, I. C., Graff, J., Linder, N., Michalon, A., . . . Mansuy, I. M. (2010). Epigenetic transmission of the impact of early stress across generations. *Biological Psychiatry, 68*(5), 408–415.

11. Dias, B. G., & Ressler, K. J. (2014). Parental olfactory experience influences behavior and neural structure in subsequent generations. *Nature Neuroscience, 17*(1), 89–96.

12. Yehuda, R., Daskalakis, N. P., Bierer, L. M., Bader, H. N., Klengel, T., Holsboer, F., & Binder, E. B. (2016). Holocaust exposure induced intergenerational effects on FKBP5 methylation. *Biological Psychiatry, 80*(5), 372–380.

13. Liu, X. S., Wu, H., Ji, X., Stelzer, Y., Wu, X., Czauderna, S., . . . Jaenisch, R. (2016). Editing DNA methylation in the mammalian genome. *Cell, 167*(1), 233–247.e17.

14. Sullivan, P. F., Daly, M. J., & O'Donovan, M. (2012). Genetic architectures of psychiatric disorders: the emerging picture and its implications. *Nature Reviews Genetics, 13*(8), 537–551.

15. Gluckman, P. D., Hanson, M. A., Cooper, C., & Thornburg, K. L. (2008). Effect of in utero and early-life conditions on adult health and disease. *New England Journal of Medicine, 359*(1), 61–73.

16. Marmorstein, N. R., Malone, S. M., & Iacono, W. G. (2004). Psychiatric disorders among offspring of depressed mothers: associations with paternal psychopathology. *American Journal of Psychiatry, 161*(9), 1588–1594.

17. Kapoor, A., Leen, J., & Matthews, S. G. (2008). Molecular regulation of the hypothalamic-pituitary-adrenal axis in adult male guinea pigs after prenatal stress at different stages of gestation. *Journal of Physiology, 586*(17), 4317–4326.

18. Thompson, W. R. (1957). Influence of prenatal maternal anxiety on emotionality in young rats. *Science, 125*(3250), 698–699.

19. Lister, R., Pelizzola, M., Dowen, R. H., Hawkins, R. D., Hon, G., Tonti-Filippini, J., . . . Ecker, J. R. (2009). Human DNA methylomes at base resolution show widespread epigenomic differences. *Nature, 462*(7271), 315–322.

20. Xie, W., Barr, C. L., Kim, A., Yue, F., Lee, A. Y., Eubanks, J., Dempster, E. L., & Ren, B. (2012). Base-resolution analyses of sequence and parent-of-origin dependent DNA methylation in the mouse genome. *Cell, 148*(4), 816–831.

21. Susser, E. S., & Lin, S. P. (1992). Schizophrenia after prenatal exposure to the Dutch Hunger Winter of 1944-1945. *Archives of General Psychiatry, 49*(12), 983–988.

22. Heijmans, B. T., Tobi, E. W., Stein, A. D., Putter, H., Blauw, G. J., Susser, E. S., . . . Lumey, L. H. (2008). Persistent epigenetic differences associated with prenatal exposure to famine in humans. *Proceedings of the National Academy of Sciences of the USA, 105*(44), 17046–17049.

23. Tobi, E. W., Goeman, J. J., Monajemi, R., Gu, H., Putter, H., Zhang, Y., . . . Heijmans, B. T. (2014). DNA methylation signatures link prenatal famine exposure to growth and metabolism. *Nature Communications, 5,* 5592.

24. Jaffe, A. E., Gao, Y., Deep-Soboslay, A., Tao, R., Hyde, T. M., Weinberger, D. R., & Kleinman, J. E. (2016). Mapping DNA methylation across development, genotype and schizophrenia in the human frontal cortex. *Nature Neuroscience, 19*(1), 40–47.

25. Waalwijk, C., & Flavell, R. A. (1978). DNA methylation at a CCGG sequence in the large intron of the rabbit beta-globin gene: tissue-specific variations. *Nucleic Acids Research, 5*(12), 4631–4634.

26. Irizarry, R. A., Ladd-Acosta, C., Wen, B., Wu, Z., Montano, C., Onyango, P., . . . Feinberg, A. P. (2009). The human colon cancer methylome shows similar hypo- and hypermethylation at conserved tissue-specific CpG island shores. *Nature Genetics, 41*(2), 178–186.

27. Ladd-Acosta, C., Pevsner, J., Sabunciyan, S., Yolken, R. H., Webster, M. J., Dinkins, T., . . . Feinberg, A. P. (2007). DNA methylation signatures within the human brain. *American Journal of Human Genetics, 81*(6), 1304–1315.

28. Horvath, S., Zhang, Y., Langfelder, P., Kahn, R. S., Boks, M. P., K. van Eijk, . . . Ophoff, R. A. (2012). Aging effects on DNA methylation modules in human brain and blood tissue. *Genome Biology, 13*(10):R97.

29. Davies, M. N., Volta, M., Pidsley, R., Lunnon, K., Dixit, A., Lovestone, S., . . . Mill, J. (2012). Functional annotation of the human brain methylome identifies tissue-specific epigenetic variation across brain and blood. *Genome Biology, 13*(6):R43.

30. Smith, A. K., Kilaru, V., Klengel, T., Mercer, K. B., Bradley, B., Conneely, K. N., . . .Binder, E. B. (2015). DNA extracted from saliva for methylation studies of psychiatric traits: evidence [of] tissue specificity and relatedness to brain. *American Journal of Medical Genetics B, Neuropsychiatric Genetics* 168b (1), 36–44.

31. Sekar, A., Bialas, A. R., de Rivera, H., Davis, A., Hammond, T. R., Kamitaki, N., . . . McCarroll, S. A. (2016). Schizophrenia risk from complex variation of complement component 4. *Nature, 530*(7589), 177–183.

32. Iwamoto, K., Bundo, M., Ueda, J., Oldham, M. C., Ukai, W., Hashimoto, E., T. . . . Kato, T. (2011). Neurons show distinctive DNA methylation profile and higher interindividual variations compared with non-neurons. *Genome Research, 21*(5), 688–696.

33. Guintivano, J., Aryee, M. J., & Kaminsky, Z. A. (2013). A cell epigenotype specific model for the correction of brain cellular heterogeneity bias and its application to age, brain region and major depression. *Epigenetics, 8*(3), 290–302.

34. Houseman, E. A., Accomando, W. P., Koestler, D. C., Christensen, B. C., Marsit, C. J., Nelson, H. H., . . . Kelsey, K. T. (2012). DNA methylation arrays as surrogate measures of cell mixture distribution. *BMC Bioinformatics, 13*, 86.

35. Wilson, M. A., Grillo, C. A., Fadel, J. R., & Reagan, L. P. (2015). Stress as a one-armed bandit: Differential effects of stress paradigms on the morphology, neurochemistry and behavior in the rodent amygdala. *Neurobiology of Stress, 1*, 195–208.

36. Niwa, M., Jaaro-Peled, H., Tankou, S., Seshadri, S., Hikida, T., Matsumoto, Y., . . . Sawa, A. (2013). Adolescent stress-induced epigenetic control of dopaminergic neurons via glucocorticoids. *Science, 339*(6117), 335–339.

37. Boersma, G. J., Lee, R. S., Cordner, Z. A., Ewald, E. R., Purcell, R. H., Moghadam, A. A., & Tamashiro, K. L. (2014). Prenatal stress decreases Bdnf expression and increases methylation of Bdnf exon IV in rats. *Epigenetics, 9*(3), 437–447.

38. Lee, R. S., Tamashiro, K. L., Yang, X., Purcell, R. H., Harvey, A., Willour, V. L., . . . Potash, J. B. (2010). Chronic corticosterone exposure increases expression and decreases deoxyribonucleic acid methylation of Fkbp5 in mice. *Endocrinology, 151*(9), 4332–4343.

39. Morris, T. J., & Beck, S. (2015). Analysis pipelines and packages for Infinium HumanMethylation450 BeadChip (450k) data. *Methods, 72*, 3–8.

40. Lee, J. H., Park, S. J., & Kenta, N. (2015). An integrative approach for efficient analysis of whole genome bisulfite sequencing data. *BMC Genomics, 16*(Suppl 12), S14.

41. Chen, H., Smith, A. D., & Chen, T. (2016). WALT: fast and accurate read mapping for bisulfite sequencing. *Bioinformatics, 32*(22):3507-3509.

42. Prezza, N., Vezzi, F., Kaller, M., & Policriti, A. (2016). Fast, accurate, and lightweight analysis of BS-treated reads with ERNE 2. *BMC Bioinformatics, 17*(Suppl 4), 69.

43. Titus, A. J., Houseman, E. A., Johnson, K. C., & Christensen, B. C. (2016). methyLiftover: cross-platform DNA methylation data integration. *Bioinformatics, 32*(16), 2517–2519.

44. Grayson, D. R., Jia, X., Chen, Y., Sharma, R. P., Mitchell, C. P., Guidotti, A., & Costa, E. (2005). Reelin promoter hypermethylation in schizophrenia. *Proceedings of the National Academy of Sciences of the USA, 102*(26), 9341–9346.

45. Mill, J., Tang, T., Kaminsky, Z., Khare, T., Yazdanpanah, S., Bouchard, L., . . . Petronis, A. (2008). Epigenomic profiling reveals DNA-methylation changes associated with major psychosis. *American Journal of Human Genetics, 82*(3), 696–711.

46. Montano, C., Taub, M. A., Jaffe, A., Briem, E., Feinberg, J. I., Trygvadottir, R., . . . Feinberg, A. P. (2016). Association of DNA methylation differences with schizophrenia in an epigenome-wide association study. *JAMA Psychiatry, 73*(5), 506–514.

47. Sabunciyan, S., Aryee, M. J., Irizarry, R. A., Rongione, M., Webster, M. J., Kaufman, W. E., . . . Potash, J. B. (2012). Genome-wide DNA methylation scan in major depressive disorder. *PLoS One, 7*(4):e34451.

48. Numata, S., Ishii, K., Tajima, A., Iga, J., Kinoshita, M., Watanabe, S., . . . Ohmori, T. (2015). Blood diagnostic biomarkers for major depressive disorder using multiplex DNA methylation profiles: discovery and validation. *Epigenetics, 10*(2), 135–141.

49. Ressler, K. J., Mercer, K. B., Bradley, B., Jovanovic, T., Mahan, A., Kerley, K., . . . May, V. (2011). Post-traumatic stress disorder is associated with PACAP and the PAC1 receptor. *Nature, 470*(7335), 492–497.

50. Smith, A. K., Conneely, K. N., Kilaru, V., Mercer, K. B., Weiss, T. E., Bradley, B., . . . Ressler, K. J. (2011). Differential immune system DNA methylation and cytokine regulation in post-traumatic stress disorder. *American Journal of Medical Genetics B, Neuropsychiatric Genetics, 156B*(6), 700–708.

51. Weaver, I. C., Cervoni, N., Champagne, F. A., A. C. D'Alessio, Sharma, S., Seckl, J. R., . . . Meaney, M. J. (2004). Epigenetic programming by maternal behavior. *Nature Neuroscience, 7*(8), 847–854.

52. McGowan, P. O., Sasaki, A., A. C. D'Alessio, Dymov, S., Labonte, B., Szyf, M., . . . Meaney, M. J. (2009). Epigenetic regulation of the glucocorticoid receptor in human brain associates with childhood abuse. *Nature Neuroscience, 12*(3), 342–348.

53. Turecki, G., & Meaney, M. J. (2016). effects of the social environment and stress on glucocorticoid receptor gene methylation: A systematic review. *Biological Psychiatry, 79*(2), 87–96.

54. Klengel, T., Mehta, D., Anacker, C., M. Rex-Haffner, Pruessner, J. C., Pariante, C. M., . . . Binder, E. B. (2013). Allele-specific FKBP5 DNA demethylation mediates gene–childhood trauma interactions. *Nature Neuroscience, 16*(1), 33–41.

55. Tang, B., Dean, B., & Thomas, E. A. (2011). Disease- and age-related changes in histone acetylation at gene promoters in psychiatric disorders. *Translational Psychiatry, 1*, e64.

56. Ruzicka, W. B., Subburaju, S., & Benes, F. M. (2015). Circuit- and diagnosis-specific DNA methylation changes at gamma-aminobutyric acid-related genes in postmortem human hippocampus in schizophrenia and bipolar disorder. *JAMA Psychiatry, 72*(6), 541–551.

57. Sharma, R. P., Grayson, D. R., & Gavin, D. P. (2008). Histone deactylase 1 expression is increased in the prefrontal cortex of schizophrenia subjects: analysis of the National Brain Databank microarray collection. *Schizophrenia Research, 98*(1–3), 111–117.

58. Sun, H., Kennedy, P. J., & Nestler, E. J. (2013). Epigenetics of the depressed brain: role of histone acetylation and methylation. *Neuropsychopharmacology, 38*(1), 124–137.

59. Schroeder, F. A., Lin, C. L., Crusio, W. E., & Akbarian, S. (2007). Antidepressant-like effects of the histone deacetylase inhibitor, sodium butyrate, in the mouse. *Biological Psychiatry, 62*(1), 55–64.

60. Covington, H. E. 3rd, Maze, I., LaPlant, Q. C., Vialou, V. F., Ohnishi, Y. N., Berton, O., . . . Nestler, E. J. (2009). Antidepressant actions of histone deacetylase inhibitors. *Journal of Neuroscience, 29*(37), 11451–11460.

61. Tsankova, N. M., Berton, O., Renthal, W., Kumar, A., Neve, R. L., & Nestler, E. J. (2006). Sustained hippocampal chromatin regulation in a mouse model of depression and antidepressant action. *Nature Neuroscience*, *9*(4), 519–525.

62. Lee, R. S., Pirooznia, M., Guintivano, J., Ly, M., Ewald, E. R., Tamashiro, K. L., . . . Potash, J. B. (2015). Search for common targets of lithium and valproic acid identifies novel epigenetic effects of lithium on the rat leptin receptor gene. *Translational Psychiatry*, *5*, e600.

63. Kumar, A., Choi, K. H., Renthal, W., Tsankova, N. M., Theobald, D. E., Truong, H. T., . . . Nestler, E. J. (2005). Chromatin remodeling is a key mechanism underlying cocaine-induced plasticity in striatum. *Neuron*, *48*(2), 303–314.

64. Maze, I., Covington, H. E., 3rd, Dietz, D. M., LaPlant, Q., Renthal, W., Russo, S. J., . . . Nestler, E. J. (2010). Essential role of the histone methyltransferase G9a in cocaine-induced plasticity. *Science*, *327*(5962), 213–216.

65. Network and Pathway Analysis Subgroup of Psychiatric Genomics Consortium. (2015). Psychiatric genome-wide association study analyses implicate neuronal, immune and histone pathways. *Nature Neuroscience*, *18*(2), 199–209.

66. Huang, H. S., Matevossian, A., Whittle, C., Kim, S. Y., Schumacher, A., Baker, S. P., & Akbarian, S. (2007). Prefrontal dysfunction in schizophrenia involves mixed-lineage leukemia 1-regulated histone methylation at GABAergic gene promoters. *Journal of Neuroscience*, *27*(42), 11254–11262.

67. Beveridge, N. J., Tooney, P. A., Carroll, A. P., Gardiner, E., Bowden, N., Scott, R. J., . . . Cairns, M. J. (2008). Dysregulation of miRNA 181b in the temporal cortex in schizophrenia. *Human Molecular Genetics*, *17*(8), 1156–1168.

68. Whalley, H. C., Papmeyer, M., Romaniuk, L., Sprooten, E., Johnstone, E. C., Hall, J., . . . McIntosh, A. M. (2012). Impact of a microRNA MIR137 susceptibility variant on brain function in people at high genetic risk of schizophrenia or bipolar disorder. *Neuropsychopharmacology*, *37*(12), 2720–2729.

69. Hauberg, M. E., Roussos, P., Grove, J., Borglum, A. D., Mattheisen, M., & Consortium Schizophrenia Working Group of the Psychiatric Genomics. (2016). Analyzing the role of microRNAs in schizophrenia in the context of common genetic risk variants. *JAMA Psychiatry*, *73*(4), 369–377.

70. Booth, M. J., Branco, M. R., Ficz, G., Oxley, D., Krueger, F., Reik, W., & Balasubramanian, S. (2012). Quantitative sequencing of 5-methylcytosine and 5-hydroxymethylcytosine at single-base resolution. *Science*, *336*(6083), 934–937.

71. Lister, R., Mukamel, E. A., Nery, J. R., Urich, M., Puddifoot, C. A., Johnson, N. D., . . . Ecker, J. R. (2013). Global epigenomic reconfiguration during mammalian brain development. *Science*, *341*(6146), 1237905.

72. Booth, M. J., Ost, T. W., Beraldi, D., Bell, N. M., Branco, M. R., Reik, W., & Balasubramanian, S. (2013). Oxidative bisulfite sequencing of 5-methylcytosine and 5-hydroxymethylcytosine. *Nature Protocols*, *8*(10), 1841–1851.

73. Yu, M., Hon, G. C., Szulwach, K. E., Song, C. X., Jin, P., Ren, B., & He, C. (2012). Tet-assisted bisulfite sequencing of 5-hydroxymethylcytosine. *Nature Protocols*, *7*(12), 2159–2170.

74. Guo, J. U., Su, Y., Shin, J. H., Shin, J., Li, H., Xie, B., . . . Song, H. (2014). Distribution, recognition and regulation of non-CpG methylation in the adult mammalian brain. *Nature Neuroscience*, *17*(2), 215–222.

Table References

Abdolmaleky, H. M., Cheng, K. H., Faraone, S. V., Wilcox, M., Glatt, S. J., Gao, F., . . . Thiagalingam, S. (2006). Hypomethylation of MB-COMT promoter is a major risk factor for schizophrenia and bipolar disorder. *Human Molecular Genetics, 15*(21), 3132–3145.

Aberg, K. A., McClay, J. L., Nerella, S., Clark, S., Kumar, G., Chen, W., . . . van den Oord, E. J. (2014). Methylome-wide association study of schizophrenia: identifying blood biomarker signatures of environmental insults. *JAMA Psychiatry, 71*(3), 255–264.

Bavamian, S., Mellios, N., Lalonde, J., Fass, D. M., Wang, J., Sheridan, S. D., . . . Haggarty, S. J. (2015). Dysregulation of miR-34a links neuronal development to genetic risk factors for bipolar disorder. *Molecular Psychiatry, 20*(5), 573–584.

Bharadwaj, R., Peter, C. J., Jiang, Y., Roussos, P., Vogel-Ciernia, A., Shen, E. Y., . . . Akbarian, S. (2014). Conserved higher-order chromatin regulates NMDA receptor gene expression and cognition. *Neuron, 84*(5), 997–1008.

Chandrasekar, V., & Dreyer, J. L. (2009). microRNAs miR-124, let-7d and miR-181a regulate cocaine-induced plasticity. *Molecular & Cellular Neuroscience, 42*(4), 350–362.

Cheung, I., Shulha, H. P., Jiang, Y., Matevossian, A., Wang, J., Weng, Z., & Akbarian, S. (2010). Developmental regulation and individual differences of neuronal H3K4me3 epigenomes in the prefrontal cortex. *Proceedings of the National Academy of Sciences of the USA, 107*(19), 8824–8829.

Cordova-Palomera, A., Fatjo-Vilas, M., Gasto, C., Navarro, V., Krebs, M. O., & Fananas, L. (2015). Genome-wide methylation study on depression: differential methylation and variable methylation in monozygotic twins. *Translational Psychiatry, 5*, e557.

Costa, E., Chen, Y., Davis, J., Dong, E., Noh, J. S., Tremolizzo, L., . . . Guidotti, A. (2002). REELIN and schizophrenia: a disease at the interface of the genome and the epigenome. *Molecular Interventions, 2*(1), 47–57.

Dempster, E. L., Pidsley, R., Schalkwyk, L. C., Owens, S., Georgiades, A., Kane, F., . . . Mill, J. (2011). Disease-associated epigenetic changes in monozygotic twins discordant for schizophrenia and bipolar disorder. *Human Molecular Genetics, 20*(24), 4786–4796.

Dempster, E. L., Wong, C. C., Lester, K. J., Burrage, J., Gregory, A. M., Mill, J., & Eley, T. C. (2014). Genome-wide methylomic analysis of monozygotic twins discordant for adolescent depression. *Biological Psychiatry, 76*(12), 977–983.

Deng, J. V., Rodriguiz, R. M., Hutchinson, A. N., Kim, I. H., Wetsel, W. C., & West, A. E. (2010). MeCP2 in the nucleus accumbens contributes to neural and behavioral responses to psychostimulants. *Nature Neuroscience, 13*(9), 1128–1136.

Elliott, E., Ezra-Nevo, G., Regev, L., A. Neufeld-Cohen, & Chen, A. (2010). Resilience to social stress coincides with functional DNA methylation of the Crf gene in adult mice. *Nature Neuroscience, 13*(11), 1351–1353.

Forstner, A. J., Hofmann, A., Maaser, A., Sumer, S., Khudayberdiev, S., Muhleisen, T. W., . . . Nothen, M. M. (2015). Genome-wide analysis implicates microRNAs and their target genes in the development of bipolar disorder. *Translational Psychiatry, 5*, e678.

Ghadirivasfi, M., Nohesara, S., Ahmadkhaniha H., Eskandari M., Mostafavi S., Thiagalingam S., & Abdolmaleky H. M. (2011). Hypomethylation of the serotonin receptor type-2A gene (HTR2A) at T102C polymorphic site in DNA derived from the saliva of patients with schizophrenia and bipolar disorder. *American Journal of Medical Genetics B, Neuropsychiatric Genetics, 156*(5), 536–545.

Hahn, M. A., Qiu, R., Wu, X., Li, A. X., Zhang, H., Wang, J., . . . Lu, Q. (2013). Dynamics of 5-hydroxymethylcytosine and chromatin marks in mammalian neurogenesis. *Cell Reports, 3*(2), 291–300.

Hollander, J. A., Im, H. I., Amelio, A. L., Kocerha, J., Bali, P., Lu, Q., . . . Kenny, P. J. (2010). Striatal microRNA controls cocaine intake through CREB signalling. *Nature, 466*(7303), 197–202. doi:10.1038/nature09202.

Im, H. I., Hollander, J. A., Bali, P., & Kenny, P. J. (2010). MeCP2 controls BDNF expression and cocaine intake through homeostatic interactions with microRNA-212. *Nature Neuroscience, 13*(9), 1120–1127.

Kaas, G. A., Zhong, C., Eason, D. E., Ross, D. L., Vachhani, R. V., Ming, G. L., . . . Sweatt, J. D. (2013). TET1 controls CNS 5-methylcytosine hydroxylation, active DNA demethylation, gene transcription, and memory formation. *Neuron, 79*(6), 1086–1093.

Kaminsky, Z., Tochigi, M., Jia, P., Pal, M., Mill, J., Kwan, A., . . .Petronis, A. (2012). A multi-tissue analysis identifies HLA complex group 9 gene methylation differences in bipolar disorder. *Molecular Psychiatry, 17*, 728-740.

Kundakovic, M., Gudsnuk, K., Herbstman, J. B., Tang, D., Perera, F. P., & Champagne, F. A. (2015). DNA methylation of BDNF as a biomarker of early-life adversity. *Proceedings of the National Academy of Sciences of the USA, 112*(22), 6807–6813.

Levenson, J. M., O'Riordan, K. J., Brown, K. D., Trinh, M. A., Molfese, D. L., & Sweatt, J. D. (2004). Regulation of histone acetylation during memory formation in the hippocampus. *Journal of Biological Chemistry, 279*(39), 40545–40559.

Li, J., Meng, H., Cao, W., & Qiu, T. (2015). MiR-335 is involved in major depression disorder and antidepressant treatment through targeting GRM4. *Neuroscience Letters, 606*, 167–172.

Lin, T., Simchovitz, A., Shenhar-Tsarfaty, S., Vaisvaser, S., Admon, R., Hanin, G., . . . Soreq, H. (2016). Intensified vmPFC surveillance over PTSS under perturbed microRNA-608/AChE interaction. *Translational Psychiatry, 6*, e801.

Matsumoto, Y., Morinobu, S., Yamamoto, S., Matsumoto, T., Takei, S., Fujita, Y., & Yamawaki, S. (2013). Vorinostat ameliorates impaired fear extinction possibly via the hippocampal NMDA-CaMKII pathway in an animal model of posttraumatic stress disorder. *Psychopharmacology (Berlin), 229*(1), 51–62.

Miller, B. H., Zeier, Z., Xi, L., Lanz, T. A., Deng, S., Strathmann, J., . . . Wahlestedt, C. (2012). MicroRNA-132 dysregulation in schizophrenia has implications for both neurodevelopment and adult brain function. *Proceedings of the National Academy of Sciences of the USA, 109*(8), 3125–3130.

Renthal, W., Maze, I., Krishnan, V., Covington, H. E., 3rd, Xiao, G., Kumar, A., . . . Nestler, E. J. (2007). Histone deacetylase 5 epigenetically controls behavioral adaptations to chronic emotional stimuli. *Neuron, 56*(3), 517–529.

Rubin, L. H., Connelly, J. J., Reilly, J. L., Carter, C. S., Drogos, L. L., H. Pournajafi-Nazarloo, . . . Sweeney, J. A. (2016). Sex and diagnosis specific associations between DNA methylation of the oxytocin receptor gene with emotion processing and temporal-limbic and prefrontal brain volumes in psychotic disorders. *Biological Psychiatry Cognitive Neuroscience Neuroimaging, 1*(2), 141–151.

Ruggeri, B., Nymberg, C., Vuoksimaa, E., Lourdusamy, A., Wong, C. P., Carvalho, F. M., . . . Imagen Consortium. (2015). Association of protein phosphatase PPM1G with alcohol use disorder and brain activity during behavioral control in a genome-wide methylation analysis. *American Journal of Psychiatry*, *172*(6), 543–552.

Sando, R. 3rd, Gounko, N., Pieraut, S., Liao, L., Yates, J. 3rd, & Maximov, A. (2012). HDAC4 governs a transcriptional program essential for synaptic plasticity and memory. *Cell*, *151*(4), 821–834.

Santarelli, D. M., Beveridge, N. J., Tooney, P. A., & Cairns, M. J. (2011). Upregulation of dicer and microRNA expression in the dorsolateral prefrontal cortex Brodmann area 46 in schizophrenia. *Biological Psychiatry*, *69*(2), 180–187.

Shi, J., Levinson, D. F., Duan, J., Sanders, A. R., Zheng, Y., Pe'er, I., . . . Gejman, P. V. (2009). Common variants on chromosome 6p22.1 are associated with schizophrenia. *Nature*, *460*(7256), 753–757.

Siegert, S., Seo, J., Kwon, E. J., Rudenko, A., Cho, S., Wang, W., . . . Tsai, L. H. (2015). The schizophrenia risk gene product miR-137 alters presynaptic plasticity. *Nature Neuroscience*, *18*(7), 1008–1016.

Sterrenburg, L., Gaszner, B., Boerrigter, J., Santbergen, L., Bramini, M., Elliott, E., . . . Kozicz, T. (2011). Chronic stress induces sex-specific alterations in methylation and expression of corticotropin-releasing factor gene in the rat. *PLoS One*, *6*(11), e28128.

Tamura, Y., Kunugi, H., Ohashi, J., & Hohjoh, H. (2007). Epigenetic aberration of the human REELIN gene in psychiatric disorders. *Molecular Psychiatry*, *12*(6), 519, 593–600.

Ursini, G., Cavalleri, T., Fazio, L., Angrisano, T., Iacovelli, L., Porcelli, A., . . . Bertolino, A. (2016). BDNF rs6265 methylation and genotype interact on risk for schizophrenia. *Epigenetics*, *11*(1), 11–23.

Van Erp, T. G., Guella, I., Vawter, M. P., Turner, J., Brown, G. G., McCarthy, G., . . . Potkin, S. G. (2014). Schizophrenia miR-137 locus risk genotype is associated with dorsolateral prefrontal cortex hyperactivation. *Biological Psychiatry*, *75*(5), 398–405.

Wingo, A. P., Almli, L. M., Stevens, J. J., Klengel, T., Uddin, M., Li, Y., . . . Ressler, K. J. (2015). DICER1 and microRNA regulation in post-traumatic stress disorder with comorbid depression. *Nature Communication*, *6*, 10106.

Wright, C., Gupta, C. N., Chen, J., Patel, V., Calhoun, V. D., Ehrlich, S., . . . Turner, J. A. (2016). Polymorphisms in MIR137HG and microRNA-137-regulated genes influence gray matter structure in schizophrenia. *Translational Psychiatry*, *6*, e724.

Chapter 13

Next-Generation Sequencing in Genetic Studies of Psychiatric Disorders

Shweta Ramdas and Jun Z. Li

Take-Home Points

1. NGS provides cost-effective and unbiased survey of DNA variants, transforming disease gene hunting for both population-based and family-based study designs.
2. Many specialized analytical methods have been developed to take advantage of these power data, especially in defining the contribution of rare variants to disease risks in different cases/families.
3. More progress is expected with integrated analysis of DNA, gene expression, and other omics data, along with increasingly rich phenotypical data that capture dynamic gene–environment interactions.

Introduction

Next-generation sequencing (NGS) refers to the series of technologies emerged in the last 15 years that can determine DNA sequence (the order of nucleotides in DNA fragments) with ultra-high throughput.[1,2] While exploiting a variety of assay chemistries and designs, these technologies share a common feature: they read 10^7 to 10^8 DNA molecules in a massively parallel fashion, and this is achieved by dramatic improvements in multiplexing, miniaturization, automated imaging, and high-performance computing. Currently (early 2017), NGS can sequence a full copy of human genome 200 times per instrument per day. The cost of a 30X human genome has been reduced to ~$1,000, and is expected to decrease further. Meanwhile, multiple specialized platforms support custom resequencing of targeted regions, sequencing of longer reads (10–200 kb) or single DNA molecules, or assembled phase-resolved long reads (100 kb). Together, these advances have transformed genetic research by enabling *ab initio* variant discovery for either the entire genome or any predefined subset of the genome for 100s–1000s of subjects with a moderate budget. In this chapter, we will provide a condensed account of how the application of NGS has impacted the pursuit of an genetic explanation of complex diseases such as psychiatric disorders. We will review relevant concepts in study design, basic data types produced by NGS, and analysis strategies that often build on linkage analysis (see Chapter 4 or 5) and genome-wide association studies (GWAS) (Chapter 4 or 5). We will conclude with a discussion of current limitations and future outlook.

Co-evolution of Genomic Technology and Gene Identification Methods

In recent decades, the prevailing approach to understanding the heritable variation of human traits has undergone several major shifts, each time driven by the arrival of new technologies that not only bring new types of DNA variants, but also survey such variants on dramatically larger and finer scales. In the 1990s, when it was possible to determine short tandem repeats at 4–20 cM intervals, the principal method for disease gene mapping was *linkage analysis*, which examines the co-segregation of marker alleles with disease status in human pedigrees. Since the mid-2000s, with the ability to genotype 10^5–10^6 single-nucleotide polymorphisms (SNPs) accurately and inexpensively, geneticists adopted a more powerful approach, *association study*, which searches for case-control differences of allele frequencies using unrelated samples that can be collected much more easily than pedigrees. By focusing on common variants that each "tag" a region of linkage disequilibrium (LD), this method can test candidate regions, but it is most powerful when used to scan the entire genome.[3] Continuing this technology-driven forward rush, NGS expanded gene hunting from common variants to rare variants. Much of this expansion is still under way, and is expected to accelerate disease gene discovery for both pedigree-based and population-based studies.

Genetic Heterogeneity and Rare Variants

To understand how NGS sets off the new round of exploration, one only need recall that the previous leading approach, genome-wide association study (GWAS), relies on genotyping known variants, which are chosen mainly as positional markers—they do not need to be coding or otherwise functional variants. In GWAS, a positive signal highlights an *associated region* of tens of kilobases, which usually contains many variants, few of which, if any, have a "causal" allele that directly alters biological function and leads to the disease. Thus a GWAS finding is no more than a statistical signpost marking a genomic region to begin searching for the actual causal variants. This often involves fine mapping and resequencing of patient samples to identify plausible high-risk alleles. In contrast, sequencing the genomes at the outset not only determines the genotype at known variant loci, but also enables unbiased identification of all variants, both common and rare, in all the regions of interest and in all subjects. The benefit of such comprehensive variant detection is especially notable in terms of allelic heterogeneity vis-à-vis locus heterogeneity. If common variants from many different loci contribute to disease risk, there is *locus heterogeneity* in the population; and GWAS is well suited to identify these loci, especially if it has sufficient power to detect small effects. However, if there is extensive allelic heterogeneity, such that the causal variants at a given locus are individually rare—carried by different people and occurring on different haplotype backgrounds—GWAS will be underpowered because LD-based association signals from different patients could contradict each other. In such a scenario, having the knowledge of all the rare variants allows us to recognize different damaging alleles in different individuals or families, and accumulate such per-gene variant burden information over many subjects or across families. In other words, sequencing creates a complete catalog of low-frequency, potentially high-risk alleles acting in different individuals/families. With this information in hand, if a positional signal has already been found in GWAS, one can more quickly prioritize the potential causal variants. Or, in family-based studies, loci with risk allele heterogeneity can still be detected. The detailed strategy to aggregate rare variant signals differs between case-control studies and family-based studies; and we will describe them separately later. But first we will provide a brief overview of genome coverage, variant detection, quality assessment, and annotation.

Scope of Genome Coverage

For cost reasons, many studies have focused on sequencing the coding regions of the genome; namely, all the exons and their flanking regions of all known genes. This is called *whole-exome sequencing* (WES), usually targeting 230,000–300,000 exons for a total length of 30–60 Mb. The main rationale for WES is that rare variants that directly affect protein structure are more likely to produce a biochemical effect in the cell; and non-coding variants, even after being discovered by *whole-genome sequencing* (WGS), will still be difficult to interpret (see *variant annotation* in the section "Functional Annotation"). WES requires an additional target capture step to selectively enrich the 1–2% of the genome corresponding to the exons. This is done by synthesizing a large pool of oligonucleotides specifically designed to "pull down" the targeted DNA fragments by hybridization, whereas the >98% of un-hybridized fragments are washed away. One of the drawbacks of WES is the non-uniform coverage across the exome due to differential capture and amplification. Consequently, some targeted exons will be poorly represented; and calling copy number variations (CNVs) is more challenging than using WGS data. Different capturing designs and reagents, supplied by different commercial vendors, often show varying coverage patterns, requiring further care when one tries to merge different WES datasets in combined analyses. With decreasing costs and more uniform coverage, WGS has increasingly become the method of choice. Some variants in non-coding regions the genome may serve important regulatory roles; thus, having the complete inventory of all variants in a genome facilitates future reinterpretation.

Variant Calling and Quality Control

To date, most sequencing-based analyses of human diseases have relied on short-read sequencing platforms such as those from Illumina. The pipeline for calling single-nucleotide variants involves read alignment to the reference human genome, removal of duplicate reads arising from PCR amplification, identifying variant sites among the sequenced samples, and determining the most likely genotypes at these sites for each sample, along with probability-based confidence scores. The best practices for implementing a robust variant calling pipeline have become increasingly standardized.[4] Meanwhile, specialized algorithms have been developed to detect other types of variation from the same data: short insertions and deletions ("indels"),[5–7] copy number variants,[8,9] structural variation such as inversions and complex translocations,[10,11] or short tandem repeats.[12,13] Some groups have developed tools to simultaneously ascertain multiple classes of variants.[14]

A rigorous data analysis plan must also include quality control routines. This is implemented by calculating quality scores to evaluate if a read is aligned with confidence, if a site is truly variable among the samples sequenced, if a genotype call is reliable, or if the calling confidence has batch-to-batch variation. The variant data of each individual are also used to identify samples that may have low-level contamination of other samples, to confirm the sex of the subjects, their ethnicity, and the expected familial relationship.

Functional Annotation

Variant annotation refers to the task of managing the evolving knowledge of functional attributes of each variant, while evaluating the quality of experimental evidence and prediction accuracy. It is essential for interpreting the variants and genes identified by statistical ranking, and for producing such a ranking; i.e., using informatics algorithms to prioritize the most likely causal variants/genes. Each variant discovered by NGS can be annotated along at least three principal dimensions.

The first dimension is the *population frequency* of the newly discovered alleles, ranging from common, rare, and extremely rare, to private—i.e., those not seen in any other individual in the existing database, and are sometimes called "singletons." As public repositories of DNA variants will contain increasingly larger samples with every passing year,[15,16] the allele frequency estimates will become increasingly accurate; some of the singletons will sometimes be seen in a second individual; and in cases of concomitant sequencing of parent–child trios, some private variants in the child will be determined as *de novo*; that is, present in the child but in neither parent, probably having arisen in the parents' gametes or during early embryonic development.

The allele frequency information is an important aspect of potential function, because it is expected that deleterious variants will be passed on less often to offspring and will thus tend to be rarer in the population. A caveat to this general trend is that population demography in the recent past also affects allele frequency. For example, rapidly expanding populations have a surplus of rare variants.[17] A damaging variant might rise to high frequency by chance alone, especially in isolated groups with a small number of founding members. Population-specific allele frequency databases are thus highly valued by the research community.

The second dimension is the known or predicted *functional effect* of a variant allele. At the molecular level, variants falling within a protein-coding gene can be immediately classified by their location within that gene (intronic, exonic, etc.), their impact on the protein (e.g., nonsynonymous variants that change the coded amino acids), and the degree to which the amino acid substitution resulting from a nonsynonymous variant is conserved across species. Many algorithms have appeared that combine the evolutionary conservation, protein structure, physical property of the amino acid, and/or prior catalog of damaging variants to infer the probable pathogenicity of a given allele. Popular prediction algorithms have been reviewed recently.[18]

Variants that fall into non-coding regions of the genome can also be annotated, but this is more challenging. Regulatory functions of some non-coding variants may be inferred from the rich data resources being developed across numerous tissues and cell types.[19–21] These also include molecular quantitative trait loci (QTL)[22,23] that impact the expression level of a gene (called eQTL) and segments of inferred chromatin states[24,25] that may reveal long-range regulatory effects.

The third level of annotation relates to prior biological knowledge of the gene. These include whether the gene was implicated in similar disorders, especially those documented in OMIM,[26] ClinVar,[27] and Human Gene Mutation Database(HGMD)[28]; whether the gene is considered *essential*[29,30] or intolerant of mutations[16,31]; whether the gene is expressed at the relevant tissues or developmental stages; and whether the gene has been implicated in prior linkage or association studies. Such gene-level annotation naturally extends to sets of interacting genes,[32,33] co-expression modules,[34–36] or pre-curated regulatory networks.[37,38]

Population-Based vs. Family-Based Studies

In case-control studies, the conventional method is to calculate association statistics one variant marker at a time. However, for rare variants, the single-marker approach has very low power, especially with the need to adjust for an increased number of variants tested. This is usually addressed by comparing the per-gene cumulative rare variant frequency between cases and controls, essentially collapsing rare variants' burden over each functional unit. The functional unit can also be a segment of non-coding region with presumed function (e.g., enhancer or promoter), or a set of such genes/segments with shared biological function. The simplest method to aggregate variants is to calculate the total count of rare alleles and compare this index between cases and controls. This index can be generalized by (1) focusing on rare variants by applying an allele frequency cutoff, or giving higher weights to variants of lower allele frequencies; (2) using predicted degree of pathogenicity as another selection criterion or weight; (3) using variant component methods to allow both directions of variant effect: either deleterious or protective; or (4) adaptively select the best weighing scheme among many combinations of variant frequency cutoffs and degrees of damaging effect. The frequently used algorithms for collapsing rare variants have been reviewed.[39,40] Across studies, the per-gene statistics can be combined using tools such as *RAREMETAL*.[41,42]

Family-based studies usually follow a different set of assumptions. Rare multiplex families, especially those with cases in multiple generations, may transmit one or a few high-penetrance variants that alter the function of key developmental or signaling genes. These extended pedigrees may represent a near-Mendelian or at least a highly penetrant subset of the cases, such that one or a few high-impact variants cause the disease in each family. Under this hypothesis, there is a high likelihood that affected relatives in one family would share the same causative variants that are rarely seen in other families. The test of this kind of hypothesis begins with unbiased discovery of rare damaging variants in each family, followed by per-family selection of variants shared among cases and not among unaffected family members. This usually highlights a short list of candidate genes for each family, allowing subsequent aggregation of gene-level or pathway-level signals across families. The list of high-value variants can either be derived from a series of hard filters or be weighted by allele frequency, pathogenicity scores, or linkage scores under a range of genetic models and phenotypical subgroups.

Per-family lists of variants and genes can be evaluated for patterns of recurrence across families and in increasingly larger sample collections. If different families carry causative variants in different genes, linkage or association studies would not effectively accrue statistical signals between families, yet the integration of sequencing–based variant discovery and analysis might still allow us to identify common biological pathways across high-risk families, thereby accumulating evidence for shared functional changes. Such higher-level analyses include pathway enrichment, overlap with past GWAS findings, epigenetic features, eQTLs, or other candidate genes.

Recent and Ongoing Studies of Psychiatric Disorders

Many large collaborative groups (see Chapter 4 or 5 on GWAS) have moved from GWAS towards sequencing-based approaches, sometimes using the same samples previously used in GWAS. Some early findings support the value of this approach. Sequencing studies of autism have revealed an increased rate of *de novo* variants in autism patients. Rare and de novo variants together account for 10–30% of people with autism spectrum disorders.[43,44] Exome sequencing studies of schizophrenia have identified a new risk gene (*SET1DA*)[45] along with an increased role of rare variants in calcium channels and those found in postsynaptic density.[46,47] Sequencing studies on major depression disorder (MDD) and bipolar disorder have produced fewer "hits" at this point. A recent study with >5,000 MDD cases found two genetic loci associated with the disorder,[48] but sequencing was "low pass"—carried out as a cost-saving alternative to genotyping common variants or deep sequencing—and the associated alleles are common in people of Asian ancestry. These and other studies have been reviewed elsewhere.[49-51]

Challenges and Future Opportunities

As NGS technologies continue to improve, future studies are likely to exploit long-read sequencing to provide phasing information (i.e., knowing whether two nearby variants came from the same or different parents, which is especially useful when a compound heterozygote leads to loss of function in the gene) and more sensitive detection of structural variations. In parallel, single-cell sequencing of RNA or epigenetic modifications will be adopted widely to reveal cellular heterogeneity at a finer granular level than ever before, with the potential to create a new generation of brain cell taxonomy and derive highly specific markers for use in high-resolution measurements of connectivity, movement of brain cells, and abnormal signaling. As a most recent example, McConnell et al.[52] described new initiatives to study somatic mosaicism among neurons and its relevance in neuropsychiatric disorders. NGS also enables cost-effective assays of epigenomic (see Chapters 11–12) features that could reflect potential impacts of early-life history and recent medication use.

While NGS technology has been a significant advance in our ability to collect ever bigger sets of genetic/genomic data, this same technology has thrown other limits in psychiatric genetics research into sharper relief. Brain disorders are inherently complex: they tend to implicate many variants in many genes, as well as gene–environment (G-E) interactions. It is in the latter that we continue to lack rich data: G-E interactions are likely to be dynamic, influenced by neurodevelopment in the embryo and stressful events in both early life and adulthood, all of which are difficult to measure. For this reason, the field is poised for significant future growth with inexpensive technologies for real-time logging of mood and physiology, and better access to electronic health records. Another direction to enhance the value of genetic data is simultaneous probing of brain function at multiple levels: individual cells, small-circuit connectivity, microanatomy, and large-ensemble behavior, including strength and timing of signaling among different brain foci.

Psychiatric genetic studies stand at an exciting crossroads. Significant progress can be made by designing multi-technology and multi-scale studies to collect the most useful data, followed by creative synthesis of such data to arrive at an integrated understanding of the biological underpinnings of psychiatric traits.

References

1. Goodwin, S., McPherson, J. D., & McCombie, W. R. (2016). Coming of age: Ten years of next-generation sequencing technologies. *Nature Reviews Genetics, 17*(6), 333–351.

2. Shendure, J., Mitra, R. D., Varma, C., & Church, G. M. (2004). Advanced sequencing technologies: Methods and goals. *Nature Reviews Genetics, 5*(5), 335–344.

3. Risch, N., & Merikangas, K. (1996). The future of genetic studies of complex human diseases. *Science, 273*(5281), 1516–1517.

4. DePristo, M. A., Banks, E., Poplin, R., Garimella, K. V., Maguire, J. R., Hartl, C., Philippakis, A. A., et al. (2011). A framework for variation discovery and genotyping using next-generation DNA sequencing data. *Nature Genetics, 43*(5), 491–498.

5. Albers, C. A., Lunter, G., MacArthur, D. G., McVean, G., Ouwehand, W. H., & Durbin, R. (2011). Dindel: Accurate indel calls from short-read data. *Genome Research, 21*(6), 961–973.

6. Chen, K., Wallis, J. W., McLellan, M. D., Larson, D. E., Kalicki, J. M., Pohl, C. S., McGrath, S. D., et al. (2009). BreakDancer: An algorithm for high-resolution mapping of genomic structural variation. *Nature Methods, 6*(9), 677–681.

7. Ye, K., Schulz, M. H., Long, Q., Apweiler, R., & Ning, Z. (2009). Pindel: A pattern growth approach to detect break points of large deletions and medium sized insertions from paired-end short reads. *Bioinformatics, 25*(21), 2865–2871.

8. Handsaker, R. E., Korn, J. M., Nemesh, J., & McCarroll, S. A. (2011). Discovery and genotyping of genome structural polymorphism by sequencing on a population scale. *Nature Genetics, 43*(3), 269–276.

9. Mills, R. E., Walter, K., Stewart, C., Handsaker, R. E., Chen, K., Alkan, C., Abyzov, A., et al. (2011). Mapping copy number variation by population-scale genome sequencing. *Nature, 470*(7332), 59–65.

10. Sudmant, P. H., Rausch, T., Gardner, E. J., Handsaker, R. E., Abyzov, A., Huddleston, J., Zhang, Y., et al. (2015). An integrated map of structural variation in 2,504 human genomes. *Nature, 526*(7571), 75–81.

11. Zhao, X., Emery, S. B., Myers, B., Kidd, J. M., & Mills, R. E. (2016). Resolving complex structural genomic rearrangements using a randomized approach. *Genome Biology, 17*(1), 126.

12. Fungtammasan, A., Ananda, G., Hile, S. E., Su, M. S., Sun, C., Harris, R., Medvedev, P., et al. (2015). Accurate typing of short tandem repeats from genome-wide sequencing data and its applications. *Genome Research, 25*(5), 736–749.

13. Gymrek, M., & Erlich, Y. (2013). Profiling short tandem repeats from short reads. *Methods in Molecular Biology, 1038*, 113–135.

14. Korn, J. M., Kuruvilla, F. G., McCarroll, S. A., Wysoker, A., Nemesh, J., Cawley, S., Hubbell, E., et al. (2008). Integrated genotype calling and association analysis of SNPs, common copy number polymorphisms and rare CNVs. *Nature Genetics, 40*(10), 1253–1260.

15. Huang, J., Howie, B., McCarthy, S., Memari, Y., Walter, K., Min, J. L., Danecek, P., et al. (2015). Improved imputation of low-frequency and rare variants using the UK10K haplotype reference panel. *Nature Communications, 6*, 8111.

16. Lek, M., Karczewski, K. J., Minikel, E. V., Samocha, K. E., Banks, E., Fennell, T., O'Donnell-Luria, A. H., et al. (2016). Analysis of protein-coding genetic variation in 60,706 humans. *Nature, 536*(7616), 285–291.

17. Keinan, A., & Clark, A. G. (2012). Recent explosive human population growth has resulted in an excess of rare genetic variants. *Science, 336*(6082), 740–743.

18. Cooper, G. M., & Shendure, J. (2011). Needles in stacks of needles: Finding disease-causal variants in a wealth of genomic data. *Nature Reviews Genetics, 12*(9), 628–640.

19. Boyle, A. P., Hong, E. L., Hariharan, M., Cheng, Y., Schaub, M. A., Kasowski, M., Karczewski, K. J., et al. (2012). Annotation of functional variation in personal genomes using RegulomeDB. *Genome Research, 22*(9), 1790–1797.

20. Ward, L. D., & Kellis, M. (2012). Interpreting noncoding genetic variation in complex traits and human disease. *Nature Biotechnology, 30*(11), 1095–1096.

21. Kundaje, A., Meuleman, W., Ernst, J., Bilenky, M., Yen, A., Heravi-Moussavi, A., Kheradpour, P., et al. (2015). Integrative analysis of 111 reference human epigenomes. *Nature, 518*(7539), 317–330.

22. Liang, L., Morar, N., Dixon, A. L., Lathrop, G. M., Abecasis, G. R., Moffatt, M. F., & Cookson, W. O. (2013). A cross-platform analysis of 14,177 expression quantitative trait loci derived from lymphoblastoid cell lines. *Genome Research, 23*(4), 716–726.

23. Nica, A. C., Montgomery, S. B., Dimas, A. S., Stranger, B. E., Beazley, C., Barroso, I., & Dermitzakis, E. T. (2010). Candidate causal regulatory effects by integration of expression QTLs with complex trait genetic associations. *PLoS Genetics, 6*(4), e1000895.

24. Ernst, J., & Kellis, M. (2012). ChromHMM: Automating chromatin-state discovery and characterization. *Nature Methods, 9*(3), 215–216.

25. Hoffman, M. M., Buske, O. J., Wang, J., Weng, Z., Bilmes, J. A., & Noble, W. S. (2012). Unsupervised pattern discovery in human chromatin structure through genomic segmentation. *Nature Methods, 9*(5), 473–476.

26. Amberger, J. S., Bocchini, C. A., Schiettecatte, F., Scott, A. F., & Hamosh, A. (2015). OMIM.org: Online Mendelian Inheritance in Man (OMIM®), an online catalog of human genes and genetic disorders. *Nucleic Acids Research, 43*(Database issue), D789–D798.

27. Harrison, S. M., Riggs, E. R., Maglott, D. R., Lee, J. M., Azzariti, D. R., Niehaus, A., Ramos, E. M., et al. (2016). Using ClinVar as a resource to support variant interpretation. *Current Protocols in Human Genetics, 89*, 8 16 1-8 16 23.

28. Stenson, P. D., Mort, M., Ball, E. V., Evans, K., Hayden, M., Heywood, S., Hussain, M., et al. (2017). The Human Gene Mutation Database: Towards a comprehensive repository of inherited mutation data for medical research, genetic diagnosis and next-generation sequencing studies. *Human Genetics, 136*(6), 665–677. doi:10.1007/s00439-017-1779-6.

29. Georgi, B., Voight, B. F., & Bucan, M. (2013). From mouse to human: Evolutionary genomics analysis of human orthologs of essential genes. *PLoS Genetics, 9*(5), e1003484.

30. Wang, T., Birsoy, K., Hughes, N. W., Krupczak, K. M., Post, Y., Wei, J. J., Lander, E. S., et al. (2015). Identification and characterization of essential genes in the human genome. *Science, 350*(6264), 1096–1101.

31. Petrovski, S., Gussow, A. B., Wang, Q., Halvorsen, M., Han, Y., Weir, W. H., Allen, A. S., et al. (2015). The intolerance of regulatory sequence to genetic variation predicts gene dosage sensitivity. *PLoS Genetics, 11*(9), e1005492.

32. Luo, X., Huang, L., Jia, P., Li, M., Su, B., Zhao, Z., & Gan, L. (2014). Protein–protein interaction and pathway analyses of top schizophrenia genes reveal schizophrenia susceptibility genes converge on common molecular networks and enrichment of nucleosome (chromatin) assembly genes in schizophrenia susceptibility loci. *Schizophrenia Bulletin, 40*(1), 39–49.

33. Cappi, C., Brentani, H., Lima, L., Sanders, S. J., Zai, G., Diniz, B. J., Reis, V. N., et al. (2016). Whole-exome sequencing in obsessive-compulsive disorder identifies rare mutations in immunological and neurodevelopmental pathways. *Translational Psychiatry, 6*, e764.

34. Willsey, A. J., Sanders, S. J., Li, M., Dong, S., Tebbenkamp, A. T., Muhle, R. A., Reilly, S. K., et al. (2013). Coexpression networks implicate human midfetal deep cortical projection neurons in the pathogenesis of autism. *Cell, 155*(5), 997–1007.

35. Gulsuner, S., Walsh, T., Watts, A. C., Lee, M. K., Thornton, A. M., Casadei, S., Rippey, C., et al. (2013). Spatial and temporal mapping of *de novo* mutations in schizophrenia to a fetal prefrontal cortical network. *Cell, 154*(3), 518–529.

36. Parikshak, N. N., Luo, R., Zhang, A., Won, H., Lowe, J. K., Chandran, V., Horvath, S., et al. (2013). Integrative functional genomic analyses implicate specific molecular pathways and circuits in autism. *Cell, 155*(5), 1008–1021.

37. Goes, F. S., Pirooznia, M., Parla, J. S., Kramer, M., Ghiban, E., Mavruk, S., Chen, Y. C., et al. (2016). Exome sequencing of familial bipolar disorder. *JAMA Psychiatry, 73*(6), 590–597.

38. Jansen, A., Dieleman, G. C., Smit, A. B., Verhage, M., Verhulst, F. C., Polderman, T. J. C., & Posthuma, D. (2017). Gene-set analysis shows association between FMRP targets and autism spectrum disorder. *European Journal of Human Genetics, 25*(7), 863–868. doi:10.1038/ejhg.2017.55

39. Bomba, L., Walter, K., & Soranzo, N. (2017). The impact of rare and low-frequency genetic variants in common disease. *Genome Biology, 18*(1), 77.

40. Lee, S., Abecasis, G. R., Boehnke, M., & Lin, X. (2014). Rare-variant association analysis: Study designs and statistical tests. *American Journal of Human Genetics, 95*(1), 5–23.

41. Feng, S., Liu, D., Zhan, X., Wing, M. K., & Abecasis, G. R. (2014). RAREMETAL: Fast and powerful meta-analysis for rare variants. *Bioinformatics, 30*(19), 2828–2829.

42. Liu, D. J., Peloso, G. M., Zhan, X., Holmen, O. L., Zawistowski, M., Feng, S., Nikpay, M., et al. (2014). Meta-analysis of gene-level tests for rare variant association. *Nature Genetics, 46*(2), 200–204.

43. Vorstman, J. A. S., Parr, J. R., Moreno-De-Luca, D., Anney, R. J. L., Nurnberger, J. I., Jr., & Hallmayer, J. F. (2017). Autism genetics: Opportunities and challenges for clinical translation. *Nature Reviews Genetics, 18*(6), 362–376. doi:10.1038/nrg.2017.4.

44. Sanders, S. J., He, X., Willsey, A. J., Ercan-Sencicek, A. G., Samocha, K. E., Cicek, A. E., Murtha, M. T., et al. (2015). Insights into autism spectrum disorder genomic architecture and biology from 71 risk loci. *Neuron, 87*(6), 1215–1233.

45. Singh, T., Kurki, M. I., Curtis, D., Purcell, S. M., Crooks, L., McRae, J., Suvisaari, J., et al. (2016). Rare loss-of-function variants in SETD1A are associated with schizophrenia and developmental disorders. *Nature Neuroscience, 19*(4), 571–577.

46. Purcell, S. M., Moran, J. L., Fromer, M., Ruderfer, D., Solovieff, N., Roussos, P., O'Dushlaine, C., et al. (2014). A polygenic burden of rare disruptive mutations in schizophrenia. *Nature, 506*(7487), 185–190.

47. Genovese, G., Fromer, M., Stahl, E. A., Ruderfer, D. M., Chambert, K., Landen, M., Moran, J. L., et al. (2016). Increased burden of ultra-rare protein-altering variants among 4,877 individuals with schizophrenia. *Nature Neuroscience, 19*(11), 1433–1441.

48. CONVERGE Consortium. (2015). Sparse whole-genome sequencing identifies two loci for major depressive disorder. *Nature*, *523*(7562), 588–591.

49. Goes, F. S. (2016). Genetics of bipolar disorder: Recent update and future directions. *Psychiatric Clinics of North America*, *39*(1), 139–155.

50. Kato, T. (2015). Whole genome/exome sequencing in mood and psychotic disorders. *Psychiatry & Clinical Neurosciences*, *69*(2), 65–76.

51. Gratten, J. (2016). Rare variants are common in schizophrenia. *Nature Neuroscience*, *19*(11), 1426–1428.

52. McConnell, M. J., Moran, J. V., Abyzov, A., Akbarian, S., Bae, T., Cortes-Ciriano, I., Erwin, J. A., et al. (2017). Intersection of diverse neuronal genomes and neuropsychiatric disease: The Brain Somatic Mosaicism Network. *Science*, *356*(6336), 395. doi:10.1126/science.aal1641

Chapter 14

Animal Models

Tadafumi Kato

> ## Take-Home Points
>
> 1. Animal models of psychiatric disorders are crucial for drug develop-
>   ment, and psychiatric genetics can contribute to the generation of new
>   animal models.
> 2. Modeling copy number variations is a suitable strategy to model autism
>   and schizophrenia.
> 3. Stress-induced depression models are controversial.
> 4. A new animal model of bipolar disorder showing recurrent spontan-
>   eous depression-like episodes was proposed.
> 5. Neural circuit models show new directions.

Introduction

Animal models are indispensable to translating the findings in psychiatric
genetics into basic sciences such as the elucidation of neurobiological bases of
psychiatric disorders, the development of new treatment, and the discovery
of new biomarkers. In this chapter, issues related to animal models relevant to
psychiatric genetics are discussed.

Validity Criteria

Requisites for animal models of diseases are construct, face, and predictive
validities.[1] *Construct validity* refers to the common etiology shared by a disease
and the model. Animals with genetic and/or non-genetic factors that confer
a risk of psychiatric disorders can satisfy this validity. *Face validity* is common
signs and symptoms shared by a disease and the model. *Predictive validity* refers
to the common effect of drugs on a disease and the model. Ideal animal models should satisfy all three of these criteria.

In modeling genetic factors by an animal model, an effect size of the
genetic variation should be large enough. The variant that confers a risk of a
disease should be directly modeled in animals. For example, knockout mice
do not recapitulate the biological consequence caused by a single-nucleotide

polymorphism (SNP) that does not disrupt the function of the gene. When face validity is considered, behavioral differences between humans and other animals make it difficult to completely model human diseases.

Species

Various species have been utilized to model psychiatric disorders—macaque, marmoset, rat, mouse, fish, fly, and even nematode (Table 14.1). It can be argued which species can have the "mind." However, in that sense, no animal can have the same higher order mental function as humans. Thus, any animal model suffers from this difficulty. On the other hand, any species can potentially be useful at certain degrees. Thus, these animals are used, depending on the purposes of a given study. For example, macaques would be better than other small animals in simulating mental symptoms, and actually hallucination might be observed in the macaque.[2,3] Gene-targeting strategy is feasible in marmosets[4] and macaques.[5] These two non-human primates are phylogenetically close to humans, and would better model humans in behavioral and genetic dimensions than rodents would. However, ethics is also a matter of concern when using these species. Rodents such as rats and mice are widely used experimental animals, and genetic manipulation is well established, especially for the mouse. Thus, the mouse is the most widely used for generation of animal models of psychiatric disorders. In the drug development studies, these two species of rodents are used as the de facto standard. Fish, especially zebrafish, have been revealed to be useful for behavioral analysis, and are used for the study of the neural circuit basis of social defeat–associated behavior[6] or the genetic model of autism.[7] Transparency at early life is also a feature of zebrafish, which enables direct observation of the brain through their skin. In contrast to these vertebrates, use of invertebrates has not been a matter of interest in psychiatry.[8] However, as these species have clear benefit for genetic manipulation and genetic screening based on behavior, they are also feasible for the screening of candidate compounds based on behavioral effects.

Autism Spectrum Disorder

In autism spectrum disorder (ASD), where no effective therapy is available, predictive validity cannot be satisfied in any model. The first mouse model of autism that satisfied construct and face validities was published in 2009.[9] In this study, three aspects of autism—impairment in social behavior, communication, and stereotyped behavior—were observed in a mouse model simulating the 15q11-13 duplication in humans. Since then, model mice of other autism-associated copy number variations (CNVs)[10] such as 17p11.2 duplication[11] or 15q13.3 deletion,[12] as well as candidate genes such as *CNTNAP2, NLGN1/3/4*,

Table 14.1 Species for Animal Model of Psychiatric Disorders

Species	Behavioral Similarity	Feasibility of Genetic Manipulation	Throughput
Macaque	++++	+	+
Marmoset	++++	+	+
Rat	+++	+	++
Mouse	+++	+++	++
Fish	++	++++	+++
Fly	+	++++	++++
Nematode	+	++++	++++

NRXN1, SHANK1-3, and *PTEN*,[13] have been analyzed, and some of them showed the three domains of behavioral abnormalities. For non-genetic factors, perinatal valproate administration is most commonly used.[14]

Schizophrenia

Since the role of copy number variations in schizophrenia was established, model mice of chromosomal abnormality have been used for the animal models of schizophrenia. Animals exposed to environmental risk factors such as perinatal immune activation are also used as animal models. Most established models include model mice of DISC1[15], which is disrupted by chromosome 1:11 translocation, and 22q11 deletion.[16] Recently, other model mice of a CNV that confers a risk of schizophrenia, 15q13.3,[12] have also been generated.

More recently, association of loss-of-function mutations of a single gene, *SETD1A* (*KMT2F*), and schizophrenia has been reported.[17,18] Such gene would be a promising target of model mice by genome-editing technique such as CRISPR/Cas9 in rodents and primates.

Depression

Heritability of depression is not high, and the role of environmental factors is larger in major depression. Thus, for animal models of depression, environmental stressors have been used. Although forced swimming and tail suspension tests have been used to screen antidepressants, they are not genuine animal models. Because rodents floating on the water look like they are "giving up" swimming, some researchers think that they are behavioral despair and model depression. However, it can also be interpreted as a coping strategy to save energy.[19]

Stress-induced animal models include social defeat,[20] learned helplessness,[21] chronic unpredictable stress,[22] maternal separation,[23] and prenatal stress.[24] Response to antidepressants is different among models.[25]

Bipolar Disorder

Bipolar disorder is the least studied area of model animals. Though amphetamine-induced hyperactivity that has been used as an animal model of mania does not model recurrent spontaneous manic episodes, it is useful when combined with genetic models.[26] Though genome-wide association studies (GWAS) showed candidate genes, the effect size was small, and there has been no established gene with a large effect for bipolar disorder.[27]

In this situation, the authors are focusing on brain-specific mutant mice modeling Mendelian diseases that show bipolar disorder as a pleiotropic effect. Such diseases include Darier's disease,[28] Wolfram disease,[29] and chronic progressive external ophthalmoplegia.[30] Causative genes of these diseases are expressed in the endoplasmic reticulum and mitochondria, which accumulate calcium.[31] Model mice expressing mutant polymerase γ in neurons show recurrent spontaneous depression-like episodes that satisfy *Diagnostic and Statistical Manual of Mental Disorders, 5th ed.* (DSM-5) criteria for major depressive episode. They were improved by a selective serotonin reuptake inhibitor, worsened by a tricyclic antidepressant,[32] and triggered by withdrawal of lithium. Together with atypical features such as hypersomnia and hyperphagia, the model might be relevant to bipolar spectrum depression.

Neural Circuit Models

Recent development of the neuroscience of mental disorders makes it possible to model mental disorders at the circuit level. Optogenetic manipulation of midbrain dopamine neurons can simulate depression-like behavior in mice.[33] Optogenetic activation of cortico-striatal circuit caused excessive grooming, possibly modeling obsessive compulsive disorder.[34]

Conclusion

Animal models of mental disorders are still their infancy. Nevertheless, discovery of CNVs conferring a risk for autism spectrum disorder and schizophrenia greatly promoted the research in this area, and several animal models of CNVs are now established. Progress in psychiatric genetics will further promote the research of animal models of psychiatric disorders.

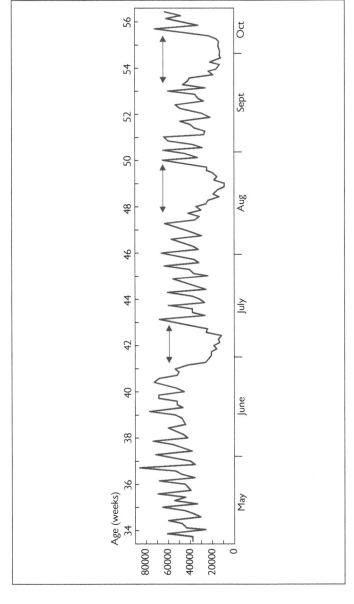

Figure 14.1 Recurrent spontaneous depression-like episodes seen in a neuron-specific mutant polymerase γ (*Polg1*) transgenic mouse. Vertical axis represents wheel running activity; horizontal axis shows the age of the mouse. The episodic changes of wheel-running activity with the duration of 4–5 days correspond to the estrous cycle. Depression-like episodes are indicated by double-headed arrows. Behavioral analysis during the episode showed that the episodes satisfied the A and B items of the DSM-5 criteria of major depressive episodes (Kasahara et al., 2016).

References

1. Nestler, E. J., & Hyman, S. E. (2010). Animal models of neuropsychiatric disorders. *Nature Neuroscience*, *13*, 1161–1169.

2. Castner, S. A., & Goldman-Rakic, P. S. (2003). Amphetamine sensitization of hallucinatory-like behaviors is dependent on prefrontal cortex in nonhuman primates. *Biological Psychiatry*, *54*, 105–110.

3. Sakai, M., Kashiwahara, N., Kakita, A., & Nawa, H. (2014). An attempt of non-human primate modeling of schizophrenia with neonatal challenges of epidermal growth factor. *Journal of Addiction Research & Therapy*, *5*, 170.

4. Okano, H., Miyawaki, A., & Kasai, K. (2015). Brain/MINDS: Brain-mapping project in Japan. *Philosophical Transactions of the Royal Society of London. Series B: Biological Sciences*, *370*.

5. Liu, Z., Li, X., Zhang, J. T., Cai, Y. J., Cheng, T. L., Cheng, C., . . . Qiu, Z. (2016). Autism-like behaviours and germline transmission in transgenic monkeys overexpressing MeCP2. *Nature*, *530*, 98–102.

6. Chou, M. Y., Amo, R., Kinoshita, M., Cherng, B. W., Shimazaki, H., Agetsuma, M., . . . Okamoto, H. (2016). Social conflict resolution regulated by two dorsal habenular subregions in zebrafish. *Science*, *352*, 87–90.

7. Hoffman, E. J., Turner, K. J., Fernandez, J. M., Cifuentes, D., Ghosh, M., Ijaz, S., . . . Giraldez, A. J. (2016). Estrogens suppress a behavioral phenotype in zebrafish mutants of the autism risk gene, CNTNAP2. *Neuron*, *89*, 725–733.

8. Burne, T., Scott, E., Van Swinderen, B., Hilliard, M., Reinhard, J., Claudianos, C., . . . Mcgrath, J. (2011). Big ideas for small brains: What can psychiatry learn from worms, flies, bees and fish? *Molecular Psychiatry*, *16*, 7–16.

9. Nakatani, J., Tamada, K., Hatanaka, F., Ise, S., Ohta, H., Inoue, K., . . . Takumi, T. (2009). Abnormal behavior in a chromosome-engineered mouse model for human 15q11-13 duplication seen in autism. *Cell*, *137*, 1235–1246.

10. Shishido, E., Aleksic, B., & Ozaki, N. (2014). Copy-number variation in the pathogenesis of autism spectrum disorder. *Psychiatry and Clinical Neurosciences*, *68*, 85–95.

11. Lacaria, M., Spencer, C., Gu, W., Paylor, R., & Lupski, J. R. (2012). Enriched rearing improves behavioral responses of an animal model for CNV-based autistic-like traits. *Human Molecular Genetics*, *21*, 3083–3096.

12. Kogan, J. H., Gross, A. K., Featherstone, R. E., Shin, R., Chen, Q., Heusner, C. L., . . . Matsumoto, M. (2015). Mouse model of chromosome 15q13.3 microdeletion syndrome demonstrates features related to autism spectrum disorder. *Journal of Neuroscience*, *35*, 16282–16294.

13. Kazdoba, T. M., Leach, P. T., & Crawley, J. N. (2016). Behavioral phenotypes of genetic mouse models of autism. *Genes, Brain & Behavior*, *15*, 7–26.

14. Ergaz, Z., Fudim-Weinstein, L., & Ornoy, A. (2016). Genetic and non-genetic animal models for Autism Spectrum Disorders (ASD). *Reproductive Toxicology*, *64*, 116–140.

15. Hikida, T., Jaaro-Peled, H., Seshadri, S., Oishi, K., Hookway, C., Kong, S., . . . Sawa, A. (2007). Dominant-negative DISC1 transgenic mice display schizophrenia-associated phenotypes detected by measures translatable to humans. *Proceedings of the National Academy of Sciences of the United States of America*, *104*, 14501–14506.

16. Stark, K. L., Xu, B., Bagchi, A., Lai, W. S., Liu, H., Hsu, R., . . . Gogos, J. A. (2008). Altered brain microRNA biogenesis contributes to phenotypic deficits in a 22q11-deletion mouse model. *Nature Genetics, 40*, 751–760.

17. Takata, A., Xu, B., Ionita-Laza, I., Roos, J. L., Gogos, J. A., & Karayiorgou, M. (2014). Loss-of-function variants in schizophrenia risk and SETD1A as a candidate susceptibility gene. *Neuron, 82*, 773–780.

18. Singh, T., Kurki, M. I., Curtis, D., Purcell, S. M., Crooks, L., Mcrae, J., . . . Barrett, J. C. (2016). Rare loss-of-function variants in SETD1A are associated with schizophrenia and developmental disorders. *Nature Neuroscience, 19*, 571–577.

19. West, A. P. (1990). Neurobehavioral studies of forced swimming: The role of learning and memory in the forced swim test. *Progress in Neuro-Psychopharmacol & Biological Psychiatry, 14*, 863–877.

20. Henry, J. P., Meehan, J. P., & Stephens, P. M. (1967). The use of psychosocial stimuli to induce prolonged systolic hypertension in mice. *Psychosomatic Medicine, 29*, 408–432.

21. Maier, S. F., & Seligman, M. E. P. (1976). Learned helplessness—Theory and evidence. *Journal of Experimental Psychology—General, 105*, 3–46.

22. Willner, P., Towell, A., Sampson, D., Sophokleous, S., & Muscat, R. (1987). Reduction of sucrose preference by chronic unpredictable mild stress, and its restoration by a tricyclic antidepressant. *Psychopharmacology (Berlin), 93*, 358–364.

23. Plotsky, P. M., & Meaney, M. J. (1993). Early, postnatal experience alters hypothalamic corticotropin-releasing factor (CRF) mRNA, median eminence CRF content and stress-induced release in adult rats. *Brain Res Mol Brain Res, 18*, 195–200.

24. Mueller, B. R., & Bale, T. L. (2008) Sex-specific programming of offspring emotionality after stress early in pregnancy. *J Neurosci, 28*, 9055–9065.

25. Berton, O., & Nestler, E. J. (2006). New approaches to antidepressant drug discovery: Beyond monoamines. *Nature Reviews Neuroscience, 7*, 137–151.

26. Gould, T. D., O'Donnell, K. C., Picchini, A. M., & Manji, H. K. (2007). Strain differences in lithium attenuation of d-amphetamine-induced hyperlocomotion: A mouse model for the genetics of clinical response to lithium. *Neuropsychopharmacology, 32*, 1321–1333.

27. Kato, T. (2015). Whole genome/exome sequencing in mood and psychotic disorders. *Psychiatry & Clinical Neurosciences, 69*, 65–76.

28. Nakamura, T., Kazuno, A. A., Nakajima, K., Kusumi, I., Tsuboi, T., & Kato, T. (2016). Loss of function mutations in ATP2A2 and psychoses: A case report and literature survey. *Psychiatry and Clinical Neurosciences, 70*, 342–350.

29. Kato, T., Ishiwata, M., Yamada, K., Kasahara, T., Kakiuchi, C., Iwamoto, K., . . . Oka, Y. (2008). Behavioral and gene expression analyses of Wfs1 knockout mice as a possible animal model of mood disorder. *Neuroscience Research, 61*, 143–158.

30. Kasahara, T., Takata, A., Kato, T. M., Kubota-Sakashita, M., Sawada, T., Kakita, A., . . . Kato, T. (2016). Depression-like episodes in mice harboring mtDNA deletions in paraventricular thalamus. *Molecular Psychiatry, 21*, 39–48.

31. Kato, T. (2008). Molecular neurobiology of bipolar disorder: A disease of "mood-stabilizing neurons"? *Trends in Neuroscience, 31*, 495–503.

32. Kasahara, T., Kubota, M., Miyauchi, T., Noda, Y., Mouri, A., Nabeshima, T., & Kato, T. (2006). Mice with neuron-specific accumulation of mitochondrial DNA mutations show mood disorder-like phenotypes. *Molecular Psychiatry, 11*, 577–593, 523.

33. Chaudhury, D., Walsh, J. J., Friedman, A. K., Juarez, B., Ku, S. M., Koo, J. W., . . . Han, M. H. (2013). Rapid regulation of depression-related behaviours by control of mid-brain dopamine neurons. *Nature*, *493*, 532–536.

34. Ahmari, S. E., Spellman, T., Douglass, N. L., Kheirbek, M. A., Simpson, H. B., Deisseroth, K., . . . Hen, R. (2013). Repeated cortico-striatal stimulation generates persistent OCD-like behavior. *Science*, *340*, 1234–1239.

Chapter 15

Biobanking of Human Induced Pluripotent Stem Cells for Psychiatric Research

Jennifer C. Moore, Michael Sheldon, and Jay A. Tischfield

Take-Home Points

1. For identification purposes and to provide a unique genetic "signature" for revealing possible cross-contamination in the future, all banked bio-samples, especially cell lines, should be profiled by either form.
2. Human induced pluripotent cell lines (hiPSC) can be produced from many different source cell types such as cultured skin fibroblasts or blood cells, but the latter have advantages in that nucleated blood cells from large numbers of subjects can be easily cryopreserved for future reprogramming to hiPSC.
3. hiPSC can be differentiated into different types of neurons, which may express altered cellular phenotypes reflecting the psychiatric disorder of the subject from whom they were taken.
4. Proper informed consent from subjects must be obtained at the outset of a project so that their cells can be reprogrammed to iPSC at a future date for use in research on the genetic etiology of psychiatric disorders.

Introduction

The broad technical aspects of biobanking in support of different types of research and clinical activity have been described in numerous publications.[1] Our immediate goal is not to provide yet another review, but rather to discuss how scientific and technological progress have placed greater and novel demands on biobanking in support of psychiatric research and functional genomics research in particular. We will concentrate on the production and banking of induced pluripotent stem cells (iPSC) from blood cells or skin fibroblasts, the two most common source tissues. The differentiation of iPSC to produce neuronal cells that can be used as surrogates for the study of brain tissue is proving to be a powerful tool for the elucidation of normal and pathological gene function in brain. We include a brief description of the production

203

and distribution of research-grade iPSCs from a biobanking perspective and the unusual demands that they place on biobanking resources.

The expertise and insight for this writing stems from our experience in establishing and growing biorepositories for the National Institute of Mental Health (NIMH), the National Institute of Drug Abuse (NIDA), the National Institute on Alcohol Abuse and Alcoholism (NIAAA), the Simons Foundation for Autism Research Initaitive (SFARI), the National Institute of Neurological Disorders and Stroke (NINDS), and other groups. Diverse services for these groups are provided through RUCDR Infinite Biologics® (Rutgers University Cell and DNA Repository [RUCDR], www.rucdr.org), located on the New Brunswick campus of Rutgers, the State University of New Jersey.

General Biobanking Issues

Biobanks maintained by individuals or small groups of researchers are at inherent risk of sample loss and/or compromise of sample quality. There have been several well-publicized incidents involving the loss of many samples that could have been avoided by adherence to best biobanking practices described in well-vetted and practiced, documented standard operating procedures (SOPs) and checklists. Biobanks in the United States and Canada with continuing College of American Pathologists (CAP) accreditation (http://www.cap.org/web/oracle/webcenter/portalapp/pagehierarchy/biorepository_accreditation_program.jspx?_afrLoop=1703393618729742#!%40%40%3F_afrLoop%3D1703393618729742%26_adf.ctrl-state%3D17fdcke37w_4) must meet clearly defined standards and undergo continuing and rigorous assessments and prompt remediation of any deficiencies determined by objective inspection. CAP serves as an interface with the International Society for Biological and Environmental Repositories (ISBER; http://www.isber.org/), which has published proficiency tests, assessment tools, and a detailed monograph on best practices for repositories (http://www.isber.org/?page=BPR). In general, CAP accreditation is an indicator of appropriately robust infrastructure and biobanking processes that include the accessioning, processing, storage, retrieval, and distribution of biosamples.

There are many documented examples of immortal human cell lines that were not the cell lines that researchers believed them to be, sometimes actually being widely grown human cell lines such as HeLa, or not even human cells.[2,3] In response to such errors and lack of experimental reproducibility consequent to cell line misidentification or contamination, the National Institutes of Health and many leading journals have now published guidelines for the authentication of key biological resources, requiring a description of methods used to ensure the identity and validity of cell lines, biologics, and specialty chemicals (NOT-OD-16-011: Implementing Rigor and Transparency in NIH & AHRQ Research Grant Applications) in order to qualify for grant funding or publication. While it is beyond the scope of this brief review to discuss all of the factors that can influence the reliability and quality of cultured cell lines, authentication of the identity of human cell lines such as lymphoblastoid cell lines (LCLs) or iPSCs is of critical importance to psychiatric research where each subject has a unique phenotype and genotype and mix-ups can be disastrous. The most widely used method for human cell line authentication is short tandem repeat (STR) DNA profiling, a multiplexed Polymerase Chain Reaction (PCR)-based assay that measures tetranucleotide repeats at up to 16 loci[4] and provides unambiguous identification of an individual by comparison to blood or other tissue from that individual. STR genotyping has the disadvantage of high cost of use on very large numbers of samples, and it is not easily automated. RUCDR introduced a 96 single-nucleotide polymorphism (SNP) panel that provides unambiguous data defining subject identity and sex in addition to limited data on ethnicity, and has very high correlation with subject self-report (unpublished). This panel, commercially known as SNP Trace®, is easily automated and much more cost effective than STR profiling for large sample numbers, while sacrificing little if any certainty of identification, and detecting cross-contamination at the 2% level. Direct comparison of STR and SNP Trace data from the same samples shows the SNP Trace panel discriminated among identical, related, and unrelated pairs of samples with a high degree of confidence, equivalent to STR profiling, at significantly lower cost and higher throughput.[5] Furthermore, SNP Trace results in the database can be compared to data from SNP microarrays (which contain many of the same SNPs) or DNA sequencing data, providing a simple means of authenticating the subject origin from genotype or sequence data without additional laboratory testing.

A secondary but important concern is mycoplasma contamination of cell cultures, which is known to change the chromosomal and biochemical properties of cell lines.[6] While most fungal or bacterial contamination is visible to the naked eye, or may kill cells after a short time, most mycoplasma contamination is cryptic and only detected through genomic testing involving PCR amplification of mycoplasma ribosomal DNA sequences,[7] or through microbiological culturing,[8] or by culturing on "reporter" mammalian cell lines and visualization through staining, (reviewed in endnote 9). Given the costs of mycoplasma testing and the workflow considerations involved in testing large numbers of cell lines, RUCDR routinely tests using automated PCR-based methods, submitting random or suspicious samples for microbiological testing. Prior to the routine utilization of this approach, there were a few limited outbreaks of mycoplasma contamination, and in most cases the mycoplasma species were determined to be bovine in origin. This finding mandates that all sera and similar biologicals be screened for mycoplasma before use. While much of recent iPSC culture does not require bovine or human serum, the source cells for reprogramming (e.g., fibroblasts) are likely to have been cultured in bovine serum.

Stem Cell Biobanking Methodologies in Psychiatric Research

The ability to generate iPSCs from somatic cells has changed the way human diseases, particularly psychiatric diseases, can be modeled. Previously, the cellular understanding of these diseases relied mainly on three different types of models: cadaver tissue, animal models, or human cell lines. In addition to potentially being difficult to obtain, donated cadaver tissue may be poorly preserved and may have been collected years after disease onset. While animal models are good at recapitulating some aspects of human psychiatric disorders, they can have significant drawbacks, including lack of genome homology,[10] non-human behaviors, and very divergent physiology.[11] Transformed cell lines have also been used extensively due to their relative abundance in biobanks (e.g., LCLs) and inexpensive culture conditions, but these cells can undergo changes in long-term culture that affect their functional and phenotypical validity.

In 2006 and 2007, mouse[12] and human fibroblasts,[13,14] respectively, were reprogrammed to a pluripotent state by the use of a combination of transcription factors consisting of OCT4, SOX2, NANOG, LIN28, KLF4, and MYC. The transcription factors required for reprogramming have since been delivered in many different ways, including via lentiviral vectors,[14–16] retroviral transduction,[17] episomes,[18] Sendai viral vectors,[19] mRNA,[20] or adenovirus.[21] Although all of these methods result in iPSCs, it is generally accepted that "footprint-free" methods that cause the least amount of alteration to the source cell genome are preferred, such as mRNA, episomes, or Sendai viral vectors. Even though episomes and Sendai are non-integrating, there is recently published evidence that suggests that they may result in some changes to the recipient cell DNA.[22] However, the use of mRNA requires multiple rounds of electroporation and can be detrimental to sensitive cells. At RUCDR, we deliver reprogramming factors by either episomes or Sendai viral vectors and test to ensure that the research-grade iPSCs are free from non-endogenous transcription factors.

The iPS cells thus derived, or "reprogrammed," by these methodologies express markers associated with the pluripotent state (Oct4, Tra-1-60, Tra1-81, and SSEA-4, among many others) and are capable of differentiating into all three developmental germ layers.[13,14] When exposed to different combinations of growth factors, these cells can be differentiated into many different types of neurons, such as cortical,[23,24] motor,[25,26] dopaminergic,[25,27] serotonergic,[28] and cerebellar,[29] among others. These neurons (or indeed, any other cell differentiated from iPSC) can provide a living system to study neural development (reviewed in endnotes 4, 30) or be used for drug screening (reviewed in endnotes 31, 32) or understand the toxicological effects of various compounds (reviewed in endnotes 33, 34).

While DNA for genomics studies can be extracted from saliva, blood, or other tissues (e.g., skin), if there is the intention of producing iPSCs immediately or at some future time, collection and processing of the latter two are preferred.

Although fibroblasts were the first cell type to be reprogrammed, they have some disadvantages. First, their collection requires a skin punch biopsy, which is invasive, less likely to be consented to by subjects than blood draw, and may raise institutional review board (IRB) concerns, especially when it involves patients with mental illnesses, or children. If IRB permission is obtained, they may specify such a small size biopsy that the quality of the resulting fibroblast culture is compromised. It has also been demonstrated that in order for cells to be reprogrammed, they need to be undergoing robust division,[35] and that reduction of p53 protein results in a higher reprogramming efficiency.[36] Also, primary fibroblasts have an inherent division limit that can be even further shortened by poor culture conditions such as allowing the cells to become contact inhibited. Experienced biorepositories culture these cells in a highly consistent manner, leading to higher quality fibroblasts without compromised proliferation potential.

Since the initial publications detailing the reprogramming of fibroblasts, many other cell types including dental pulp,[37] cord blood,[38] peripheral T cells,[4,28,29,32] LCLs,[39] and erythroblasts[40,41] have been reprogrammed. Because of the availability of cryopreserved blood cells stored in biobanks around the world, much attention has been given to reprogramming these excellent source cells. Cord blood was first reprogrammed by Haase et al., in 2009.[38] They found that the resulting iPSCs expressed markers associated with the pluripotent state in cells and were able to be differentiated into all three germ layers. Because the number of CD34+ stem cells circulating in adult peripheral blood is very low, representing only 0.01—0.1% of the total cell number, the utility of other cell types in blood has been investigated. Several groups have demonstrated that CD4+ T cells undergo very efficient reprogramming[28,29,42] and can be readily stimulated to proliferate by interleukin-2 (IL-2) and anti-CD3/CD28 microbeads,[42] but their usefulness is theoretically hampered by the fact that as part of their maturation, they undergo T cell receptor recombination and contain only a single T cell receptor. In addition to cryopreserved lymphocytes, many biorepositories also store immortalized B cells or LCLs. These cells, which are immortalized by infection with Epstein-Barr virus, are also capable of being reprogrammed to iPSCs.[39,43] An advantage of these cell lines is that they proliferate in continuous culture and can be cryopreserved, stored, and thawed for reprogramming whenever needed. However, analogous to T cells, B cell-derived LCLs have undergone immunoglobulin locus recombination and as such may not completely recapitulate immunological aspects of disease modeling.

Biorepositories are increasingly opting to induce proliferation of the erythroblast population from cryopreserved lymphocyte preparations for reprogramming to iPSCs.[41] Unlike T and B cells, erythroblasts have not undergone any immune cell genomic recombination, thus producing iPSCs that have an unaltered somatic genome. Erythroblasts can be readily isolated from cryopreserved lymphocytes (CPLs) and exist in peripheral blood at a concentration of 10–40 cells per 100,000 CPLs.[44] These progenitor cells can be isolated without the use of column or bead purification and only require several soluble factors in the medium to induce proliferation, the most important of which are stem cell factor (SCF), thrombopoietin

(TPO), and interleukin-3 (IL-3).[44] Since these cells are a progenitor cell type, they can be more easily expanded than other more differentiated cell types and can also be frozen and activated for later use without loss of proliferative capacity.

In general, all of these aforementioned blood cells suitable for iPSC derivation can be found in small lymphocyte preparations separated from whole blood as either buffy coat or, better yet, the small lymphocyte fraction obtained through the use of a Ficoll-type gradient. RUCDR has always routinely cryopreserved and banked the Ficoll-derived fraction for use as a backup if initial Epstien Barr Virus (EBV) transformation to LCLs failed. Few of these samples were required as backup for LCL transformation, so there is now a large collection of these cells from well over 100,000 individuals in the NIMH, Simons Foundation, NIDA, and other repositories at RUCDR that are suitable for reprogramming into iPSCs. This has already proven to be a very useful psychiatric genetics resource that will undoubtedly become more valuable in the future.

Biorepositories play a critical role in providing subject material for these types of assays because they contain very large numbers of well-characterized samples, often represented by multiple cell types collected from the same subject. For example, many biobanks house a large amount of clinical and genetic data associated with their subjects, allowing investigators to choose the subject that best fits their research parameters. Biorepositories also help investigators determine the number of samples necessary to reach statistical power when studying polygenic disorders such as schizophrenia, autism, and bipolar disorder by having multiple subjects with the same clinical phenotype or genotype, or by having additional affected or unaffected family members. The large number of subjects in biorepositories also makes it easier to find age- and/or gender-matched controls. Biobanks can also provide significant support either by providing source cells for reprogramming or by providing a consistent, characterized source of iPSCs, thereby reducing the costs associated with collecting samples *de novo* for each study.

Now that investigators can use the resources provided by biorepositories for obtaining either iPSCs or the source cells that can be reprogrammed to iPSC, in vitro modelling of human psychiatric disorders becomes a possibility (see, e.g., endnote 50) and a challenge. The biggest challenge may be the difficulty faced when trying to model the interactions that occur between neurons in a three-dimensional brain with a two-dimensional cell culture model. Thus far, neurons with the characteristics of all six cortical layers have been shown to exist in two-dimensional cultures, but there is no organization of these neurons into the characteristic brain layers observed in vivo.[45] This lack of anatomical and developmental structure and clinically relevant organization may be partially overcome by the use of brain organoids—rudimentary organ structures formed during suspension culture of pluripotent stem cells with neural inducing factors. Methods have been described that lead to the development of cerebral organoids that closely mimic an embryonic cortex,[23,46-48] which may be particularly relevant for the modelling of psychiatric diseases of congenital origin. An additional hurdle is the need to generate more mature neurons characteristic of the fetal and postnatal brain. Currently, iPSC-derived neurons need 8–12 weeks to mature in culture[49] and even then may need to be cultured with astrocytes to achieve full maturation. With the well-characterized biomaterials provided by biorepositories, we are entering an era when these challenges will be overcome, and tools to produce culture systems that can serve as better models of normal and pathologic brain function will emerge. Additionally, these models will probably be used as initial screening platforms to test new drugs or repurpose existing drugs, thereby shortening the time and decreasing the expense of bringing to market new and highly effective treatments for psychiatric disorders.

Informed Consent and Sample Availability

Biobanks should always address the issue of informed consent from individuals submitting samples. Laws and practices concerning informed consent often vary between countries, regions and even institutions, so it is difficult to generalize in the context of this review. In our view, however, the situation is optimal when all biobank samples are de-identified and biobank employees have no information that could link individual identities with biosamples. In our biobanks, the identities and personal information of the participants are held in confidence by those obtaining the primary samples and submitting them to the biobank; i.e., the researchers interacting with the subjects and drawing blood. Additionally, the phenotypical data management section of a biobank must receive sex, age (birth date) and pertinent diagnostic information, as much as possible in standardized formats. Should a secondary researcher requesting the sample from the biobank wish to obtain an additional sample from a subject, and if the informed consent allows recontact, it is then necessary to relay the request to the primary researcher, who decides whether or not to recontact the subject. The prime directive should always be the protection of human subjects and adherence to their wishes, as stated in the informed consent documents.

For biobanking purposes, the informed consent must stipulate, and the participant agrees, that their samples will be shared with other researchers studying either a certain disorder, a group of disorders, or diseases in general, the latter allowing the greatest future flexibility. Some informed consent documents allow participants to stipulate the exact level of sharing. In addition, the informed consent should indicate the types of materials that may be derived from the participant's sample. For example, the document should state that nucleic acids and proteins will be extracted from the blood sample and/or live cells from the sample may be used to create cell lines and DNA. In most instances it may be wise or necessary to stipulate that stem cell lines may be produced. At the time our biobanks were established, we did not contemplate the induction of stem cell lines from blood cells, but we were fortunate in that the consent forms stipulated that cell lines would be created from the sample.

Informed consent must also provide the subject with the option of permanently withdrawing their sample from the biobank. In such cases, biosamples must be destroyed, and authorized individuals within the biobank must attest to their destruction and the removal of all records. However, the subject must be informed that results obtained from their sample could appear in publications whose research was begun before the withdrawal request. An example of an informed consent document that meets these general requirements but can be modified as needed may be found on the NIMH website (https://www.nimhgenetics.org/documents/NIMH%20Human%20Genetics%20Initiative%20Consent.pdf).

RUCDR houses a wide variety of human sample types. Since its inception 19 years ago, it has received and processed over 1.6 million biospecimens (e.g., blood and saliva), distributed more than 1.8 million derivative biosamples, and banked over 13 million aliquots of DNA, plasma, urine, cryopreserved lymphocytes, iPS cell lines, lymphoblastoid cells, and other biosamples. Most of these biosamples are available for request by the global academic and commercial research communities through the auspices of the agencies whose repositories are managed by RUCDR, such as National Institutes of Health (NIH) institutes and assorted private and public foundations. The RUCDR website (www.RUCDR.org) can direct investigators to the cumulative numbers for different types of biosamples for different classes of disorders, or they can be directly assessed through supporting agency websites (e.g., www.NIMHgenetics.org, https://nindsgenetics.org/ and www.NIDAgenetics.org).

In the past five years, RUCDR has established a Stem Cell Resource for providing iPSC lines and related services such as reprogramming, characterization of pluripotency, and quality control. As a result, RUCDR was awarded grants to maintain stem cell repositories for NIMH (www.nimhgenetics.org), NINDS (www.nindsgenetics.org), the NIH Regenerative Medicine Program (NIH-RMP: www.commonfund.nih.gov/stemcells/lines), and the Target ALS (Amyotrophic Lateral Sclerosis) Foundation (www.targetals.org/).

Each agency has its own requirements for approving investigator requests to obtain biosamples as well as access to associated phenotypical and genetic data. Interested investigators can contact RUCDR (support@rucdr.org) for specific details for each collection and assistance with the request process.

References

1. Moore, J. S. M., & Hart, R. (2012). Biobanking in the era of the stem cell: A technical and operational guide. Colloquium Series on Stem Cell Biology [Internet].

2. American Type Culture Collection Standards Development Organization Workgroup ASN-0002 (2010). Cell line misidentification: the beginning of the end. Nature Reviews Cancer, 10(6), 441–448. Epub 2010/05/08. doi:10.1038/nrc2852 nrc2852 [pii]. PubMed PMID: 20448633.

3. Chatterjee, R. (2007). Cell biology. Cases of mistaken identity. Science, 315(5814), 928–931. Epub 2007/02/17. doi:315/5814/928 [pii] 10.1126/science.315.5814.928. PubMed PMID: 17303729.

4. Barral, S., & Kurian, M. A. (2016). Utility of induced pluripotent stem cells for the study and treatment of genetic diseases: Focus on childhood neurological disorders. *Frontiers in Molecular Neuroscience, 9*, 78. doi:10.3389/fnmol.2016.00078. PubMed PMID: 27656126; PMCID: PMC5012159.

5. Liang-Chu, M. M., Yu, M., Haverty, P. M., Koeman, J., Ziegle, J., Lee, M., . . . Neve, R. M. (2015). Human biosample authentication using the high-throughput, cost-effective SNPtrace(TM) system. *PLoS One, 10*(2), e0116218. Epub 2015/02/26. doi:10.1371/journal.pone.0116218   PONE-D-14-45036   [pii].   PubMed PMID: 25714623; PMCID: 4340925.

6. McGarrity, G. J., Vanaman, V., & Sarama, J. (1984). Cytogenetic effects of mycoplasmal infection of cell cultures: a review. *In Vitro, 20*(1), 1–18. Epub 1984/01/01. PubMed PMID: 6199287.

7. Hopert, A., Uphoff, C. C., Wirth, M., Hauser, H., & Drexler, H. G. (1993). Mycoplasma detection by PCR analysis. *In Vitro Cellular & Developmental Biology, Animals, 29*A(10), 819–821. Epub 1993/10/01. PubMed PMID: 8118618.

8. Masover, G. K., & Becker, F. A. (1998). Detection of mycoplasmas in cell cultures by cultural methods. *Methods in Molecular Biology, 104*, 207–215. Epub 1998/08/26. doi:10.1385/0-89603-525-5:207. PubMed PMID: 9711656.

9. Young, L., Sung, J., Stacey, G., & Masters, J. R. (2010). Detection of mycoplasma in cell cultures. *Nature Protocols, 5*(5), 929–934. Epub 2010/05/01. doi:10.1038/nprot.2010.43 nprot.2010.43 [pii]. PubMed PMID: 20431538.

10. Church, D. M., Goodstadt, L., Hillier, L. W., Zody, M. C., Goldstein, S., She, X., . . . Mouse Genome Sequencing Consortium. (2009). Lineage-specific biology revealed by a finished genome assembly of the mouse. *PLoS Biology, 7*(5), e1000112. doi:10.1371/journal.pbio.1000112. PubMed PMID: 19468303; PMCID: PMC2680341.

11. Hamlin, R. L., & Altschuld, R. A. (2011). Extrapolation from mouse to man. *Circulation: Cardiovascular Imaging, 4*(1), 2–4. doi:10.1161/CIRCIMAGING.110.961979. PubMed PMID: 21245362.

12. Takahashi, K., & Yamanaka, S. (2006). Induction of pluripotent stem cells from mouse embryonic and adult fibroblast cultures by defined factors. *Cell, 126*(4), 663–676. doi:10.1016/j.cell.2006.07.024. PubMed PMID: 16904174.

13. Takahashi, K., Tanabe, K., Ohnuki, M., Narita, M., Ichisaka, T., Tomoda, K., & Yamanaka, S. (2007). Induction of pluripotent stem cells from adult human fibroblasts by defined factors. *Cell, 131*(5), 861–872. doi:10.1016/j.cell.2007.11.019. PubMed PMID: 18035408.

14. Yu, J., Vodyanik, M. A., Smuga-Otto, K., Antosiewicz-Bourget, J., Frane, J. L., Tian, S., . . . Thomson, J. A. (2007). Induced pluripotent stem cell lines derived from human somatic cells. *Science, 318*(5858), 1917–1920. doi:10.1126/science.1151526. PubMed PMID: 18029452.

15. Loh, Y. H., Hartung, O., Li, H., Guo, C., Sahalie, J. M., Manos, P. D., . . . Daley, G. Q. (2010). Reprogramming of T cells from human peripheral blood. *Cell Stem Cell, 7*(1), 15–19. doi:10.1016/j.stem.2010.06.004. PubMed PMID: 20621044; PMCID: 2913590.

16. Staerk, J., Dawlaty, M. M., Gao, Q., Maetzel, D., Hanna, J., Sommer, C. A., . . . Jaenisch, R. (2010). Reprogramming of human peripheral blood cells to induced pluripotent stem cells. *Cell Stem Cell, 7*(1), 20–24. doi:10.1016/j.stem.2010.06.002. PubMed PMID: 20621045; PMCID: 2917234.

17. Brown, M. E., Rondon, E., Rajesh, D., Mack, A., Lewis, R., Feng, X., . . . Nuwaysir, E. F. (2010). Derivation of induced pluripotent stem cells from human peripheral blood T lymphocytes. PLoS One, 5(6), e11373.

18. Chou, B. K., Mali, P., Huang, X., Ye, Z., Dowey, S. N., Resar, L. M., . . . Cheng, L. (2011). Efficient human iPS cell derivation by a non-integrating plasmid from blood cells with unique epigenetic and gene expression signatures. Cell Research, Epub 2011/01/19. doi:cr201112 [pii] 10.1038/cr.2011.12. PubMed PMID: 21243013.

19. Seki, T., Yuasa, S., Oda, M., Egashira, T., Yae, K., Kusumoto, D., . . . Fukuda, K. (2010). Generation of induced pluripotent stem cells from human terminally differentiated circulating T cells. Cell Stem Cell, 7(20621043), 11–14.

20. Warren, L., Manos, P. D., Ahfeldt, T., Loh, Y. H., Li, H., Lau, F., . . . Rossi, D. J. (2010). Highly efficient reprogramming to pluripotency and directed differentiation of human cells with synthetic modified mRNA. Cell Stem Cell, 7(5), 618–630. doi:10.1016/j.stem.2010.08.012. PubMed PMID: 20888316; PMCID: PMC3656821.

21. Stadtfeld, M., Nagaya, M., Utikal, J., Weir, G., & Hochedlinger, K. (2008). Induced pluripotent stem cells generated without viral integration. Science, 322(5903), 945–949. Epub 2008/09/27. doi:1162494 [pii] 10.1126/science.1162494. PubMed PMID: 18818365.

22. Choi, J., Lee, S., Mallard, W., Clement, K., Tagliazucchi, G. M., Lim, H., . . . Hochedlinger, K. (2015). A comparison of genetically matched cell lines reveals the equivalence of human iPSCs and ESCs. Nature Biotechnology, 33(11), 1173–1181. doi:10.1038/nbt.3388. PubMed PMID: 26501951; PMCID: PMC4847940.

23. Eiraku, M., Watanabe, K., Matsuo-Takasaki, M., Kawada, M., Yonemura, S., Matsumura, M., . . . Sasai, Y. (2008). Self-organized formation of polarized cortical tissues from ESCs and its active manipulation by extrinsic signals. Cell Stem Cell, 3(5), 519–532. doi:10.1016/j.stem.2008.09.002. PubMed PMID: 18983967.

24. Shi, Y., Kirwan, P., & Livesey, F. J. (2012). Directed differentiation of human pluripotent stem cells to cerebral cortex neurons and neural networks. Nature Protocols, 7(10), 1836–1846. doi:10.1038/nprot.2012.116. PubMed PMID: 22976355.

25. Kirkeby, A., Grealish, S., Wolf, D. A., Nelander, J., Wood, J., Lundblad, M., . . . Parmar, M. (2012). Generation of regionally specified neural progenitors and functional neurons from human embryonic stem cells under defined conditions. Cell Report, 1(6), 703–714. doi:10.1016/j.celrep.2012.04.009. PubMed PMID: 22813745.

26. Wada, T., Honda, M., Minami, I., Tooi, N., Amagai, Y., Nakatsuji, N., & Aiba, K. (2009). Highly efficient differentiation and enrichment of spinal motor neurons derived from human and monkey embryonic stem cells. PLoS One, 4(8), e6722. doi:10.1371/journal.pone.0006722. PubMed PMID: 19701462; PMCID: PMC2726947.

27. Kriks, S., Shim, J. W., Piao, J., Ganat, Y. M., Wakeman, D. R., Xie, Z., . . . Studer, L. (2011). Dopamine neurons derived from human ES cells efficiently engraft in animal models of Parkinson's disease. Nature, 480(7378), 547–551. doi:10.1038/nature10648. PubMed PMID: 22056989; PMCID: PMC3245796.

28. Erceg, S., Lainez, S., Ronaghi, M., Stojkovic, P., Perez-Arago, M. A., Moreno-Manzano, V., . . . Stojkovic, M. (2008). Differentiation of human embryonic stem cells to regional specific neural precursors in chemically defined medium conditions. PLoS One, 3(5), e2122. doi:10.1371/journal.pone.0002122. PubMed PMID: 18461168; PMCID: PMC2346555.

29. Erceg, S., Ronaghi, M., Zipancic, I., Lainez, S., Rosello, M. G., Xiong, C., . . . Stojkovic, M. (2010). Efficient differentiation of human embryonic stem cells into functional

cerebellar-like cells. *Stem Cells & Development*, *19*(11), 1745–1756. doi:10.1089/scd.2009.0498. PubMed PMID: 20521974.

30. Haggarty, S. J., Silva, M. C., Cross, A., Brandon, N. J., & Perlis, R. H. (2016). Advancing drug discovery for neuropsychiatric disorders using patient-specific stem cell models. *Molecular & Cellular Neuroscience*, *73*,104–115. doi:10.1016/j.mcn.2016.01.011. PubMed PMID: 26826498.

31. Hunsberger, J. G., Efthymiou, A. G., Malik, N., Behl, M., Mead, I. L., Zeng, X., . . . Rao, M. (2015). Induced pluripotent stem cell models to enable in vitro models for screening in the central nervous system. *Stem Cells & Development*, *24*(16), 1852–1864. doi:10.1089/scd.2014.0531. PubMed PMID: 25794298; PMCID: PMC4533087.

32. Zhang, N., Bailus, B. J., Ring, K. L., & Ellerby, L. M. (2016). iPSC-based drug screening for Huntington's disease. *Brain Research*, *1638*(Pt A), 42–56. doi:10.1016/j.brainres.2015.09.020. PubMed PMID: 26428226; PMCID: PMC4814369.

33. Kumar, K. K., Aboud, A. A., & Bowman, A. B. (2012). The potential of induced pluripotent stem cells as a translational model for neurotoxicological risk. *Neurotoxicology*, *33*(3), 518–529. doi:10.1016/j.neuro.2012.02.005. PubMed PMID: 22330734; PMCID: PMC3358591.

34. Laustriat, D., Gide, J., & Peschanski, M. (2010). Human pluripotent stem cells in drug discovery and predictive toxicology. *Biochemical Society Transactions*, *38*(4), 1051–1057. doi:10.1042/BST0381051. PubMed PMID: 20659002.

35. Li, H., Collado, M., Villasante, A., Strati, K., Ortega, S., Canamero, M., . . . Serrano, M. (2009). The Ink4/Arf locus is a barrier for iPS cell reprogramming. *Nature*, *460*(7259), 1136–1139. doi:10.1038/nature08290. PubMed PMID: 19668188; PMCID: PMC3578184.

36. Zhao, Y., Yin, X., Qin, H., Zhu, F., Liu, H., Yang, W., . . . Deng, H. (2008). Two supporting factors greatly improve the efficiency of human iPSC generation. *Cell Stem Cell*, *3*(5), 475–479. doi:10.1016/j.stem.2008.10.002. PubMed PMID: 18983962.

37. Tamaoki, N., Takahashi, K., Tanaka, T., Ichisaka, T., Aoki, H., Takeda-Kawaguchi, T., . . . Tezuka, K. (2010). Dental pulp cells for induced pluripotent stem cell banking. *Journal of Dental Research*, *89*(8), 773–778. doi:10.1177/0022034510366846. PubMed PMID: 20554890.

38. Haase, A., Olmer, R., Schwanke, K., Wunderlich, S., Merkert, S., Hess, C., . . . Martin, U. (2009). Generation of induced pluripotent stem cells from human cord blood. *Cell Stem Cell*, *5*(4), 434–441. doi:10.1016/j.stem.2009.08.021. PubMed PMID: 19796623.

39. Rajesh, D., Dickerson, S. J., Yu, J., Brown, M. E., Thomson, J. A., & Seay, N. J. (2011). Human lymphoblastoid B-cell lines reprogrammed to EBV-free induced pluripotent stem cells. *Blood*, *118*(21708888), 1797–1800.

40. Soares, F. A., Pedersen, R. A., & Vallier, L. (2015). Generation of human induced pluripotent stem cells from peripheral blood mononuclear cells using Sendai virus. *Methods in Molecular Biology*. doi:10.1007/7651_2015_202. PubMed PMID: 25687300.

41. Yang, W., Mills, J. A., Sullivan, S., Liu, Y., French, D. L., & Gadue, P. (2008). *iPSC reprogramming from human peripheral blood using Sendai Virus Mediated Gene Transfer.* In *StemBook*. Cambridge, MA: Harvard Stem Cell Institute.

42. Okita, K., Yamakawa, T., Matsumura, Y., Sato, Y., Amano, N., Watanabe, A., . . . Yamanaka, S. (2013). An efficient nonviral method to generate integration-free

human-induced pluripotent stem cells from cord blood and peripheral blood cells. *Stem Cells*, *31*(3), 458–466. doi:10.1002/stem.1293. PubMed PMID: 23193063.

43. Choi, S. M., Liu, H., Chaudhari, P., Kim, Y., Cheng, L., Feng, J., . . . Jang, Y.-Y. (2011). Reprogramming of EBV-immortalized B-lymphocyte cell lines into induced pluripotent stem cells. *Blood*, *118*(21628406), 1801–1805.

44. Migliaccio, A. R., Campisi, S., & Migliaccio, G. (2001). Standardization of progenitor cell assay for cord blood banking. *Annali dell'Istituto Superiore Di Sanita*, *37*(4), 595–600. PubMed PMID: 12046230.

45. Espuny-Camacho, I., Michelsen, K. A., Gall, D., Linaro, D., Hasche, A., Bonnefont, J., . . . Vanderhaeghen, P. (2013). Pyramidal neurons derived from human pluripotent stem cells integrate efficiently into mouse brain circuits in vivo. *Neuron*, *77*(3), 440–456. doi:10.1016/j.neuron.2012.12.011. PubMed PMID: 23395372.

46. Lancaster, M. A., Renner, M., Martin, C. A., Wenzel, D., Bicknell, L. S., Hurles, M. E., . . . Knoblich, J. A. (2013). Cerebral organoids model human brain development and microcephaly. *Nature*, *501*(7467), 373–379. doi:10.1038/nature12517. PubMed PMID: 23995685; PMCID: PMC3817409.

47. Nasu, M., Takata, N., Danjo, T., Sakaguchi, H., Kadoshima, T., Futaki, S., . . . Sasai, Y. (2012). Robust formation and maintenance of continuous stratified cortical neuroepithelium by laminin-containing matrix in mouse ES cell culture. *PLoS One*, *7*(12), e53024. doi:10.1371/journal.pone.0053024. PubMed PMID: 23300850; PMCID: PMC3534089.

48. Pasca, A. M., Sloan, S. A., Clarke, L. E., Tian, Y., Makinson, C. D., Huber, N., . . . Pasca, S. P. (2015). Functional cortical neurons and astrocytes from human pluripotent stem cells in 3D culture. *Nature Methods*, *12*(7), 671–678. doi:10.1038/nmeth.3415. PubMed PMID: 26005811; PMCID: PMC4489980.

49. Verpelli, C., Carlessi, L., Bechi, G., Fusar Poli, E., Orellana, D., Heise, C., . . . Sala, C. (2013). Comparative neuronal differentiation of self-renewing neural progenitor cell lines obtained from human induced pluripotent stem cells. *Frontiers in Cellular Neuroscience*, *7*, 175. doi:10.3389/fncel.2013.00175. PubMed PMID: 24109433; PMCID: PMC3791383.

50. Oni, E. N., Halikere, A., Li, G., Toro-Ramos, A. J., Swerdel, M. R., Verpeut, J. L., . . . Hart, R. P. (2016). Increased nicotine response in iPSC-derived human neurons carrying the CHRNA5 N398 allele. *Scientific Reports*, Oct 4, *6*, 34341. doi:10.1038/srep34341. PubMed PMID: 27698409; PMCID: PMC5048107.

Index

Page references for figures are indicated by *f* and for tables by *t*.